Charity Law and Social Inclusion

Social inclusion for marginalized groups is among the most important challenges facing western governments today. The existence of alienated groups within a state impacts disproportionately on efforts to build and sustain civil society and the difficulties are set to increase as population displacement continues to impact upon developed nations.

Profiling national and international social inclusion agendas, *Charity Law and Social Inclusion* examines the fit between the charity law framework and the needs of the socially marginalized in some leading common law nations – the US, England and Wales, Ireland, Australia, New Zealand and Canada. The book:

*   examines the concepts of philanthropy, inclusion, alienation and justice;
*   considers the competing claims of philanthropy, legal rights and politics as appropriate methods of pursuing social justice;
*   explains how weaknesses in charity law obstruct philanthropic intervention; and
*   makes recommendations for changes to the legal framework governing philanthropy.

O'Halloran argues that our common charity law heritage must be updated and co-ordinated to be capable of addressing social inclusion in the twenty-first century. It will be of interest to academics and students in social policy, sociology and law, as well as professionals in community and voluntary work.

Kerry O'Halloran is Adjunct Professor at the Centre of Philanthropy and Nonprofit Studies, Queensland University of Technology, Australia.

Charity Law and Social Inclusion

An international study

Kerry O'Halloran

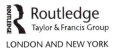
Routledge
Taylor & Francis Group

LONDON AND NEW YORK

First published 2007 by Routledge
2 Park Square, Milton Park, Abingdon, Oxon OX14 4RN

Simultaneously published in the USA and Canada
by Routledge
270 Madison Avenue, New York, NY 10016

Routledge is an imprint of the Taylor & Francis Group, an informa business

Typeset in Baskerville by RefineCatch Limited, Bungay, Suffolk
Printed and bound in Great Britain by
MPG Books Ltd, Bodmin, Cornwall

British Library Cataloguing in Publication Data
A catalogue record for this book is available from the British Library

Library of Congress Cataloging-in-Publication Data
O'Halloran, Kerry.
Charity law and social inclusion : an international study / Kerry O'Halloran.
p. cm.
Includes bibliographical references and index.
1. Charity laws and legislation. 2. Charitable uses, trusts, and
foundations. 3. Social service. 4. Social integration. I. Title.
K797.O353 2006
344.03′17–dc22
2006014251

ISBN10: 0–415–34722–X (hbk)
ISBN10: 0–415–34723–8 (pbk)
ISBN10: 0–203–64014–4 (ebk)

ISBN13: 978–0–415–34722–8 (hbk)
ISBN13: 978–0–415–34723–5 (pbk)
ISBN13: 978–0–203–64014–2 (ebk)

This book is dedicated to my mother Mavis Sancho
(15 August 1920–10 March 2000), whose balancing of
love, principles and authority was accompanied by a
wariness of all things political

Contents

Acknowledgements

Charity Law and Social Inclusion owes a great deal to Professor Myles McGregor-Lowndes[1] who not only wrote the chapter on Australia, read and made thoughtful comments on all other chapters, but also provided a warm and generous welcome for author and wife at the Centre of Philanthropy and Nonprofit Studies. For his support and companionship and that of all other colleagues at the Centre – particularly Anita Green Kellett, Rhonda Richards, Laloma Dawn, Kym Madden, Ted Flack, Annie Liu, Peter Walsh, Dot Summerfield, Dawn Butler, Margaret Steinberg and Wendy Scaife – I remain extremely grateful.

The book itself leans heavily on the more scholarly work of Myles and of the many others who have trudged this road before me, including Hubert Picarda,[2] Gino dal Pont,[3] Geoffrey Shannon,[4] Diana Leat,[5] and on the excellent charity law reports commissioned and now published by several governments. The process of writing benefited greatly from correspondence and conversations with a variety of people too numerous to risk attempting to list here but to all of whom I acknowledge a deep personal debt of gratitude. In particular, the charitable contribution of several specialists, inveigled into reading and commenting on the jurisdiction-specific chapters, has been most helpful in broadening my understanding of variations in the way national law relates to social inclusion and this cannot be allowed to pass without specific mention. Sincere thanks are due to Paul Bater[6] and Gareth Morgan[7] who kindly read and commented on the chapter dealing with England and Wales. I am also most grateful to Bob Wyatt,[8] Blake Bromley[9] and Kathryn Chan[10] for their similar contributions in respect of the chapter on Canada. Michael Gousmett[11] provided advice in relation to the New Zealand chapter and his published articles on the charity law reform process in that country were insightful. Jill Manny,[12] very kindly and at short notice, read and offered guidance on the US chapter. Without their generous help this would have been a weaker book.

At this point it is customary and indeed standard practice to exonerate all the aforementioned, and anyone else who may have been involved with the project, from guilt by association with the views expressed by the author in the following pages. In this instance it is perhaps particularly important to state that such views and all other comments, points made, positions taken up, etc., are mine alone. Responsibility for such, and of course for all mistakes, inconsistencies and omissions, etc., must unfortunately rest exclusively with me.

I am most grateful to Routledge for the vote of confidence that resulted in the publishing of this book.

Finally, thank you, Elizabeth, for giving me the strength to see this through to completion.

Introduction

Poverty and charity have an unequal relationship. Asymmetries of scale and values have ensured the persistence of the former despite millennia of the latter. For at least the past four centuries charity law has provided a frame of reference for channelling charitable activity towards the alleviation of poverty in particular and issues of social inclusion in general but it is no longer the primary frame of reference for doing so, nor indeed has charity law ever been exclusively concerned with such matters. Only good government can invest public resources on the scale necessary to ensure that safety nets catch the vulnerable and the marginalized. Moreover, charity law does not function in isolation. Social justice, human rights and other perspectives are also clearly relevant while the benefits of charity are as always left to fall in accordance with the whim of donors. So a sense of perspective is needed when considering the role of charity in relation to poverty and social inclusion.

Charity, however, has its place and charity law more so than any other legal framework is explicitly stamped with the obligation to address the needs of the socially disadvantaged. If it's not to fail in its central mission, the law governing philanthropy in all its modern guises must now be made to fit contemporary manifestations of need, domestic and global. The legal framework regulating the philanthropic environment could facilitate a more effective contribution of charitable resources for the alleviation of poverty and the encouragement of social inclusion. At the very least, existing obstructions should be removed. The resulting public benefit dividend in both the domestic and international arenas would be considerable.

On the domestic front, the social inclusion agenda presents a fundamental political challenge to the governments of modern western nations – how can our concerns to give other countries the benefits of democracy be taken seriously when after several centuries we have failed to deal with the poverty, racism, discrimination and other indicators of social exclusion that are now manifestly prevalent in all our democracies? As they pursue the probably ephemeral holy grail of civil society, governments would now seem to be enthusiastically forging partnerships with the third sector (voluntary and community sector, or not-for-profit sector) of which charities form the cutting edge. In the common law nations the terms of such partnerships are being set within the structure provided by a reformed charity law, and in some cases specific reference is made in that law to the needs of the socially disadvantaged groups that typically feature on the domestic social inclusion agenda of those nations (e.g. the poor, the mentally ill, the disabled, the elderly, ethnic minorities, etc.). This partnership approach does bring with it certain challenges, not least of which is the uncertainty surrounding the principles that should govern the distribution of public benefit responsibilities between government and charity. There can be little doubt, however, that these new formal arrangements offer the best chance of building more stable, cohesive and engaged societies within which the needs of the socially disadvantaged can be readily acknowledged and accountability for failure to address them swiftly ascertained.

On the international front also, the social inclusion agenda presents a fundamental political challenge to the same governments – how can we square the co-ordinated investment of resources and the efficiency of our coercive intervention in countries like Iraq with the inadequacy of our consensual intervention in places like Kashmir? As legislatures make time to process rafts of anti-terrorism laws, what evidence is there of a proportionate legislative interest in addressing poverty? The current 'global war against terrorism' (GWAT) in conjunction with the minefield of international trade has undoubtedly combined to constrain the overseas activity of charities. Government pursuit of terrorists and maintenance of subsidies for domestic produce, often in conjunction with other governments, can result in charities being regarded with some suspicion; they may be viewed as muddying the water at a time when governments are giving urgent priority to safeguarding national interests. However, the presence of such third parties, as they manoeuvre between polarized ideologies to reach the more vulnerable and demonstrate good faith by their charitable activity, has perhaps never been more necessary. Again there is some evidence that charity law reform together with adherence to human rights provisions may prevail to allow charities the freedom to go on developing their unique role as western ambassadors of goodwill. Because they can go where governments often cannot and because of their experience and credibility, sometimes earned over decades if not centuries, charities are well placed to build bridges with foreign cultures and perhaps forestall or offset the alienation of marginalized groups such as the more radical adherents of Islam.

Both domestically and internationally there are growing pressures on charity law to provide an appropriate framework for modern philanthropy. Some of these emanate from its essentially fiscally driven nature and push for greater regulatory control in matters of transparency, accountability and effectiveness. Others press for fiscal concerns to be balanced by mechanisms that facilitate a development of charitable purposes in keeping with contemporary patterns of social need; a function previously performed by the courts until factors of costs, delay and adverse publicity fatally undermined their traditional role. There is also pressure to develop legal structures that blend trust principles with company law and are better fitted to strategically co-ordinate the resources of government, charities and for-profit bodies.

Clearly any adjustment to the legal framework regulating the role of philanthropy on a national and international basis to ensure a better fit with contemporary circumstances is the business of legislatures. This, however, is an area of law where legislatures seldom venture. The fact, therefore, that the leading common law nations – each wrestling with much the same agenda of social inclusion issues and all doing so in a not dissimilar political context – are now committed to charity law reform would seem to present a unique legislative opportunity.

Many of the world's largest, most modern and powerful democracies including the USA, and Commonwealth countries such as Australia, Canada and New Zealand – alongside some of the smallest and most undeveloped such as the Seychelle Islands and the island kingdom of Tonga – all share the same legacy of institutional infrastructure, laws and legal principles inherited from Great Britain. In particular they share the same charity law heritage. The Statute of Charitable Uses 1601, the Preamble to it and an ever burgeoning body of related case law have underpinned and guided the development of the legal framework governing philanthropy in each of these nations. For 400 years they and some 60 other members of the Commonwealth (and other post-empire nations such as Ireland) have all found it equally unnecessary to introduce formative legislation to define 'charity' and broaden its purposes to meet contemporary patterns of need.[1] Coincidentally, or not, many of these nations are now engaged at various stages in charity law review processes designed to achieve that end.

This book asserts that the reviews do provide a window of opportunity. In the aftermath of a sequence of natural disasters and acts of terrorism, in the shadow of the unfolding tragedy of AIDS and poverty in sub-Saharan Africa and faced with the violent consequences of cultural estrangement on a national and international basis, it is clearly time for the developed nations to pause and reflect. The charity law framework that binds so many of the wealthiest nations in a shared heritage of compassionate values could provide a basis for strategically addressing issues of poverty and social inclusion both nationally and internationally. The reviews offer a space and a platform for the governments of many modern western nations to co-ordinate their efforts and produce a concerted response to the challenges presented by the contemporary social inclusion agenda.

Failure to co-ordinate, or at least to take fully into account, the law reform processes of other nations will have consequences for all that share the same common law legacy. The singular strength of this heritage, as a shared platform for formulating and applying the principles that relate private resources to public need, may not survive. As each nation translates its particular common law experience into legislative parameters there is a serious danger that one or more will put in place new definitions, or will otherwise structurally alter the common law architecture, and so make it difficult if not impossible for the 400-year-old web of judicial precedents to continue to loosely bind some 70 nations as they develop a compassionate response to social need. The consequences of failure will as always impact most grievously upon those already in need. Failure to make a better fit between the shared charity law infrastructure of the developed nations and their particular patterns of need and also with the greater need of those that remain underdeveloped is to risk further alienating those already marginalized by poverty, cultural dissonance and other issues of social inclusion.

Charity Law and Social Inclusion takes an analytical look at the meaning of charity and philanthropy within the common law tradition. It identifies and assesses the functions of charity law and examines the appropriateness of the regulatory framework as a means of giving effect to the new approaches of modern philanthropy. It considers issues of poverty and social inclusion on a national and international basis and explores the nature and effect of the lack of fit between contemporary social need and the charity law framework. It provides a comparative evaluation of the current regulatory environment for philanthropy in a number of the more developed common law nations. As it holds focus on the functions of charity law and their implications for issues of social inclusion within the common law nations, it avoids the temptation to digress by exploring matters such as governance, administration, company law and the wilder shores of modern philanthropy. The book concludes with a summary of the main themes to emerge and with some tentative suggestions for the future relationship between charity law and social inclusion.

Part I, 'Philanthropy, social inclusion and the law', begins the book with two chapters that consider some core concepts, basic parameters and fundamental dilemmas. Using the Titmus theory of 'the gift relationship' as a touchstone, it explores matters such as, Where did 'charity' come from? What is it for? How does the law relate to it? How do charity, the law and social inclusion interrelate? Where does philanthropy fit in?

Part II, 'Charity law: the common law legacy', consisting of three chapters, examines in some detail the origins, characteristics and the regulatory framework of charity law in a common law context. It provides a chronological overview of the process whereby charity law emerged from the law of trusts in the courts of Chancery and subsequently developed in England and Wales. It considers the meaning, role and weighting of the 'public benefit' test in relation to other important principles. Charitable status, as awarded by the State, is considered in terms of the resulting profit and loss to the public. The various legal structures available to give effect to charities are identified and explained, as is the related institutional infrastructure. It identifies the distinctive hallmarks of this body of law as formed in England and Wales and as they have transferred to and endured in the common law nations.

Part III, 'Legal rights and functions: a framework for philanthropy', again consisting of two chapters, identifies and considers benchmarks for an appropriate, effective and sufficient charity law system and is central to the book. One chapter formulates a template for identifying and assessing the functions of charity law and for conducting the comparative jurisdictional analysis that follows in Part IV. The other considers the provisions and related case law of international conventions, particularly the European Convention for the Protection of Human Rights and Fundamental Freedoms 1950, and assesses their significance for charity law and practice.

Part IV, 'Contemporary law and practice', presents a jurisdiction-specific profile of contemporary charity law in six prominent common law nations chosen because they are each engaged in or have recently completed a process of law reform. In template form, it provides an outline of law and the regulatory framework, relates this to the social inclusion agenda of each nation, highlighting areas of commonality and difference, thereby permitting a degree of comparative analysis. Attention is paid to social inclusion as manifested in a nation's domestic agenda, in its policies toward indigenous people (where relevant), the threat of terrorism and to international aid. It notes how the law measures up against the benchmarks identified in Part III and it considers any implications arising for interpreting and applying the 'public benefit' test. In broad terms, it identifies the characteristic features of charity law in each jurisdiction.

Finally, *Charity Law and Social Inclusion* concludes with a brief summary of the main points to emerge from the comparative survey. Central to the book's thesis is the assertion that having inherited the common law legacy from England and Wales, and thereafter been guided by the precedents established by the judiciary of that jurisdiction, the nations concerned (including India and others in the Commonwealth) have perpetuated much the same legal framework for charity, with similar structural faults, which may now be amenable to the same type of adjustment, thereby permitting modern philanthropy to uniformly address contemporary social inclusion issues in the common law jurisdictions more appropriately and effectively than they do at present. Accordingly, the conclusion focuses on the following main areas of sensitivity in the relationship between the charity law framework and social inclusion as these occur within the six common law jurisdictions:

- partnership with government;
- restrictions on advocacy/political activity;
- human rights and anti-terrorism;
- international aid;
- issues relating to indigenous people/multicultural matters;
- fiscal issues, particularly tax orientation;
- roles of the court and Attorney General;
- forums for developing charitable purposes;
- legal structures; and
- public benefit issues.

Kerry O'Halloran,
White Park Bay,
Spring 2006

Part I

Philanthropy, social inclusion and the law

Chapter 1

The gift relationship
Charity and the law

Introduction

This chapter suggests that 'the gift relationship'[1] provides an appropriate leitmotif and convenient starting point for a book on charity and social inclusion. It uses the dynamics of that relationship to introduce and explain the key parties, concepts and principles underpinning the themes that interplay throughout the book. It then considers the central axis around which the themes turn: charity and charity law.

The concept and practice of charity, in a common law context, would seem to have been formed in pre-Reformation England at a time when Church and King were the twin institutions governing society. For both, charity served to some extent as the default position for hierarchical authorative powers that prescribed the rights and duties of all loyal subjects within the realm. Those too poor, infirm or otherwise incapacitated to play a useful role in a heavily structured society would be cared for and maintained, and kept in their place, by services paid for by parish tithes imposed and administered by worthy men of both institutions. This system provided for the inbuilt reciprocity of two sets of needs: those who wished to be fed in this life and those who by feeding them hoped to save their souls in the next, the dutiful role conformity of both contributing to maintaining the compliant status quo necessary for continuing the established authority of lord and bishop. The gift relationship then worked as a necessary solvent for an otherwise rather inflexible society.

The law, when it eventually arrived, provided a framework that fitted around these relationships and was designed primarily to prevent abuses of charitable funds and taxes while pragmatically allowing the concept of charity to extend to more general public service provision including such items of social infrastructure as bridges for the use of rich and poor alike. As the saintly were displaced by the secular so charity became more aligned with the agenda of government, though never quite losing its deference to religious institutions. Whether supplementing or substituting for government provision, charity continued to deal mainly with the effects of poverty; persons of means had little need to concern themselves with issues regarding ownership of schools, hospitals and other public utilities. Gradually, the stream of charity was judicially broadened to engulf more esoteric aspects of social provision, such as concert halls and art galleries, that previous generations might have been puzzled to find alongside the usual traditional rudimentary public benefit charitable institutions, particularly when poverty and its effects were still very much in evidence. The emphasis in the gift relationship had shifted from the alleviation of poverty to filling in the gaps in an ever more sophisticated society. Its social function, however, was arguably much the same: to work alongside the powers that be to provide such palliative services as were required to improve social infrastructure, ease points of stress and facilitate social cohesion.

The impact of globalization has further stretched the gift relationship and poses a more fundamental challenge for the modern role of charity. If it is to continue its role attending to gaps in the social fabric then it will have to deal with the fact that both power and the threat of disruption now often lie outside the society in question: it is no longer possible for modern western societies to look only internally and address the effects of social stress. Governments and charities will need to clarify their respective roles and address social inclusion, the root cause of the greatest threat to the future stability of such societies, on a domestic and international basis.

This chapter explores the evolution of charity and the law and explores the roles of the principal parties involved to consider the question, What is charity for?

The gift relationship

Charity involves donors, recipients, charitable organisations and the State in a complex set of transactions governed by common law and legislation; other interests such as business, politics and international Conventions are also represented and call for examination at a later stage. The legal intricacies thus generated are explored throughout the book but it may be helpful to begin by examining the roles played by the main players.

Giving and the 'gift relationship'

At the heart of charity lies what has been termed the 'gift relationship'. It was Titmus who, in his seminal and much quoted work under that title,[2] first brought sociological expertise to bear on the nature of the relationship between donor and recipient in the context of philanthropic exchange. He examined the act of 'giving', seeing it as the voluntary and altruistic act of an individual, and compared it with a commercial system in a study which focused on blood donors. The contrast, as he saw it, was between ethically based behaviour and behaviour motivated by self-interest. In the former instance, the National Blood Transfusion Service in the UK provided a service to which blood donors made anonymous contributions without financial or other reward and from which recipients took according to need incurring no cost and without knowing the identity of the donor. In Titmus's view, this free gift of blood left the relationship between giver and recipient uncompromised by any 'contract of custom; legal bond; functional determinism; situations of discriminatory power; nor by domination, constraint or compulsion'. On the other hand, he considered that the alternative approach to the same service in the US reduced people's willingness to donate blood because the transaction had become tarnished by commercialism causing such adverse consequences as the repression of expressions of altruism and an erosion of a sense of community.

Since then much academic attention has been drawn to philanthropy in general.[3] As has been said: 'The very voluntariness and optionality of private philanthropy gives it an important moral status ... a society without private philanthropy would be a morally impoverished society.'[4] The gift relationship, it has been argued, is something that can bond us as a society

The giver

Titmus considered that the reason why people donated blood without direct reward, at a cost of their own time and effort, to another with whom they have no direct contact, was altruism. A regard for the needs of others was the principle that motivated their action. Donors showed a high sense of awareness of belonging to a community and of social responsibility. It followed that it was important for the State to provide the opportunity for individuals to express their commitment to the community in which they lived; indeed, he developed this theme in his final chapter 'The Right to Give'. He argued that the submersion of such opportunities within a market economy inhibited the freedom to give or not to give, that material incentives destroyed rather than complemented moral incentives. The freedom of choice, enabling an individual to select the class of persons or type of cause to benefit from his or her gift, and to do so on a basis that may discriminate on grounds of country, religion, gender, locality, etc., was to be valued in a democracy for its own sake and because it demonstrated altruism it would encourage others to become givers. The act of giving modelled ethical conduct and generated a sense of shared morality and civic responsibility in communities.

Titmus acknowledged that the altruistic motive of the giver could also be accompanied by a degree of self-interest. The fact of anonymity in the blood donation process removed the possibility of donors being motivated by the desire for social approval; though clearly this could be a factor in other forms of giving. The concern to help another, however, may, to a varying extent, be attributable to a desire to see that person lead an independent and useful life and relieve the giver of further concern for their welfare. Whether utility or unalloyed altruism was the driving factor for a particular giver in relation to the equally particular gift and recipient was not a significant issue for Titmus. They were compatible, conducive to promoting socially responsible behaviour and at risk of negation by blanket market forces.

The gift

The gift is twofold: from the donor and from the State. The first is uncontroversial: in a democracy, any person of sound mind (subject to the rights of dependants) is free to give their property to whomsoever they choose; this can, but need not be, by way of charity. The second, when the charity vehicle is used and the State adds considerably to the value of the gift by exempting it from tax, is hedged about with conditions that can give rise to controversy (see p. 96). The gift, intended to meet a need, also provides a measure and social confirmation of inadequacy while its nature and the manner of giving are clearly matters that ultimately affect its utility.

The recipient

In a common law context, the categories of those from whom requests may legitimately be received have long since been embedded in charity law. *Pemsel*,[5] together with such new categories as can fit within the 'spirit and intendment' rule[6] has served to identify charitable purposes, the bodies upon which charitable status is to be conferred and ultimately those entitled to charitable resources (see p. 82).

The position of the recipient in the gift relationship is complicated and clearly not confined to responding with expressions of gratitude and satisfaction in respect of needs that to some degree have been met. The gift is always an acknowledgement of the recipient's functional deficit; to receive is to accept not just the benevolence of others but that your failure to provide for yourself has acquired a level of social exposure. The fact that the recipient recognizes and is comforted by the inherent virtue of the giver, who may well have given anonymously, and values and uses the gift as intended, does not necessarily mean that they thereby become better equipped to cope. For the recipient, the psychological dynamics of the gift relationship can all too often serve to confirm their inadequacy and enduce long-term compliant dependency.

The charitable organization

The infinite variety of not-for-profit organizations together represent the collective moral strength of a sector that makes a non-exploitive contribution to society. Within that range of organizations, charities are distinctive because they cleave to the public benefit principle as their *raison d'être* and have the capacity to channel the value of donors' gifts to their intended purposes across many generations. The trust and specialist knowledge that charities build up in the process of mediating between giver and recipient places them in a crucially important strategic position between State and citizen, as broker on behalf of the socially disadvantaged, and vests them with the responsibility to work with both to further social inclusion. Their registration as such confirms the special status of charities as organizations dedicated to furthering the public benefit of the disadvantaged and in the eyes of society confers upon them a stamp of virtue.

Free from the exigencies of government, and to some extent also from the competitive pressures of the commercial market place, unaccountable to shareholders or constituency, while entrusted with funds from private donors and the public purse, the responsibility rests squarely with a charitable organization to promote the interests and publicly champion the cause of those they represent. In theory the independence, resources and knowledge of a charitable organ ation operating from within a centuries-old charitable sector of enormous v ealth should enable it to effect change in the social inclusion agenda.

The State

For the State, to endorse the gift relationship is to inculcate a value system that encourages altruism, reinforces a sense of obligation, stimulates social capital, provides a basis for community bonding and builds a more ethical society. The State can only gain from a sector that: generates a vibrant and diverse participative form of democracy; attracts the involvement of an army of volunteers; bolsters civic responsibility and thereby fosters the growth of social capital and consolidates civil society. In addition to being a catalyst for a more civil and morally based society, the encouragement of altruistic conduct also has the happy consequence of reducing State expenditure.

However, some of the criticism leveled by Titmus against the influence of commerce on altruism applies equally to that of the welfare state. They both inhibit individual acts of altruism, in the latter case because of the collective view that taxes are paid and systems exist to address the needs of the socially disadvantaged. The value of the individual gift is devalued by the collective provision of the welfare state. This in turn may well have a correspondingly negative effect on moral values as a binding social influence.

Charity

Theoretically, charity is concerned with the fact and effects of poverty and is focused on methods for directly alleviating the suffering of others. This should serve to distinguish charity from philanthropy which is primarily about respect for the civilizing effects of human endeavour and is focused on providing and promoting opportunities for bettering the human condition.[7] It should also differentiate charity from public utility provision which deals with the more institutional aspects of social infrastructure that provides generally for the security and well-being of the population. Again, it should be clearly different from the activities of religious organizations in which member benefit is essentially pursued as an aspect of worship. The difference is one represented, respectively, by soup kitchens, the Royal Opera House, hospitals and the saying of mass.

'Charity', however, has managed to accommodate all the above. For four centuries it evaded the constraints of legislative and judicial definition and remained a creature of the common law. In the process, the meaning it acquired in law diverged considerably from any social meaning that would otherwise have logically been ascribed to it. The distortions inflicted upon it by successive generations of the judiciary have left the concept of 'charity' inadequate and ill-fitted to the role of lynchpin in a modern legal framework for philanthropy.

Charity in its traditional Christian context

Charity, as it is known to the common law, has its roots in the supplicant/benefactor relationship set within a Christian social context. The relationship was initiated by a humble plea for assistance, and elicited a dutiful response in which the benefactor gave as little as was judged sufficient to forestall further requests, attract acknowledgement of their virtue in this life and safeguard their soul in the next. Both parties played to a Christian rulebook which provided for inbuilt reciprocity: their roles and relationship were preordained and affirmed by the gift, palliative in nature and nicely weighted to ensure the continuance of that dynamic.

This symbiotic relationship survived the secularization of charity, endured as a strong if increasingly anomalous theme in the world of the welfare state and now challenges our perception of the meaning and role of philanthropy in a modern western society (see, further, chapter 5). Its longevity is directly attributable to the religious connotations of personal sacrifice and compassion for the helpless being grafted onto the common law. Charity, as practised and endorsed within its Christian social context, perpetuated the patronizing approach traditionally associated with it, and is now anathema to contemporary social values and obstructs productive philanthropic engagement with those who are socially disadvantaged.

Social function

Charity and Christianity were inextricably linked in the pre-Reformation era. To subscribe to the Christian faith entailed obeying the duty to love one's neighbour, an inescapable requirement for salvation of the soul.[8] In its initial religious context, charity was thus 'more a means to the salvation of the soul of the benefactor than an endeavour to diagnose and alleviate the needs of the beneficiary'.[9] Indeed, the soul, not just of the giver but that of those already deceased, could be saved by acts of generosity to the poor: masses offered for the dead being accompanied by alms for the poor of the parish; chantries[10] by endowments for the Church and monasteries; and guilds[11] by bequests of property for the use of the Church. The duty of the individual Christian was matched by the Church as an institution as it provided shelter and succour for the poor and needy and engaged in other such charitable activity. To some extent the rise of the monastic orders in the thirteenth and fourteenth centuries largely displaced the previous parish-based charitable activities of the Church as religion focused more on the salvation of souls than on temporal welfare. Provision for the poor, however, remained primarily a matter for Church rather than State.

The role of the mediaeval Church, with its blend of saintly and secular concerns, received powerful support from the State which, through laws proclaiming that 'God's churches are entitled to their rights',[12] required taxes to be paid to the Church and imposed severe penalties for non-payment.[13] The instilling of Christian beliefs, accompanied by charitable provision for the disadvantaged, throughout society was an area of shared common interest between Church and State. As has been said:[14]

> The enormous status and prestige of the early and mediaeval Church enabled her to assume jurisdiction over whole areas of social life which today would rightly be considered the concern of secular government. Indeed not until the mid-nineteenth century did the ecclesiastical courts in England lose their jurisdiction over marriage and matters relating to the probate of wills.

The private and the public interests in charity were thus harmoniously balanced in their Christian origins.

Social endorsement

It has been argued that charity in Elizabethan England was a public act, intended and resulting in social rewards for the giver and in the humility and compliance of the recipient:[15]

> In social terms, donors helped to create a community that was both more fully Christian and less likely to be troubled by unrest or violence among the poor. If they were employers, they profited from having a trained labour force able to weather temporary hard times. Furthermore, everyone knew about their generosity. Elizabethan England had little hidden charity – the kind advocated in the early stages of the three Abrahamic religions, to be given privately between one person and another to avoid humiliating recipients or creating harmful pride in donors. In this setting, donors expected to be recognised and praised for their generosity, now and in the years to come. Almshouse dwellers, for example, usually wore a distinctive robe when they appeared in public, labeled with the name of the founder of the institution.

Charity in this view, while undoubtedly beneficial to those in need, also served as a discrete social mechanism for reinforcing the roles, relationships and status of those involved, instilling a common morality and sense of acceptance while helping to preserve the existing social structure.

The Christian legacy

In all common law countries (though in some more than others) a significant proportion of charities, charitable resources and charitable activity continue to be embedded in religious organizations. Several consequences flow from this fact.

Member benefit   The activities of religious organizations are essentially member benefit oriented and self-serving. Good deeds and proselytism are often pursued simultaneously, both motivated by the duty to save the souls of benefactor[16] and recipient and serving to emphasize religious differences. The partisan nature of such activities may generate social capital within the membership of Church or faith-based bodies but often at the price of hardening divisions in the wider community. In some jurisdictions (notably Northern Ireland) this can polarize communities and exacerbate sectarian divisions.

Social conformity   The Christian attitude of acceptance tends to instil a conformist approach to contemporary social circumstances and an attitude of acceptance towards conditions of inequity. Being inherently conservative in nature, religious organizations are never to the fore in meeting newly emerging areas of social need and on the contrary may often direct their resources in a reactionary fashion to slow if not obstruct the pace of change where this is perceived as not wholly compliant with religious values and belief.

Wealth   Given their survival over the millennia, some such organizations have accumulated great wealth (if measured only in terms of city centre property) which, if amenable to an objective public benefit test, could be available for the direct relief of deprivation.

Patronage   An attitude of discretionary benevolence on the part of the giver, coupled with the reciprocal helplessness of the recipient, leading to a gift that confirms the dependency of the latter and the corresponding virtue of the former are inescapable components of this relationship. Arguably it results in the institionalization of attitudes and responses to poverty; ensuring that the poor are indeed always with us.

Charity in a modern context

Our understanding of what charity is for, its role and functions in society, has evolved since Christianity defined it in terms of alms-giving, succour for those in need, as a palliative response to social stress and a means for saving souls. In the context of contemporary national and international experiences of alienation it would be delusionary and corrosive to believe that the patronizing approach, embodied in the legacy of charity law throughout the common law world, is an appropriate response to the needs of those who are socially marginalized. If charity is to find a credible role in modern society, one that sits respectably alongside social justice, human rights and politics, this will have to involve the realignment of 'need' and 'gift' which form the twin core components of the gift relationship.

The need

Blood, unlike money or other resources, is of little value as social currency: having more than is absolutely necessary is not going to proportionately increase personal wealth and social status; it has little buying power and is not an appreciating asset. In the Titmus theory it has the distinction of simultaneously forming both the need and the gift in equal measure to satisfy an essentially value-free exchange. Addressing contemporary social need has become somewhat more complicated.

Poverty   This, the most traditional and enduring manifestation of social need, continues to resist the efforts of charity and government to consign it to history. All modern western nations have a significant proportion of their populations subsisting at or below the poverty threshold, even if this is a relative term in comparison with its meaning for previous generations. It particularly and disproportionately afflicts the indigenous communities within such nations. In many developing countries poverty is endemic, unremitting and devastating. The failure of charity to cope with poverty at home or abroad is an inescapable indictment of its effectiveness. For this book, the fact that four centuries of charity law has left poverty firmly entrenched in the common law nations raises some basic questions (see further chapter 2 and Part IV).

Human rights   The work and reports generated by the United Nations, the judgments of the European Court of Human Rights and the evidence provided by such other organizations as Amnesty International testify to the continued worldwide abuse of basic human rights (see, further, chapter 7). While addressing that abuse is a responsibility that generally falls more to government than charity, certain rights such as freedoms of expression and assembly, the right to private family life and to a cultural identity represent needs that lie at the heart of the charitable modus operandi.

Alienation   Cultural dissonance has become a serious threat to social stability. Whether within families and communities, between indigenous people and others, between immigrant ethnic groups, or between nations, a lack of mutual understanding and willingness to respect and value cultural difference is causing destructive tensions. Similar tensions are also evident on a more domestic social level in terms of inequities rooted in such differentiating factors as gender, disability, mental health, age, etc. Where the fact or perception of inequity caused by such differences is not acknowledged or is unaccompanied by actions demonstrating good faith in dealing with them, then the disadvantaged can quickly become alienated with long-lasting destructive consequences, as evidenced by the pattern of deterioration in places such as Northern Ireland. Charities, as mediating agencies and power brokers between 'the haves and the have-nots', should have a crucial role to play in bridging cultural gaps and forestalling alienation whether within or between nations. Again, for this book, there are issues to be faced if we are to explain why, after 400 years of addressing social inequity, charity law is not more relevant to the most pressing social problem of our age and facilitating effective charitable intervention on behalf of alienated minorities.

Civil society   Even where alienated minority groups do not threaten civil strife and fragmentation, the lack of individual engagement and low level of civic responsibility can leave a society unhealthy and vulnerable to stresses that may undermine its sustainability as a true democratic nation. Consolidating civil society is a challenge facing the governments of all western nations and this book seeks to explore how those who share the common law tradition have managed to use the framework of charity law to forge an appropriate partnership with charities and advance that task.

The gift

Titmus would still recognize the altruism that underpins modern charity and his defence of the right to give remains valid. It continues to allow individuals the opportunity to practise virtuous behaviour and inculcates more generally a sense of obligation, civic responsibility and shared morality. It also generates a range of socially useful activity that serves to bond individuals and communities and contributes towards building a more vital, engaged and compassionate society. However, while the parties to the gift relationship remain the same, the gift itself has changed considerably.

Perhaps the most striking change to have occurred is that the gift, whatever form it takes, is now most usually selected with, if not by, rather than simply for the recipient.

Of capital assets   The traditional gift of funds and/or food and shelter still has its place in societies where real poverty persists but now use is increasingly made of assets with potential for achieving more long-term and sustainable improvement. The strategic value of a workshop, farm or manufacturing plant can be an effective exit gift in situations where those who are to use it and thereby secure their future independence have received the necessary preparatory training and appropriate support systems are in place. For example, some indigenous people in Australia, and presumably those in other countries, have benefited from charitable gifts of land accompanied by the incorporated legal structures, specialist support and finance systems necessary to transform it into a sustainable community farming enterprise.

Of time   A charitable gift may involve the giving of time as well as or instead of a gift of money or other forms of property. Volunteering lies at the heart of charitable activity. Indeed, the gift of personal skill, time and energy for the benefit of others is now valued as being of greater charitable worth than the giving of funds. By engaging concerned individuals to ameliorate the disadvantages of others charities generate a healthy, caring and responsible sense of community. As a consequence it is often the policy of governments to develop and support the contribution of volunteers in order to foster a sense of civic responsibility and promote the growth of social capital.[17]

Of opportunity   The provision of such tangible forms of assistance as time and money is seldom sufficient to lift a person, family or community from circumstances of dependency. Providing opportunities for the unemployed to acquire appropriate skills and training, followed by sequenced opportunities to enter the job market and receive the support necessary to sustain that achievement, has become a particularly important development in charitable activity. Similarly, creating opportunities for private business and government bodies to join in partnership with charities to formulate and implement programmes designed to comprehensively address circumstances of rural and urban deprivation is now accepted as good practice.

Of information   Many large charities now run or fund very professional research departments which generate and disseminate authoritative data to identify, measure and assess causal relationships between social need and effective resource deployment. The archives of such data, sometimes accumulated over many generations and available on a jurisdiction-specific and on a global basis, equip charities to advise governments and lead the development of socially disadvantaged communities in a more informed manner than ever before. The responsibility that comes with information places a heavy onus on both charities and governments to give or intervene in ways that effect enduring change.

Charity law

Charity in law has a technical meaning[18] but not a statutory definition.[19] As understood within the terms of the Preamble to the Statute of Charitable Uses 1601[20] and as organized under the four *Pemsel*[21] heads, it is an activity undertaken by bodies that vary greatly in type, size, legal form, longevity and in resources. Charities predate the 1601 Act and have existed for at least the last millennium.[22] The law relating to charities is also of ancient origin, most probably its origins lie in the *parens patriae*[23] responsibilities of the King (protecting the interests of charities, wards and lunatis), and over the past four centuries it has continued to judicially evolve within the common law tradition with very little legislative interference (see, further, chapter 3). During this time it has taken root throughout nations formerly comprising the former British Empire, which have contributed to forming a body of jurisprudence that now, with varying emphases and subject to certain jurisdictional differences, constitutes charity law in the common law tradition.

Public/private

On the face of it individual acts of charity, and by extension the activities of charities, are essentially private matters to be governed by private rather than public law. For the most part charity has been regarded in that way. The law, in keeping with its treatment of other subjects of the ancient *parens patriae* jurisdiction, has tended to respect the *inter partes* nature of the issues, restrict itself to protecting the interests of donors, appointing officials to monitor, supervise and prevent abuse but to otherwise leave the parties concerned to their own devices. The steady migration of charity into public law has to a large extent been due to charitable organizations becoming enveloped by the tax regime: fundamentally, private/public interests are reflected in the balance struck between charitable purposes and tax liability – as evidenced by the extent to which the tax collection agency determines charitable exemption.

The regulatory framework and the public interest

The public law dimension is also attributable to the regulatory machinery put in place by the State to safeguard donors and to facilitate supervision, transparency and accountability in the management of charities and their activities. A number of government bodies and mandatory administrative requirements now intrude into the affairs of charities.

The outcome is that in all common law countries, though in some more than others, charities and their activities are now increasingly becoming creatures of public law.

Tax exemption and the public/private interest

Taxation is an essential tool for redistributing wealth in the context of societies that permit inherited fortunes: it funds public service infrastructure for all and welfare benefits for the few. The cost of maintaining levels of public service provision has to be met through taxes and any exemption from tax liability simply means shifting the tax burden elsewhere. Tax concessions for charities are broadly justified on the basis that as they do what government would otherwise have to do so the public interest is served by facilitating their altruistic activities. The strength of this argument, however, varies according to the perceived usefulness of the charity, the prevailing politics and socio-economic conditions and does not always produce a logically sound result. The argument becomes most contentious in the context of full welfare state provision when the equation is less convincing for charities dedicated to providing hospitals and schools: tax concessions to defray the cost of services, that can only be extra to the full complement of government services, defy economic argument, particularly when service access is limited by fee-paying ability. On the other hand where, as in most modern western nations, the State is withdrawing from full public service provision then tax concessions that facilitate the filling of gaps in that provision make sound economic sense. Again, it can be disputed whether a charity expending all its resources for the benefit of people in another country is providing value for those within the jurisdiction who having contributed the resources now also have to make up the tax shortfall. In computing public benefit the State must take into account the longevity and enormous resources of some charities and of the charitable sector as a whole: a short-term gain of tax revenue may be at the price of sustaining long-term charitable investment.

Charity and the public/private partnership

Tax exemption is ultimately a political issue. Whether, in relation to any organization, the public interest is best served by imposing or exempting tax liability must turn on a political judgement as to which will earn a better rate of public benefit for society. The taxation system in play reflects the politics of the government in office and forms the cutting edge of its policy towards the voluntary sector in general and charities in particular. On one level this will be apparent in the particular institutional arrangements of that system: particularly by the presence of a body (e.g. the Charity Commission in England and Wales) to counterbalance the remit of the tax collecting agency and further the development of charitable purposes. At another level, it will be evident in government policy towards the sector: whether it favours a representative or participative model of democracy. If the former, then it will distance itself from the sector, rely on formal regulatory legislation to govern it and on elected politicians to represent its interests and negotiate with it. Where, however, it favours a more participative manner of engagement this will be demonstrated by an explicit policy declaring a commitment to working in partnership with the sector to achieve mutually agreed strategic goals (as recommended by the UN in its 'pillars of society' approach). In such a context the terms of engagement will be set by charity law and played out through the tax system. Charity, in short, then becomes much more a matter of public law. It is no coincidence that many common law nations have witnessed both the forming of a strategic partnership between government and voluntary sector followed closely by a charity law review the outcome of which can be read as a political statement of organizational activities now deemed to be matters of public law.

The parties

Charity law is concerned with the interests of donor, charitable organization and the State: defining and regulating their mutual interests; preventing and detecting abuse; and facilitating the operation of the related institutional infrastructure. The recipient of charity, the ultimate end-user of a system established for centuries and generating a considerable proportion of national GDP, is not a party and has no *locus standi* within charity law. In fact it could be argued that the rules regarding political activity actually prevent the voice of the 'subject' from being heard on matters concerning their interests (see, further, chapter 4). This provides an interesting contrast to that other *parens patriae* category 'wards': until recent decades, legal proceedings were conducted for and about their interests without any requirement that they be involved or otherwise represented in the decision-making process; now their wishes must be ascertained and taken into account and in some circumstances may be determinative of issues concerning them.

The donor

The basis for exempting a charitable trust from certain tax and other financial impositions rests on the fact that, in deciding to make a gift, a donor has chosen not to confer a private benefit upon a personally selected recipient but to instead make an altruistic gift for the public good. The right to voluntarily redistribute private wealth for the public benefit and the ancillary need to protect the value of that gift underpins charity law. The right of donor choice is subject to certain constraints if it is to be exercised in the form of a charitable gift.

The charity

An organization established and registered as dedicated to the pursuit of charitable purposes provides the conduit for channelling a donor's gift to the recipient. Such an organization, by virtue of its charitable status as being dedicated to public benefit activities and thereby supplementing or displacing the need for State service provision, will be eligible for tax exemption. Charities, being exempt from the rule against perpetuities (see, further, chapter 3), may in theory exist in perpetuity. Many have existed for centuries and in the process accumulated vast assets, data bases of irreplaceable worth and close bonds of mutual understanding with those socially disadvantaged whose interests they serve.

The State

The State's interest in relation to the charitable sector is mainly to ensure that, by facilitating the involvement of charities in public service provision that it would otherwise be obliged to fund, it gets good value to compensate for lost taxes. To that end its role has traditionally been entrusted to the tax collection agency which has arbitrated on entitlement to charitable status. Ancillary to that is the need to supervise to prevent abuse and for that reason alone the State would have an interest in maintaining an involvement in sector affairs.

However, the State has another interest in the sector. Developing sector capacity is an investment in social stability. The government can moderate the balance between its tax and support functions to achieve political outcomes by various means: interposing an agency to determine charitable purposes and status, quite separate and independent of the tax collection agency; and by manipulating tax concessions and donation incentives. It can also do so by direct statutory intervention. For example, the governments of many common law nations have accorded charitable status to sport, play and recreation activities by introducing legislation to that effect on the grounds that such activities contribute to the forming of social capital and enhance civic responsibility.

The gift relationship in charity law

The roles of the three parties intersect when a donor makes a charitable gift conferring a benefit upon members of the public (whether made to a charitable organization or for the purposes of establishing one). The legal right to do so is among the more singular characteristics of western democracies. The component parts of a charitable gift, which will itself attract tax concessions, have been identified as follows:[24]

> The essential attributes of a legal charity are, in my opinion, that it shall be *unselfish* – ie for the benefit of persons other than the donor – that it shall be *public*, ie that those to be benefited shall form a class worthy, in numbers of importance, of consideration as a public object of generosity, and that it shall be *philanthropic* or *benevolent* – ie dictated by a desire to do good.

All components must be present for the gift to be charitable in law.

Charitable intention of the donor

Motive is important but the presence or absence of charitable intent is not itself determinative. In most common law jurisdictions the test judicially applied to ascertain a donor's intention is objective, i.e. the fact that a donor believed when making the gift that it was charitable will not prevent the courts from ruling otherwise and vice versa because 'the court cannot inquire into the motives of the donor if the gift is in its nature a charity'.[25] This contrasts with the approach in Ireland where the test is subjective, i.e. 'if he intended to advance a charitable object recognised as such by the law, his gift will be a charitable gift'.[26] In all jurisdictions and in all cases, however, charitable intent is in itself insufficient. No matter how charitable the donor's intention may be, this will not make charitable a gift which does not satisfy the common law definition of 'charity', has no intrinsic merit,[27] breaches the law or is contrary to public policy (see, further, chapter 3).

In the latter context the court may well enquire: what moves the donor to act for the good of a stranger? To be charitable the beneficiary must be a stranger to whom no legal or moral obligation is owed and the motive must be altruistic rather than spiteful or prejudicial. It must also be intended to benefit others and not designed to confer an advantage on the donor.

Moreover, it has long been a firmly established rule that to be charitable a gift must be exclusively dedicated to charitable purposes. Where the courts find any ambiguity or equivocation in a donor's expressed intention or any possibility of a gift being used partially for non-charitable purposes then they will deny the gift charitable status.

Charitable purposes to be achieved

The second element requires that the charitable donation is 'within the gift' of the donor (i.e. it must be owned by him/her), be given exclusively for purposes which are recognized in law as charitable (as per *Pemsel* and related case law) and not be contrary to public policy or otherwise illegal[28] (see, further, chapter 3). The courts have readily acknowledged that the test of what may or may not be lawful will 'vary from generation to generation as the law successively grows more tolerant'.[29] The fact that a purpose was previously judicially found to be non-charitable will not prevent it from becoming charitable in the future and vice versa.[30]

The public benefit outcome

Thirdly, the gift must satisfy both arms of the 'public benefit test'; i.e. it must both confer an objectively verifiable 'benefit' and it must do so in favour of sufficient members of the 'public' (see, further, chapter 3). The test is applied unevenly across the four *Pemsel* heads of charity, falling most onerously upon all the relatively new purposes in the last category. Essentially, it is the nature and application of this test that makes charity a matter of public law.

Public   While it is certain that a gift conferred on a very limited number of identifiable people is private and therefore not charitable it is less certain what number of persons or other criteria would be sufficient to satisfy a definition of 'public' and justify charitable status. It will not be justified where the gift is to a closed class such as the employees of a particular company, any organization with a fixed membership or where potential beneficiaries are linked by a personal nexus (subject to the poor relations anomaly). It is well established that this component of the test will not be met where the gift is solely for member benefit; a restriction which can compromise the status of self-help groups or localized community development projects.[31] Such organizations will not be compromised, however, if the private benefit is a necessary and incidental consequence of bona fide charitable activity, is not disproportionate in amount and no other criteria unrelated to the purpose are imposed to further limit potential beneficiaries.[32]

Benefit   The benefit must be one that is recognized as charitable within the *Pemsel* classification or can be found to be so on the grounds that it comes within the 'spirit and intendment' of the Preamble (see, further, chapter 3). A gift to a closed religious order, for example, was found not to be charitable because intercessory prayers and the example set by leading pious lives were viewed as being too vague in terms of their benefit to the public.[33] Benefit has been found to exist in relation to gifts for the purpose of providing homes for lost dogs or cats, which are held to be charitable not for their sake but on the grounds that such animals are useful to man.[34]

The public benefit test   Its essentially subjective quality has allowed this crucial test of charitable status to be applied in accordance with the eye of the judicial beholder. This has resulted in an accumulated baggage of disparate case law and doubtful precedent, leaving the test exposed to accusations that it is not always serving the best interests of western society in the third millenium. For example, it may be argued that providing amenities for a privileged minority such as public school education, private hospital care, opera houses and concert halls, etc is a doubtful interpretation of public benefit. Similarly, organizations which reinforce sectoral differences by ensuring affiliation to a particular religion arguably also provide only membership benefit to specified groups and are thereby discriminatory, emphasize social divisions and possibly the inequities in society as a whole. This approach, however, may be countered by a broad view argument that charitable status is an appropriate stamp of approval for the activities of organizations which enrich the texture, health and general good of society, promoting diversity rather than stultifying it by protecting homogeneity. In our sophisticated and rapidly changing society the concepts of 'poverty', 'education' and indeed 'religion' are increasingly uncertain and social inclusion is no longer synonymous with assimilation. A significant challenge for this book is to explore the public benefit test, examine how it is currently applied across the common law jurisdictions and consider its potential as a strategic device for addressing issues of social inclusion.

The overseas gift relationship in charity law

The Titmus altruism test is particularly problematic in the moral minefield of international aid. In this context there is not only the clear danger of the parties being equally trapped in the traditional supplicant/benefactor dynamic writ large, but also a distinct utility factor often emerges to tarnish the altruistic role of the donor.

Charitable intent

The donor role in the overseas gift relationship has for the most part been borne by religious organizations from modern western societies working in developing countries. To do so as charities the law required, and continues to require, that the advancement of religion be the primary purpose. This in turn means that ultimately the intention must be the traditional one of saving souls. In more recent decades, many large secular charities have undertaken the donor role and have usually done so with their primary purpose defined under the fourth *Pemsel* head. While the accompanying charitable intent undoubtedly satisfies the requirements of charity law, their activities may be constrained by other factors.

Charitable purpose

Just as the altruism in the donor role of religious organizations is compromised by the proselytism that accompanies aid so that of the secular agencies is also liable to be compromised, this time by trade concerns (see, also, chapter 2).

Government's trade policy   The government to government aid budgets of western nations dwarfs the resources of charities engaged in overseas aid and the latter are often both funded by government and used by it to channel its aid budget to developing countries. Government choice of recipient, however, is a political matter that will be at least influenced by international trade agreements, loans and tariffs. The Common Agricultural Policy of the European Union, for example, sets the trade parameters for the 25 member states in relation to trade in agricultural produce with developing nations (leading to massive distortions in the real market-place price for goods such as sugar). Charities that are not financially independent can be under considerable pressure to channel aid in directions that are compliant with government trade policies.

Charity and trade   The Fairtrade foundation is an excellent example of what charitable activity can achieve. Created in the Netherlands in the late 1980s, by September 2004 Fairtrade had grown to include 422 certified producer groups in 49 producer countries selling to hundreds of Fairtrade registered importers, licensees and retailers in 19 countries. Many international charities have developed trading arms which provide the vital service of finding and managing markets for locally produced goods. To support this service, they often have organizational infrastructure in particular developing countries. The protection of that investment may at times arise as a factor influencing choice of destination for aid.

Recipient nation's economy   Then there is the fact that whatever injection of aid is made to the fragile economies of the third world, this will have a disproportionate impact on existing patterns of commerce. The distortion caused to local supply/demand chains by gratuitous acts of benevolence can cause serious long-term disruption to established family, tribal and community networks. The irony is that this is usually coupled with crippling long-term debt repayments, often to the same developed nations that are providing the overseas aid. The net result leaves the recipient nation's economy to a considerable extent in the control of others.

The public benefit outcome

The legal requirement that the gift satisfy both arms of the 'public benefit test' is also problematic in an overseas context.

Public   In kinship-based communities it is not always possible to establish charitable structures that are not limited by a nexus of personal relationship that is fatal to charitable gifts (see, further, chapter 4).

Benefit   Difficulties could arise in the case of organizations dedicated to pursuing purposes charitable under the fourth *Pemsel* head. The public benefit test falls most rigorously upon such organizations and the settled judicial view has been that unless it could demonstrate that its activities resulted in some public benefit accruing in its home jurisdiction then such an organization would be ineligible for charitable status.

Building social capital and promoting civil society between nations

Although Titmus confined his analysis of donors and the gift relationship to within national boundaries, there would seem to be no good reason why charities should not extend their role by developing on an international basis their current function as catalysts for advancing civil society.

International altruistic activity is useful in itself and it demonstrates good faith. In the post-9/11 world it is of crucial importance that honest brokers be facilitated to forestall the drift from social marginalization to alienation and possible violent confrontation. Demonstrating altruistic conduct may well encourage such activity among other international agencies as well as helping to cultivate a more general sense of trust, shared morality and civic responsibility in the international arena. Charities, being free from the need to appease their constituents and from the constraints of pressing political considerations, are arguably better placed than governments to develop an untainted altruistic mediatory role on behalf of the socially disadvantaged whether the latter take the form of a group, community or nation.

Failure of the gift relationship in charity law

Fitting the donor's gift within the technical constraints of charity law as practised within the common law nations has proved problematic. The landscape provided by 400 years of charity case law practised over many continents is one filled with a rich spread of examples of man's humanity to man and indeed to animals. The colourful array of good intentions that failed to convince the judiciary of their charitable nature include: a sanctuary for birds and wild flowers;[35] a sanctuary or reserve for 'animals, birds or other creatures not human' was not charitable as they would only 'be free to molest and harry one another'[36] and thus was of no benefit to the community; while a hospital for hedgehogs[37] was too irrational and absurd.

It is also dotted with quirky illustrations of how donors' good intentions have failed to materialize into charitable gifts as the law sought to separate essentially charitable purposes from all others. The common law courts have exercised rigorous vigilance in policing the boundaries of charity, extinguishing any entity that strayed or could stray outside the limits of the technical legal meaning judicially assigned to it.

Beneficial

The fact that a gift is of benefit to the community does not, in the eyes of the common law, necessarily make it charitable.[38] The marrying of quantity and quality in the public benefit test has been controversial: there are those who take the view that the quality element (e.g. the restoration of a quixotic work of art) enriches the public domain whether or not a quantity of people think so – an argument that plays out in the fields of 'public schools',[39] private hospitals,[40] concert halls, etc. The alternative view that no matter what else is undertaken in its name, charity is failing to justify itself if it does not give priority to poverty, has never held much credence in common law. This is clear from the Preamble lists and is equally clear in *Pemsel* where Macnaghten L.J. explained that trusts falling under the fourth head 'are not the less charitable in the eye of the law, because incidentally they benefit the rich as well as the poor, as indeed every charity that deserves the name must do either directly or indirectly'.[41]

The legal structure of an organization can also cause problems. Even if a gift is undoubtedly beneficial to a large part of the community it may still be denied charitable status because of the legal structure or nature of the organization designated to give effect to it: self-help organizations, advocacy agencies, mutual benefit organizations and other types of bodies will be considered too inherently compromised to qualify as charities (see, further, chapter 3).

Benevolent

The lexicon of charity is replete with deceptive terminology. Benevolence, for example, is not to be construed in law as charity because 'the word "benevolent" is a word of somewhat shadowy meaning',[42] while gifts expressed for charitable or benevolent purposes have often been declared void as they are open to being interpreted in ways that may go beyond what is exclusively charitable.[43] So, in *Morice* v. *Bishop of Durham*[44] an estate left to the Bishop for him to dispose of to 'such objects of benevolence and liberality' as he at his discretion should see fit was found not to be charitable as the terms of the gift allowed for the possibility of it being used for both charitable and non-charitable purposes. As Picarda has stated:[45]

> A gift simply to 'benevolent purposes' is objectionable:[46] a benevolent purpose may be (but is not necessarily) charitable. The same is true of gifts to philanthropic purposes,[47] utilitarian purposes,[48] emigration,[49] patriotic[50] and public purposes:[51] they all go further than legal charity. Likewise gifts for encouraging undertaking of general utility,[52] for hospitality,[53] for such societies as should be in the opinion of trustees 'most in need of help'[54] and for such purposes, civil or religious, as a class of persons should appoint,[55] are too wide . . . the permutations are endless.

Where the gift for benevolent purposes is expressed as being additional, rather than as an alternative, to charitable purposes then it will be construed as charitable.[56]

Philanthropic

Just as 'benevolent' fails the technical definition of 'charity' in law, so too does 'philanthropic' even though it is 'no doubt a word of narrower meaning than "benevolent" '.[57] As has been explained 'an act may be benevolent if it indicates goodwill to a particular individual only, whereas an act cannot be said to be philanthropic unless it indicates goodwill to mankind at large'.[58] Where gifts are expressed as being for charitable or philanthropic purposes they invariably fail as was the case with: 'to such religious charitable and philanthropic objects' as three named persons might select;[59] 'for charitable, religious, educational or philanthropic purposes';[60] 'for such charitable, religious philanthropic educational or scientific institution or institutions';[61] and for 'charitable benevolent religious and educational institutions associations and objects'.[62] The rationale for adversely discriminating against philanthropy puzzled Lord Sterndale MR:[63]

> I confess I find considerable difficulty in understanding the exact reason why a gift for the benefit of animals, and for the prevention of cruelty to animals generally, should be a good charitable gift, while a gift for philanthropic purposes, which, I take it, is for the benefit of mankind generally, should be bad as a charitable gift. The gift for the benefit of animals, apparently, is held to be valid because it is educative of mankind, it being good for mankind that they should be taught not to be cruel but kind to animals, and one would quite agree with that. But if the benefit of mankind on that particular side makes that a good charitable gift it is a little difficult to see why any philanthropic purpose to benefit mankind on all sides is a bad one. But it is so.

Where the gift is expressed to be for both charitable and philanthropic[64] purposes then it will be a good charitable gift because the object to be benefited must possess both characteristics.

There are, however, some indications that in England and Wales the law relating to charity is beginning to relax its approach towards policing these distinctions. In the Charities Act 1992 a 'charitable institution' is 'a charity or an institution other than a charity which is established for charitable or philanthropic purposes'. The National Lottery Act 1993, section 44(1) provides that 'charitable expenditure' means expenditure by charities or by institutions other than charities that are established for charitable purposes (whether or not those purposes are charitable within the meaning of any rule of law), benevolent purposes or philanthropic purposes. In other common law jurisdictions, perhaps Australia in particular (see, further, Part IV) a similar trend is apparent. It remains to be seen whether the new charities legislation will take the opportunity to consolidate a broader interpretation of 'charity' in the law of England and Wales and elsewhere.

Retrieving and redirecting charitable assets

The courts have long recognized that it is advantageous to all concerned that a gift intended for charitable purposes should acquire or retain charity status. This basic concern, to ensure that where possible the charitable intentions of a donor should be respected, explains the significance of the *cy-près* doctrine (see, further, chapters 3 and 6).

Cy-près

There is an equitable presumption[65] that the charitable intentions of a donor should not be allowed to fail because of an inconsequential difficulty. Inevitably, however, some do so, either at the outset or much later, perhaps after centuries of successful existence as a charitable entity. This may be due to a mere technical legality, an area of uncertainty, or perhaps a fundamental failure, to construct a trust or for one of many other reasons which the donor may not have foreseen.[66] Sometimes the failure was due to judicial intervention to halt activities previously judged to be charitable.[67] The legal significance of *cy-près*, which has been in use since at least the seventeenth century, lies in its capacity to overcome such legal technicalities and give effect to a donor's charitable intent.

Also, many charities began as trusts created wholly in the private sphere by donors who placed a fund of money or property in the hands of trustees. If the beneficiaries are indefinite and the trust has a charitable purpose, the charitable purpose may exist in perpetuity. However, although a charity cannot die the purposes for which it was established may become impossible or impractical to fulfill and the law then had to find a means to deal appropriately with its assets. In such circumstances the remedy of *cy-près* has been available to protect the assets and allow them to be used for charitable purposes similar to those indicated by the donor.

Cy-près has proved to be a useful and flexible mechanism for adjusting the use of charitable assets. It allows the purposes of a defunct charity or a group of such charities to be revised and permits their assets (often very considerable, some having been left to accumulate for generations) to be released to address contemporary social need. Access to this procedure, however, can be problematic. In some jurisdictions it falls exclusively to the High Court where the entailed delay and expense can make it impractical.

Conclusion

This chapter has explored the origins of charity, considered its social function and reflected on how this has developed over time. It examined the concept of 'benefit', inquiring as to how and to whom this was distributed and how it was defined in law. As an aid to understanding the dynamics involved it suggested that the Titmus theory of 'the gift relationship' offered useful insight and could be seen as underpinning both charity and the law. In particular, his claim that altruism lay at the heart of that relationship, and that activities which allowed opportunities for altruism were of value to the individuals concerned and to society generally because ethical conduct was good in itself and generated a sense of shared morality and civic responsibility that served to bond society, seemed convincing. It could be seen as offering guidance for the role of charities in representing the interests of the socially disadvantaged within communities and nations while also justifying an extension of that role to authorize a mediatory function for charities in the international context of alienated cultures and countries.

An argument to be developed throughout this book is that the legacy of charity law, which has for centuries provided a platform for altruism among the common law nations, could now become the means for facilitating and co-ordinating a future such role for charities. Given that they share the same legal platform and are engaged in similar charity law reform processes, many of the most developed nations of the western world are now uniquely placed to adjust the law relating to altruism and thereby make a strategic and united contribution to focusing charities and their immense resources on addressing issues of social inclusion on a national and international basis. A necessary preliminary to doing so would be the identification of difficulties, inherent in the common law approach, that currently obstruct the capacity of charities to deal with such issues; a task of central importance to this book.

The Titmus theory of the gift relationship was noted to have omitted to deal with the price, in terms of self-esteem etc., that the recipient often has to pay for the 'gift'. There would seem to be a fundamental problem to do with the gift relationship as an effective means of transferring resources that enables their use by those in need to acquire sustainable self-sufficiency. To give or to intervene in the lives of others – not just without demeaning but to instil self-respect, confidence, trust and a determination to succeed while doing so – and to thereafter sustain achieved improvements, has manifestly not always been possible in the context of that relationship. Arguably, in its Christian origins, this was not even seen as desirable. Following on from the above exploration of what charity is and what it is for, the next chapter examines what it does and how it does it. It suggests that the gift relationship may need to be reworked to become more of an exchange relationship, allowing charity to assume the broad characteristics of philanthropy, if it is to effectively address social inclusion issues.

Chapter 2

Philanthropy and the challenge of social inclusion

The contemporary issues

Introduction

This chapter explains how charity, resting essentially on a supplicant/benefactor dynamic, has given way to modern philanthropy. It begins by considering charity and its limitations as a response to contemporary social issues. In the context of contemporary developed western nations, the charitable approach is considered relative to that of human rights and social justice. In that context, the strengths, weaknesses and relevance of the gift relationship underpinning charity are also identified and assessed.

The chapter then considers the complex problems presented by current social inclusion issues. Concepts such as social capital and civil society are examined and the challenges to social cohesion are explored. This leads into an examination of modern philanthropy and the legal structures needed to give effect to it. In particular, attention is given to the role played by the trust and the endowed trust/foundation. The chapter concludes by reflecting on the implications arising from the failure of the latter to fulfil its potential.

The gift relationship in a contemporary context

Charity serves and has always served an important strategic social function by mediating between the needs of the disadvantaged and the resources of the privileged. This has not always been to the long-term advantage of either; in particular charitable intervention, channelled through trusts existing in perpetuity, can confirm the dependency and marginalization of recipients while reinforcing the role of the benefactor. Nor is it always necessarily the answer to inequitable social divisions that may instead require redress through a political or rights frame of reference. There are areas in which the gift relationship has no legitimate role.

Where it has legitimacy, the vast resources and public benefit purposes of charity should make a difference. It is not itself the answer to poverty and deprivation but it does have enormous potential to address the causes and ameliorate the effects of disadvantage while also facilitating social inclusion. If charity is to be permitted to fulfil its potential and promote the social inclusion of marginalized groups it is important that a better fit be found between the law, charitable resources and the needs of the socially excluded. As a preliminary, this will entail differentiating between the different frames of reference applicable to the circumstances of the latter and being clear about what it is that falls specifically to charity.

Charity and rights

Good charity law can never be an adequate remedy for bad politics. The frameworks provided by politics and fundamental human rights must always be allowed clear application, free of obfuscation and unsullied by the perspectives of charity. While this is examined in more detail later (see, further, chapters 6 and 7) it is necessary at this stage to briefly delineate some relevant parameters.

Social justice

All modern western nations have in recent decades put in place legislative platforms providing legal recognition of and protection for social diversity and difference, whether on the basis of race, disability, religion, culture or gender. Universal programmes of law and policy appropriately underpin standards that must prevail in situations of possible injustice or social inequity; these include rights to equality of opportunity and freedom from adverse discrimination. The emphasis on collective rights provides a structural response to systemic social exclusion (e.g. racism) and a basis for the assertion of an individual's rights. It replaces a victim perspective with a situational perspective in which 'blame' for the circumstances of social disadvantage lies with society rather than with the individuals concerned.

This approach, like the welfare state ethos, is based on the assumption that 'across the board' provision is socially less divisive than targeted intervention aimed at addressing the circumstances of a particular disadvantaged group. The latter approach is one left to bodies such as trade unions which, through advocacy, negotiation and strike action, have often proved effective in redressing circumstances of social inequity, if, at times, at the price of an exposure not wholly in the best long-term interests of the group concerned. Targeted intervention has also been the traditional modus operandi of charities but has differed from the trade union approach by generally being less strategic, short-term in its effect, often demeaning to recipients and more socially stigmatizing.

Human rights

Again, all modern western nations now subscribe to the European Convention on Fundamental Human Rights or to a national equivalent. The international recognition given to such basic rights as the right to life, the right not to be tortured, to privacy of family life, etc., reinforced by the rulings and principles established in the European Court of Human Rights (ECHR), provide guarantees of protection or means of redress for the citizens of those nations and benchmarks for measuring the progress of other countries (see, further, chapter 7). Clearly, for individuals affected by issues relating to status, discrimination, invasion of privacy, etc., there can be no substitute for a rights-based approach. For charities, the fact that certain rights such as freedom of assembly and freedom of expression are now embedded in international law has given extra leverage and helped to legit-imize their role in countries without a tradition of democratic rule. However, although of enormous importance in the context of raising standards, the human rights movement with its necessarily single-issue, one-dimensional approach is an inadequate response to situations of social exclusion. Whether experienced as an individual, community or nation, social exclusion requires a comprehensive approach in which the assertion of human rights can only ever play a limited role.

Anti-terrorism

In all modern western nations the above rights-oriented approaches have in recent years been counterbalanced by an increased preoccupation with intro-ducing legislation to combat international terrorism. This has necessarily resulted in measures that curtail the democratic rights of individuals and organizations. In particular, they have added considerably to the insecurity felt by minority racial groups and by non-government organizations, especially charities, working in developing countries (see, further, chapter 6).

Charity

At the outset of the third millennium, charity is finding itself squeezed at both ends by the rights-oriented pressures of the above approaches. At one end charity is being 'capped' by rights and forced to concede ground to an expansive libertarian movement requiring legislative recognition of that which individuals should in future be entitled to receive as of right rather than as a result of acts of discretion-ary charity. At the other, established liberal principles that have long governed the activities of individuals and non-government organizations, for example the freedom of expression and freedom to conduct affairs without interference from the State, are being forced to give way to measures asserting the paramount right of national security.

Charity and government provision

Charity in the common law nations has always, to a greater or lesser extent and with varying emphases, complemented the role of government. It has never been possible, in the broad field of family and community provision, to draw a clear line between matters that fall to either and the capacity to do so has become more difficult as the level of government funding and range of tax exemptions for charities increases.

Welfare

The balance between provision by government and charity in relation to education, health and social care has altered over time. In the UK it was most clearly weighted in favour of government in the years following the Beveridge-led reforms in the 1950s and the building of comprehensive welfare state provision (see, further, chapter 5). By the close of the twentieth century, the UK and other modern western nations were experiencing the effects of State withdrawal from 'cradle to grave' services and the balance began to be redressed as charities assumed, or were pressured into, responsibility for meeting the services shortfall.

While there can be no doubt as to the value of comprehensive State service provision, a floor of basic services available and accessible to all as of right and according to need, opinion is divided as to whether charity or State is best positioned to provide for the socially excluded. The availability of non-stigmatizing services is obviously desirable but it has often fallen to charities to provide the means for the socially marginalized to access them; in terms of information, psychological and other forms of support. Moreover, the 'one size fits all' approach of State provision has never been wholly effective in meeting the needs of those who are or perceive themselves to be different. Again, the chronically socially marginalized who will not avail themselves of public services, perhaps because they reject the legitimacy of the State or have become so 'victimized' that they lack the self-confidence to claim their entitlements, need to be given recognition, acceptance and a 'voice'. Charities are then often the only acceptable agency positioned to advocate on behalf of and empower those who would otherwise be left to become alienated.

Public utility

While it is reasonably clear that the provision of basic institutions and social infrastructure is the responsibility of government and is paid for in taxes, it is less clear what aspects of ancillary provision such as museums, concert halls, etc., should or could fall to charity. Where there is an element of poverty and/or abandonment then charity has traditionally had a role (e.g. residential accommodation for animals, children, the disabled and the elderly), though whether to supplement or to substitute for government provision has never been clear. Where the need to be met is outside the standardized range of State services then regardless, or in spite of, any poverty factor, both State and charity have been content to leave provision to the latter (e.g. fee paying schools and hospitals). Also, the independence and flexibility of charities enables them to provide facilities that are targeted and acceptable because: they recognize and address links between poverty and other sources of exclusion such as racism, disability and perhaps the legacy of colonial oppression (e.g. hostels for indigenous people); can provide services that are sensitive to local demand; and can deliver these more cost effectively than government bodies.

In this uncertain territory perhaps all that can be said is that charitable provision of public utilities helps to acknowledge the diversity of social need, broadens the range of utilities available and thereby enhances the capacity of a society to act in a more inclusive manner (see, further, chapter 5).

Charity and the gift relationship

Outside the above frames of reference, the Titmus theory of the gift relationship, as explored in the previous chapter, remains valid within its own terms. It helpfully and accurately explains how the altruism of ethically motivated behaviour can benefit all involved, generate more of the same and thereby contribute to building social capital and consolidating civil society. There are, perhaps, certain circumstances to which the theory is particularly applicable and can be readily substantiated.

Poverty

Responding to the effects of poverty on individuals, communities and nations as opposed to addressing its causes, continues to represent and affirm the validity of the gift relationship. The integrity of the traditional supplicant/benefactor dynamic, revolving around a one-way transaction of resources with an essentially short-term and palliative effect, cyclically repeated in a pattern that reinforces reciprocity among the participants while leaving poverty in place, remains intact in modern western societies.

Disaster

Similar in their effect to poverty, disasters rob their victims of the resources necessary for self-sufficiency and trigger the supplicant/benefactor dynamic. The relevance of the gift relationship in this context is, however, subject to certain caveats.

Prevention of avoidable disaster   The installation of early warning systems to detect impending disaster whether caused by nature (earthquakes, tsunamis, volcanic eruptions, etc.) or man (crop failures, AIDS, war, etc.) is outside the reach of developing countries where such events most usually occur but within the gift of advanced western economies. There are many countries where there is a pressing need for systems to detect unusual earth movement or cyclonic weather patterns, or for the provision of wells for fresh water, vaccinations for HIV, spray for mosquitoes, seeds for crops, irrigation schemes, etc. Despite the best efforts of the UN, such systems are not fully in place. Advance provision, by western nations initiating the gift relationship, can prevent an event of nature or human failure from having its usual disastrous consequences and would then place management responsibility where it belongs. Not to intervene in advance, the moral equivalent of the traditional model whereby the benefactor waits until the helpless supplicant has to plead for aid, is to demonstrate unethical conduct, give permission for further inaction and is manifestly not cost-efficient.

Preparation for disaster relief   The overriding obligation on affluent western nations to give prompt unconditional assistance to developing countries at times of natural disaster extends to a responsibility to commit resources in advance for that purpose. In order to be prepared to respond quickly and efficiently to the next disaster, it is clearly necessary for a multinational task force to be established, equipped and on permanent standby (the civil equivalent, if you like, of police armed response units or the armed services' swift reaction force). Such a body would have all the known core components for prompt efficient intervention (doctors, helicopters, weatherproof tents, dried foods, water, etc.) and with the powers necessary to call upon such additional expertise and resources as the particular situation required. Again, this would require the western nations acting as benefactor to initiate the gift relationship.

Disaster relief   In circumstances where an overwhelming calamity has left its helpless victims without the basic necessities of life and assistance is urgently requested, the Titmus approach is wholly legitimate. The altruism of a one-way transaction then constitutes a clear moral imperative outweighing other considerations and does not itself present an obstacle to appropriate use of an unconditional gift. All parties recognize that intervening circumstances over which they had no control are responsible for the necessity of a gift relationship where the gift is essentially value-free and where the roles of the participants could have been reversed. Such a situation most closely approximates the context for the gift of blood upon which the Titmus theory was initially based.

The challenge of social inclusion

Social inclusion is a modern sociological concept with ancient roots. In developed western nations its contemporary origins lie in the beginnings of the retraction of the welfare state in Europe in the late 1970s and 80s and the consequent growing social divisions. As universal welfare benefits were cut, to be replaced by targeted means-tested benefits, it became apparent that the effects were disproportionately affecting those who were already disadvantaged (e.g. immigrants, racial minorities, the unemployed) leading to increased levels of urban poverty and homelessness. This was exacerbated by a gradual collapse of heavy industry and manufacturing and by revolutionary changes in agriculture, causing the disappearance of sources of employment that had sustained families and communities for generations. The resulting phenomenon of large-scale unemployment and drift to the cities triggered social inclusion policies designed to address urban poverty through retraining programmes that would equip redundant workers with service sector skills and a chance to develop a new social identity. Subsequently, the concept and policies of social inclusion were extended to address the needs of immigrants and racial minorities and then to those such as the disabled, the aged, children, lone parents, gay and lesbian groups, religious and ethnic minorities and Gypsies. It is a concept that clearly applies to relationships between the privileged and disadvantaged, between those set apart by differences or perceived differences, whether occurring on a community level, more generally between groups within a society or between nations.

Concepts and definitions

It has become customary for sociologists and others, including with increasing frequency, politicians, to refer to one or more of a clutch of interdependent concepts when dealing with what is seen as the fragility of modern society. These include: social cohesion; social capital; civil society; social inclusion and exclusion.

Social cohesion

Canadian social theorist Jane Jenson has usefully described a 'socially cohesive society' as one where all groups have a sense of 'belonging, participation, inclusion, recognition and legitimacy'.[1] Jenson also suggests that these positive attributes of cohesion are often complemented by reference to negative variables such as isolation, exclusion, non-involvement, rejection and illegitimacy as examples and perceptions of the absence of cohesion.[2] Beauvais and Jenson combine an interest in social cohesion with social capital and underline the interactive elements of:[3]

- common values and a civic culture;
- social order and social control;
- social solidarity and reductions in wealth disparities;
- social networks and social capital; and
- territorial belonging and identity.

Social cohesion can also be promoted through the permeation of explicit ethical standards into significant areas of social functioning, e.g. ethical investments by banks and big businesses, ethical foreign policy, etc. For any society, the exclusion of individuals or groups can become a major threat to its social cohesion and ultimately to its economic prosperity.

Social capital

The concept of 'social capital' has been coined to explain the motivation of individuals to engage in collective activity for altruistic purposes and refers also to the environment of mutual trust which is then necessary if that engagement is to be conducive to building the components of civil society. It has been explained by Putnam as a concept that 'refers to connections among individuals – social networks and the norms of reciprocity and trustworthiness that arise from them'.[4] He distinguishes between two forms of social capital: that which acts as a bond between communities; and that which bridges the differences between them. It is the latter which potentially has a particular significance for the role of charities in relation to social inclusion.

Willingness and trust are prerequisites if charitable activity is to successfully address the social inclusion agenda. Whether the gap to be bridged is on a local, national or international scale there must exist a mutuality of good faith, a common understanding and acceptance that means and ends are in harmony and that intended outcomes are advantageous to all concerned. This requires recognition and respect for cultural differences, a willingness and trust to engage on clear terms for specific purposes and an acceptance that the process will not result in any fudging or assimilation of the interests of either party.

Civil society

The concept of 'civil society' means different things to different people. Bothwell has usefully suggested that the literature on the subject reveals four distinctively different approaches:[5]

> First, scholars such as Robert Putnam, Larry Diamond and Francis Fukuyama focus on what they see as the results of a strong civil society – the behaviours they believe healthy civil society produces including trust, reciprocity, tolerance and inclusion (traits and networks that add to a society's social capital) ... Second, other students of civil society, such as Rajesh Tandon, David Brown and John Clark focus on the preconditions that must be met before a healthy civil society can come about (e.g. freedom of speech, freedom of association, rule of law etc) ... Third, many who have considered what is a healthy civil society have sought to define it as a desirable state of all society (e.g. free public education and health care available to all) ... Fourth, most who write about civil society define it in terms of its composition (e.g. including religious organisations, social clubs and movements, community based organisations etc but excluding family, tribe, clan, political parties etc).

These are not discrete, mutually exclusive categories, as it would be quite feasible to subscribe to some or all without losing much of the concept's egalitarian essence. As has been emphasized 'the boundaries of the space in which civil society activities take place are permeable'.[6] For the purposes of charity law, however, the concept is perhaps best seen as represented by the preconditions of the second approach leading to the goals of the first. Regardless of the approach adopted, the concept of civil society would seem to rest on the free association of people in the pursuit of aims that complement the public benefit efforts of the State and result in a more coherent and engaged body politic. It is then most usually envisaged as being given effect by a myriad of non-governmental bodies that influence, supplement or counterbalance the institutional infrastructure of the State.

The concepts of 'civil society' and 'social capital' have, in recent decades, generated a considerable body of work and have now been adopted as the modern hallmarks, or perhaps the slogans, of democracy.[7]

Social inclusion

This is best understood not simply as the antithesis of social exclusion, or as a response to it, but as a concept and a strategic approach that includes but transcends it. Social exclusion has been defined as:[8]

> A shorthand label for what can happen when individuals or areas suffer from a combination of linked problems such as unemployment, poor skills, low incomes, poor housing, high crime environments, bad health and family breakdown.

Or more precisely:[9]

> An individual is socially excluded if he or she does not participate to a reasonable degree over time in certain activities of his or her society, and (a) this is for reasons beyond his or her control, and (b) he or she would like to participate.

Social inclusion, however, while certainly indicating the need to overcome the particular obstacles constituting social exclusion, goes a good deal further. It calls for an approach that is not limited to addressing the more salient socio-economic variables but is designed to also identify and engage with whatever other factors might be creating a sense of distance between those in mainstream society and the more marginalized. It insists that differences be respected and protected, maintains that social diversity is of value in itself and is not to be subsumed in the hegemony of the majority and requires common ground to be found and developed linking the interests of majority and minority groups. Social inclusion is not just a policy it is also a process. It requires a proactive approach involving the investment of resources and the implementation of action plans necessary to make it attractive for the marginalized to join with the majority. This may involve any one or any combination of different strategies: specific adjustments to the relevant legal framework to incorporate social justice principles of equity and equality of opportunity, together with provisions ensuring universal rights; a broad focus on opportunities for capacity building and promoting social capital; a targeted multi-agency focus on service provision to improve the circumstances of a particular marginalized group (e.g. the long-term unemployed, racial/ethnic minorities, people with disabilities, the homeless, etc.); or a straightforward legal rights approach in which a policy and programme, based on fundamental human rights, are formulated and implemented in respect of matters causing exclusion.

A distinction can usefully be drawn between the concepts of 'social inclusion' and 'civil society': while the latter must always encompass the former, the reverse is not necessarily the case. A modern democratic nation cannot reasonably be regarded as such unless it has achieved a significant measure of social inclusion and has in place the policies, the law and the institutional infrastructure for addressing emerging issues. Having done so, however, it may still fall short of attaining the status of a civil society, which requires not just the inclusion but the positive engagement of minority groups in building or sustaining a fully operational democratic society (see, also, chapter 6).

The social inclusion agenda

Every modern western society is currently struggling to manage its particular configuration of issues from what is a fairly standard domestic social inclusion agenda. For each this priority is compounded by the need to simultaneously respond to international pressures: of poverty and deprivation in the third world; of trade and debt repayment arrangements with undeveloped countries; and to the social exclusion agenda of other nations as currently most graphically illustrated in the 'asylum seekers' phenomenon and in the growing political complications emanating from the war in Iraq. For the common law nations, the subjects of this book, the challenge to facilitate social inclusion also arises in a post-colonial context in which a legacy of suppression remains to be worked through. The present circumstances of many indigenous communities provide – in varying degrees – examples of unfinished business in terms of cultural imbalance, social justice and rights.

Domestic social inclusion

The internal social inclusion issues facing most modern western nations, including the common law countries that are the subject of this study, are broadly similar (see, further, Part IV).

Persistent poverty   The enduring nature of poverty in all common law nations is a challenge for government. The numbers of children born into poverty and living a childhood in conditions below the poverty threshold constitute a target for social inclusion policies in all the countries studied. They all note an over-representation of minority racial groups living in poverty in urban areas.

Immigrants and refugees   In recent decades all modern western nations have struggled to cope with the impact of refugees, 'asylum seekers' or 'economic migrants' who have arrived in large numbers seeking sanctuary and the opportunity to rebuild family life. Between 1975 and 2006 the numbers of global migrants more than doubled to almost 200 million and for the developed nations their arrival is often accompanied by human rights concerns. Many form close-knit alternative communites, within but apart from their 'host' society, prevented by mutually incomprehensible cultural barriers from access to appropriate service provision and full participation in that society. This tension was recognized in the memorable dissenting judgment of Gonthier J, articulating the rationale for opposing the decision to refuse charitable status, in *Vancouver Society of Immigrant and Visible Minority Women* v. *Minister of National Revenue*:[10]

> immigrants are often in special need of assistance in their efforts to integrate into their new home. Lack of familiarity with the social customs, language,

economy, job market, educational system, and other aspects of daily life that existing inhabitants of Canada take for granted may seriously impede the ability of immigrants to this country to make a full contribution to our national life. In addition, immigrants may face discriminatory practices which too often flow from ethnic language, and cultural differences. An organisation . . . which assists immigrants through this difficult transition is directed, in my view, towards a charitable purpose.

The 'ethnic enclaves' established by immigrants – which express the preferences, common interests, social networks and common cultural and/or religious needs of their residents – also serve to segregate urban communities. While providing support systems for women and children, for the elderly and for those not fluent in the English language, they also separate ethnic communities from ease of access to mainstream opportunities in employment, education and to social and shopping facilities. Such segregation – often associated with low incomes, poverty and poor housing – creates poor neighbourhoods and a barrier to social inclusion. In all common law nations the official policies of multiculturalism, anti-racism and immigrant citizenship acquisition, sit alongside the growing reality of social exclusion for newcomers.

Inequality   All modern western nations are struggling to address the distinctive needs of socially disadvantaged minority groups such as the disabled, the elderly, the mentally ill, the drug-dependent, disaffected youth and the gay and lesbian community (see, further, Part IV). How best to deliver targeted and preferential services in a context of welfare state withdrawal and non-discriminatory and universalist principles of social justice, and in a way that promotes equity, equality and social inclusion, is proving difficult.

The international social inclusion agenda

Increased globalization correspondingly reduces the ability of any nation to concentrate solely on its own internal social inclusion agenda. Looking simply inward is not an option when international refugees, economic migrants and terrorists are seeking host nations. Arguably, only by attending to circumstances in developing countries will developed nations be free to exercise more control over their borders, be in a position to devote more resources to their domestic agendas and be better informed as to how to build multicultural, cohesive and socially inclusive communities and nations. The challenge of the international social inclusion agenda for every developed nation is how best to balance aid, trade and terrorism concerns.

Aid   In the underdeveloped countries of the world the very poor are getting poorer.[11] In the worst affected regions – sub-Saharan Africa and Southern Asia – the number of hungry people has increased by tens of millions because of growing populations and poor agricultural productivity. Every year, almost 11 million children die – i.e. 30,000 children a day – before their fifth birthday. Five diseases – pneumonia, diarrhoea, malaria, measles and AIDS – account for half of these deaths which could be prevented by expanding low-cost prevention and treatment measures.[12] The lack of appropriate and sufficient medicines is largely due to the protectionist approach of western governments towards the patents and profits of their pharmaceutical producers.

As noted in a recent UN report,[13] most of the recent increase in aid has been used to cancel debts and meet humanitarian and reconstruction needs in the aftermath of emergencies. While a debt-relief programme for the most heavily indebted countries has reduced future debt payments for 27 nations by $54 billion, this relief often goes to countries that have ceased debt repayments and does not necessarily provide new finance for social services or poverty reduction. Similarly, emergency and disaster relief, although essential, does not address long-term development needs.

The statistics are appalling, make a convincing case for continued aid, disclose the constraints imposed by western commercial interests and reveal how the inadequate response of the western world is allowing deprivation in developing nations to continue on a scale that is devastating to it and detrimental to the bona fides of western nations. This dynamic resonates with the archetypal supplicant/benefactor relationship that characterized the role of the gift relationship within early Christian society when maintaining the status quo was perhaps the governing concern.

Trade   In the relationship between the developed and underdeveloped nations, trade is both part of the problem and yet is also crucial to the solution of overcoming the wealth imbalance and to making that relationship more socially inclusive.

As the UN has pointed out,[14] if developing countries are to realize the potential of international trade to enhance economic growth, the main barriers to their exports need to be removed. These include tariffs (taxes) imposed by developed countries on imports from developing countries and the subsidies that developed countries provide to domestic agricultural producers. The European Community is a particular offender in this area as it maintains protection and subsidies for its own producers while imposing punitive tariffs on producers in developing nations seeking to access its markets; textiles and farm produce, which are strategically important to developing economies, suffer heavy tariffs.

However, trade rather than aid provides the better basis for a long-term relationship between developed and underdeveloped nations and is infinitely more acceptable to the latter. If developing countries are to be given the opportunity to acquire economic self-sufficiency then the developed nations are going to have to be more proactive in capacity building measures that assist and protect the growth of production in developing nations.

Terrorism   The approach of western governments to developing countries associated, or alleged to be associated, with terrorism became complicated after the events of 9/11, more so after the invasion of Iraq in 2003 and shows every sign of becoming intractable as the occupation of that country continues. Countries such as Somalia, Libya, the Palestinian State and Iran unquestionably need to be drawn into a closer relationship with the developed nations of the western world if a more global civil society is to be cultivated. The threat of international terrorism, however, and the suspicion that links may exist between some such countries and the perpetrators of atrocities in western nations (and elsewhere, e.g. Bali, New Delhi and Jordan), together with the polarizing effect of the war in Iraq, have combined to inhibit consensus-building activity between western nations and some of those in the developing world. Caution and a level of mutual suspicion now permeates any such activity (see, further, chapter 6).

Indigenous people and social inclusion

Some modern western nations include within their borders distinct indigenous cultural groups, each established over many centuries and maintained in accordance with traditional customs that have survived relatively intact into the twenty-first century. This is particularly evident in relation to the indigenous people of such common law countries as Australia,[15] New Zealand, the US and Canada. These indigenous cultural groups ('the Indigenous People' or 'Aboriginal nation' as they are more properly referred to in Australia) are more or less coherent entities founded on rules and practices governing relations within and between families and applying to the functioning of their social system as a whole. They co-exist alongside and in an uneasy relationship with the prevailing western social culture; sharing time, territory and the necessities of life but often very little in the way of values, knowledge, social customs or wealth. Their circumstances – echoed to some extent by those of contemporary refugees, economic migrants and asylum seekers – often contrast harshly with those of the majority non-indigenous population. Indeed, it is interesting that those common law nations with the experience of absorbing the largest volume of newcomers (namely Canada and Australia) are also those that have had and continue to have the greatest difficulty in addressing social inclusion issues relating to their indigenous people. The challenge to facilitate social inclusion is perhaps most readily acknowledged in the stark contrast presented to a modern western country by the presence within it of a wholly different minority culture suffering chronic social disadvantage.

The problems presented by the circumstances of indigenous people cannot be seen simply as a more extreme version of those affecting the non-indigenous socially disadvantaged. Even if the profile of disadvantage was successfully tackled and their circumstances realigned to match those of the non-indigenous mainstream, this would be insufficient to provide for the social inclusion of indigenous people. Their position would remain additionally complicated by factors relating to culture and a legacy of oppression. Until some level of acknowledgement and reconciliation is achieved in respect of past injustice and a policy is formulated that offers a future in which their traditions, values and cultural icons are incorporated into the national legal and social infrastructure, their agenda of social inclusion issues will remain unresolved.

The following data is specific to the indigenous people of Australia but the broad trends are not unrepresentative of those relating to indigenous people elsewhere (see chapter 11 for the Maori of New Zealand and chapter 13 for the Inuit of Canada[16]).

Poverty   The long history of well-intentioned intervention in relation to indigenous communities has made little inroad on their generally impoverished circumstances. In Australia, for example, they are now reduced in number ; nd in average life expectancy, are comprehensively disadvantaged across many h alth, social and economic indicators and as a cultural group their collective expei ence is one of continued social exclusion.[17] Their economic circumstances clearly reveal continuing and endemic impoverishment: their unemployment rate is 22.7 per cent compared with a rate of 9.2 per cent for the general population; while the mean individual income is 65 per cent of that of the general population.

Health   In Australia, Indigenous people continue to suffer a greater burden of ill health than the rest of the population with higher levels of many mental and behavioural disorders and their susceptibility to infectious diseases is 12 times higher than the Australian average. In 1998–9, Indigenous people were more likely than others to be hospitalized for most diseases and conditions; hospital admissions for males being 71 per cent higher and for females 57 per cent higher than for their counterparts in the non-Indigenous population. Diabetes is a disease of particular importance for Indigenous people, affecting 30 per cent of the population. Babies of Indigenous mothers were nearly twice as likely as others to be of low birthweight and childhood mortality is three to five times higher; babies of Indigenous mothers are twice as likely to die at birth and during the early post-natal phase. The health of the Indigenous population is now so poor that 45 per cent of men and 34 per cent of women will die before the age of 45.

Housing   In 1999, Aboriginal and Torres Strait Islander people were more likely than the non-Indigenous population to live in conditions considered unacceptable by general Australian standards. In particular, overcrowding, high housing costs relative to income, poorly maintained buildings and facilities, and inadequate infrastructure were major issues associated with the housing of Indigenous people. Aboriginal and Torres Strait Islander people were also less likely to own their own homes than non-Indigenous Australians.

Education   Religious organizations in particular, using a combination of residential care and education provision, have for generations, in some cases for centuries, endeavoured to improve conditions in indigenous communities and extend to them the benefits and protection available in mainstream society. Sometimes, paradoxically, this intervention has been of an overtly coercive nature as when in Australia and Canada a government policy of assimilation used the residential child care facilities of religious organizations to provide compulsory education for Indigenous children. At times these endeavours simply exacerbated the difficulties of the recipients (e.g. the systemic abuse of children in residential accommodation provided by religious organizations in Canada, Ireland and elsewhere).

From charity to philanthropy

The gift relationship has its limitations. As formulated by Titmus and as represented by the altruistic, one-way transaction that typifies the traditional interpretation of charity, it provides an inadequate basis for responding to the challenges presented by the contemporary social inclusion agenda of modern western nations. It is sufficient within its own terms as a response to the effects of poverty and disaster and is also to be valued for affirming a sense of obligation, raising the bar for norms of ethical conduct in society, generating trust and social capital and contributing towards the building of civil society. In the common law nations, its present inadequacy as a means of addressing the causes of poverty and alienation in communities, nations and internationally is to a large extent due to the constraints imposed upon the interpretation of charity by the shared legacy of 400 years of restrictive judicial interpretation. Exploring the nature and effect of the common law characteristics that now generally inhibit the effectiveness of charity as a response to contemporary social inclusion issues in many modern western nations is a major theme of this book. This is given particular attention in Part II.

Before moving on to examine charity as practised within the constraints of the legal framework provided by the common law tradition, it is necessary to stay with the Titmus theory to consider the effect that 'packaging' the gift has had on the gift relationship. Arguably, the fact that the 'trust' was the basic legal device for transferring resources from donor to recipient had consequences for how the resources could then be used. The mutation of the basic trust provides something of a record illustrating the tensions between structure and content as charity law evolved from its defence of the supplicant/benefactor relationship so characteristic of traditional charity to accommodate the more modern philanthropic approach essential for addressing issues of social inclusion.

The trust/foundation

Charities originated as trusts. The gift relationship, underpinning charity in the common law tradition, revolved around a gift that was most usually legally packaged as a trust, and to a large extent this continues to be the means for giving effect to the charitable intentions of a donor. In England and Wales and in some but not all common law jurisdictions, the charitable trust and the charitable foundation are the same thing and the terms are used interchangeably; although a trust or foundation need not necessarily be a charity and vice versa (see, further, chapter 3). The gift, however, was seldom sufficient to constitute an endowment and only a small proportion of charities have ever been launched and sustained indefinitely as an endowed trust or foundation; by far the majority now and in the past have been dependent on fundraising and/or government grants and contracts. The infinite range of such organizations, large and small – necessarily in close and continuing engagement with the general public, with the socially disadvantaged and with government bodies – have been and remain representative of charitable trusts in the common law world.

However, it is the endowed trust or foundation with its unique characteristics that is best positioned to take a leadership role in furthering the development of philanthropy. For that reason, as representing the role of charitable trusts if not as a typical charity, the endowed trust/foundation deserves particular attention.

The endowed trust/foundation

The foundation, or trust, is the 'creature of the founder'.[18] The person providing the first gift, or endowment, is regarded as the founder and has the power to make directions for its use and provide for the control of it and its income in perpetuity. This is its greatest strength and, some would argue, its biggest weakness.

Strengths

The trust/foundation is a common law institution with its roots in the law of equity that has existed for at least 400 years. Some of the more characteristic aspects of the English democratic social infrastructure, and subsequently that of other common law nations, have been put in place and maintained due to the singular strengths of the trust/foundation.

Independence   A trust/foundation is always self-governing, non-profit distributing, dedicated to public purposes (whether charitable or not) and, to a varying degree, has its own resources. It need not necessarily be established by endowment but in that event it then has guaranteed long-term financial independence with no constituency that it is obliged to cultivate. The freedom of not having to fundraise and/or seek government grants or contracts means that it is not a hostage to the goodwill of government or the general public. As long as it stays within the parameters of its donor's stated purposes, a trust/foundation is free to be innovative, to take risks and to lend its support to other causes. Perhaps most importantly, its independence in theory allows it to operate without fear or favour, without having to negotiate vested interests and it is thus in a position to address the root causes of social problems, particularly those associated with more marginal or less popular groups, not just their effects. As has been said:

> The signature characteristic of foundations, namely their specific capacity to innovate, is based on their freedom from the constraints of both the market and the State. Accordingly, their lack of democratic accountability is a virtue and the source of their freedom to innovate, or to support innovation, for the common good.[19]

Wealth   A trust/foundation need not be rich but many have accumulated great wealth. In the generations that have passed since their founding endowment, some have received further endowments which, together with the proceeds of investments, have made them very rich indeed. While money in itself is by no means an answer to poverty or issues of social inclusion, the great wealth of the larger trusts/foundations does enable them to contract effective partnerships and sustain an investment in a sufficient range of resources to make a significant impact on such problems. Their size, capacity and prominent social profile makes them both difficult to ignore when they adopt an advocacy role and attractive partners for government bodies engaged in the provision of health, social care and education services.

Long-term   In addition to their independence and wealth, trusts/foundations have the great advantage over other organizations that they can exist in perpetuity. Their durability enables them to avoid the temptations of a 'quick fix' approach and adopt the long view that is needed when tackling problems of poverty and social inclusion. It means that they can build relationships with the socially disadvantaged group specified by their founder, based on mutual trust and understanding, which may endure for generations. Some trusts/foundations (e.g. Barnardo's and Help the Aged) have forged such close links with particular groups, acquiring such archives of research data and a reputation for representing their interests, that to the general public they have become synonymous with the needs of that group. This unique capacity to endure and to build relationships of knowledge and trust with the socially disadvantaged, equips trusts/foundations to exercise informed leverage on their behalf and makes them an invaluable resource for government.

Networks   One particular consequence of their independence and longevity is that trusts/foundations are in a position to cultivate a strategic network of relationships with other bodies on a regional, national and international basis. Free from the constraints of prevailing policies and politics they can exchange information, staff and other resources, compare circumstances and related methods of intervention with similar organizations elsewhere or establish duplicate versions of themselves, as seems necessary. From a position of strength, as they hold the central but neutral ground in terms of politics and religion, they are accessible to all and provide a bridge for open communication between those who would otherwise be mutually estranged. They can negotiate and broker deals where governments cannot. In an uncertain national and international context dominated by the vagaries of politics and the market place, the enduring networks established by trusts/foundations provide a thread of consistency and continuity and a platform for ongoing informed mediation between governments and the socially excluded.

Weaknesses

The fact that a private individual, or large corporation, can commit sometimes great private wealth for public benefit, indefinitely, would appear to be unequivocally beneficial for society. However, there can be problems.

Democratic deficit   Although the designated recipients are chosen entirely at donor discretion the gift nevertheless qualifies for the same level of tax exemption. Donor priority may not accord with social priority and a substantial gift to a home for abandoned dogs, a concert hall or a private school, subsidized in effect by the taxpayer for ever, may well be controversial in circumstances of considerable poverty. Arguably, the tax loss could have been more usefully invested by the government in purposes that it was elected by the taxpayers to pursue. This characteristic 'democratic deficit' of foundations arises because, unlike governments, they are unaccountable for their choice of beneficiary and they cause public money to be diverted to defray the cost of that private choice.

Donor control   As has often been pointed out, it is the fact that control over the gift is retained by the donor, and subsequently by his/her family and chosen associates, that distinguishes foundations from other forms of charitable giving and this is so whether the donor is an individual or a corporation.[20] However, the fact that a trust/foundation can exist in perpetuity (see, further, chapter 3) means that a time will come when the donor-determined purpose may no longer be necessary or perhaps be incapable of fulfilment. Over a period of many generations the initial gift may well have grown into a considerable sum which could be usefully redirected to meet other areas of social need. The law, however, has always attached great importance to protecting the expressed wishes of a donor and confining the use of the gift to the terms on which it was given. The resulting inflexibility can give rise to situations where the donor rules from the grave and resources are wasted. A charity, for example, may no longer be able to give effect to its purposes because the circumstances for which it was intended no longer exist (e.g. slavery, civil rights for black people or for the relief of those suffering from the plague). Alternatively, the circumstances may exist but the means the donor has directed should be used in relation to them are illegal,[21] or changes in public policy (anti-vivisection) or State assumption of responsibility make it impossible or impracticable for the charity to give effect to them as the donor has directed. Again, although the circumstances persist they may have shrunk to become relatively inconsequential while the charity's assigned assets have grown disproportionately large. The charity then becomes defunct and its funds lie dormant or are squandered in endless legal proceedings unless a means can be found to vary the terms of the original gift and release the assets for use in a similar purpose. In the common law nations, the *cy-près* rule (see, further, chapter 3) has existed to provide such a means, but ease of access to this facility varies considerably. It is clearly a matter of some importance that dormant funds are made available to address contemporary issues of social inclusion and close attention is paid in this book to the provision made in the different jurisdictions for expeditiously redirecting the use of dormant charitable assets.

Spending   Trusts/foundations have been accused, not without some justification, of being more interested in safeguarding and growing their wealth than in deploying it. Throughout the twentieth century they functioned almost exclusively as organized grant-making bodies, zealously guarding their particular niche funding role, and many continue to do so. They spend in accordance with statutory disbursement requirements and their own inflexible tariff of grants that relate to a menu of projects determined by the government policies then 'in fashion'. They have no direct contact with or knowledge of the needs of the socially disadvantaged and the level and frequency of their spending bears no relation to those needs. Kramer, managing partner of the Center for Effective Philanthropy, reflecting on the $435 billion tied up in US foundation assets, comments that foundations 'are insulated from performance pressures' and assuming that 'they invest and spend conservatively, foundations will almost always survive in perpetuity . . . whether their grants are effective or not'.[22]

Class privilege   Traditionally, trusts/foundations have been established by the wealthy, have been managed by them and in many cases they were established for purposes of their enjoyment. From time to time the accusation has been levelled at the bigger foundations that they show too much interest in protecting their brand name and their place in the hierarchy of rich foundations, that they in fact reflect the acquisitive, competitive, capitalist values of the social strata from which they emerged. Certainly, social status would seem to adhere to the larger foundations named after a founder's family or company and it may be that they are viewed by some as extending its social standing, to be supported and disported accordingly. It may also be the case that charitable activity from such a source carries with it implicit values and interests to be protected.

The association with wealth and privilege has not always worked to the advantage of an organization seeking to build relationships with the socially disadvantaged. At the very least the privileged genesis and ongoing social context of a trust/foundation must mean that it is not best placed to know much about the circumstances of the socially disadvantaged, nor about the methods that might be used to effect change and, at least initially, may be regarded with some mistrust by them. Where the purpose of a trust/foundation was to address poverty or issues of social inclusion, the assessment of that need and the method for dealing with it has in the main been from a perspective and on terms set by the wealthy; a generalization offset by the more recent rise of foundations pursuing goals and objectives based on empirical research. It remains broadly true, however, that 'in the case of Britain, but also for the US, one could say, with only some overstatement, that foundations are created and governed by the country's elite. They are deeply embedded in its political systems'.[23] Without overstating it, there may at some level be a connection between trusts/foundations as the main legal structure for charity and the fact that poverty and charity have continued to co-exist in the common law nations for the past four centuries.

Recent history of the endowed trust/foundation

This is a robust social institution with all the above strengths and weaknesses. Their number, size, variety and longevity enable them to contribute colour, consistency and continuity to the fabric of modern democratic societies. They also redistribute wealth. The endowed trust/foundation, when established within the boundaries of charity law, is a powerful institution within the charity family. Even when not established as a charity – and many donors choose not to accept the limitations of this legal structure (e.g. because of the constraints regarding political activity) – it is still a powerful institution. But it is not a typical charitable trust.

From its origins in the US the modern foundation movement has gradually transferred to the UK and spread unevenly throughout the rest of Europe. This social phenomenon has yet to attract much research but recently the work of Diana Leat and Helmut Anheier (to which the author is indebted for the following material) has done much to illuminate our understanding of the role and potential of endowed trusts/foundations.[24] In tracing the modern evolution of this phenomenon they have suggested that having existed primarily as a dispenser of 'charity' as traditionally understood until the mid-twentieth century, it then passed through the stages of 'scientific philanthropy' and 'new scientific philanthropy' and is now, perhaps, poised to enter a phase of 'creative philanthropy'. The recent history of the endowed trust/foundation reflects the dilemmas inherent in making the transition from charity to philanthropy.

Scientific philanthropy

The initial growth period of foundations in the US reflected the perceived social responsibilities and moral obligations of the entrepreneurs during the post-bellum reconstruction period and the rapid industrialization that followed. Importantly, in the US, foundations represented an innovation that implied a fundamental shift in their *raison d'être*: foundations refocused from the gift relationship characteristic of traditional charity to become problem-solving institutions; and they moved from responding to effects to dealing with causes.[25] It was seen by some as a prime tool and exemplar of 'knowledge-based social engineering' in modern society.[26] This, after all, was a time when the scientific approach being successfully applied to problems in medicine and industry seemed equally applicable to social problems. In the early half of the twentieth century a wave of big foundations were established including Rowntree, Nuffield, Rockefeller, Carnegie and Ford – names that were to become synonymous with the investment of funds into projects dealing with the causes of chronic social disadvantage. However, in the view of Anheier and Leat, this approach was deficient:[27]

> First, like the charity approach, scientific philanthropy fails fully to exploit the unique potential of endowed foundations. For the most part, this approach can, and is, adopted by other kinds of organisations as well, including governments. Second, it rests on assumptions that may be true in physical science but are questionable when applied to social issues. If the causes of something as complex as, say, poverty are identifiable, they may not be susceptible to scientific solutions and simple control measures. Third, while scientific

philanthropy has much wider potential impact, it often fails to appreciate the long, slow, complex and expensive path to effective problem solving.

New scientific philanthropy

In recent years, as Anheier and Leat point out, many new approaches have been added to the foundation lexicon including 'strategic philanthropy, venture philanthropy, social investment, the blended value proposition etc' of which the first two have been particularly significant.[28] They refer to these collectively as the 'new scientific philanthropy' because they see them as directly descendent from 'scientific philanthropy'.

Strategic philanthropy   This approach has been described as 'moving away from grant-making as an end in itself and beginning to think about developing strategies to solve problems and seeing grants as pieces of acivity that implement strategy'.[29] A report by the Pew Charitable Trust[30] lists ten criteria for strategic philanthropy:

1   Well-defined goal.
2   Discernible impact on a problem.
3   Responds to a ripe opportunity and is timely.
4   Has appropriate partnerships.
5   Is simple in design.
6   Allocates an appropriate amount of resources.
7   Approaches a problem on multiple fronts.
8   Is ambitious yet feasible.
9   Considers core competencies, internal as well as external.
10   Aims to show progress in three to five years.

Strategic philanthropy has been criticized by Anheier and Leat because it 'lacks a broader vision and conceptual grounding for foundations and that brings their central competencies into focus' and is 'not radical enough'.[31]

Venture philanthropy   This relatively new form of philanthropy refers to the nonprofit sector's application of certain practices used by venture capitalists when investing in new business ideas.[32] Venture philanthropy may also be used more loosely to refer to all kinds of charitable endeavours that involve risk-taking, innovation and entrepreneurship. Specifically it includes 'funding social entre-preneurs in organisations with scale-up potential. Support it long-term and the funder makes substantial commitments to a few rather than smaller commitments to many'.[33] Its adherents criticize foundations for investing in programmes and projects rather than in nonprofit infrastructure, capacity building and entre-preneurial talent. They urge foundations to borrow six strategies from venture capitalists: deploying risk management tools, creating performance measures, developing close relationships with their investments, investing more money, investing over longer periods and developing an exit strategy.[34]

The venture philanthropy approach takes donor control much further – involving participation in governance and management of funded organizations. As explained by Anheier and Leat:

> Its dual emphasis is on 'value for money and money for value' and its interest in developing the notion of 'value' in non-profit capital markets are bold steps forward. At the very least, the introduction of venture philanthropy has broadened the options available to donors; at its best it is the initial step to go beyond the philanthropic foundation that has now been the dominant model for a century.[35]

Venture philanthropists tend to focus on efficiency and effectiveness and performance but some non-profits would argue that this fails to take into account the importance of participation and process which are central to the concepts of civil society and social capital.

Anheier and Leat suggest that these approaches are all equally open to the same criticism that they:

> tend to focus on foundation processes rather than roles, let alone purposes, and do not address the question of the unique value of foundations in a democracy. They apply business models to foundation practices, with the assumption that if only foundations were run like businesses, all would be well . . . their fundamental weakness stems, in large part, from their instrumentalist, managerial assumptions . . .[36]

Creative scientific philanthropy

Having noted the limitations of the 'scientific' and 'new scientific' philanthropic approaches, Anheier and Leat suggest that:

> rather than being charitable and appeasing in the context of a society stressed by rising social inequalities and poverty, the creative philanthropists of today seek to encourage debate, social inclusion and change. The new approach to philanthropy seeks to link the distinctive characteristics of foundations to what are seen as the urgent problems of society, including the decline of civic engagement, the crisis in democracy and value crisis.[37]

Believing that the endowed, philanthropic foundation is a good and potentially vitally important institution in modern society[38] and has never been more important than it is today,[39] Anheier and Leat strongly assert that the critical challenge for philanthropic foundations is the 'lack of creativity and the lack of both knowledge and awareness of interdependence . . . creativity is the central issue for foundations today'.[40]

Conclusion

Anheier and Leat are quite rightly critical of modern philanthropy because of its underachievement. Given the importance of its role in modern society coupled with its unique strengths they suggest that the endowed trust/foundation as an institution should have achieved more than it has and that this is largely due to a failure of vision among philanthropists. This is true. However it is not the whole story. This book suggests that the failings of that institution are not wholly separable from the shortcomings of the trust as an appropriate legal form for philanthropy and that in turn is only one aspect of other fundamental weaknesses in charity law, as it is known to the common law nations. The shared legacy of the common law framework for charity law, in many respects a wonderful body of case law and judicial principles that did much to continue a sense of shared culture between nations, has carried over into the twenty-first century certain structural flaws which now obstruct the development of philanthropy. The identification and assessment of those flaws, and a comparative evaluation of how they now affect particular common law jurisdictions, is the central task of the following chapters.

Part II

Charity law

The common law legacy

Chapter 3

The common law

The emergence of principles, structures and legal functions relating to charities

Introduction

In all common law countries, the roots of the current jurisdiction in relation to charities, their property and activities, lie in the ancient *parens patriae* responsibilities of the Crown.[1] The inherent obligation resting on the King of England to safeguard the interests of wards and lunatics extended also to charities. The essentially protective nature of this jurisdiction, illustrated most clearly in the exercise of wardship, has always guided the judicial approach towards charities and their activities. Grafted onto the common law, the law relating to charities transferred with the armies of the Crown to all parts of the British Empire.

The legislative foundations for the development of modern charity law were laid with the introduction of the Statute of Charitable Uses 1601. For four centuries the 1601 Act facilitated a similar judicial approach towards charities within the jurisdictions of the UK and, to a greater or lesser extent, throughout all common law nations. A resulting body of precedents and related principles, largely shared among those countries, continues to inform the contemporary relationship between law and charities. Tracing the origins and subsequent evolution of the legal framework for charities in England reveals the distinctive common law characteristics that shaped the legal functions relating to charitable activity across the common law world.

This chapter begins by outlining the historical background to the introduction of the 1601 Act. It considers the singular significance of trusts, charitable trusts and the role of the courts in their development in the UK. It examines the rationale for the 1601 Act, the context within which it fitted, the nature of its provisions and the immediate consequences of its introduction. The focus is firmly on examining the contribution of the statute to shaping modern charitable purposes. The chapter then considers the emergence of the modern administrative system in relation to charities, the range and duties of different agencies and the significance of certain governing principles; not all of which transferred from England to its colonies. It identifies the characteristics and structures that differentiate charities from other types of not-for-profit organizations. It briefly traces the growth of the legislative process that resulted in a modern statutory framework for charities in England and Wales but leaves to later (see chapter 8) a consideration of the contemporary law reform process. The chapter concludes by summarizing the features of the common law legacy and their consequences for the development of charity law in that jurisdiction.

Historical background: the context for the introduction of the Statute of Charitable Uses 1601

Equity and the law of trusts provide the foundations for modern charity law. Many of the principles now governing charitable trusts have a history that can be traced to at least the sixteenth century and many existing charities long predate 1601 (the oldest being, perhaps, the King's School, Canterbury, founded in 597). The evolution of charitable trusts and the significance of their common law development after the 1601 Act is therefore not wholly explicable without some preliminary understanding of equity and the law of trusts.

Land, its use and the development of charitable trusts

Feudalism was based on a system of land tenure. This ensured that land could not be wholly and absolutely owned by anyone; every 'owner' held their rights as tenant to their lord. Estates in land consisted of gradations of title from serf to lord, with final authority of ownership and disposal being vested in the King as the ultimate lord and sovereign of his people and territory. This system provided the basis for imposing taxes and dues.

The transference of land to another for the latter's 'use' was intended to avoid the tax liability that attached to actual ownership. It was also employed to facilitate gifts to religious bodies which, prior to the Statute of Mortmain 1391, would have been prohibited. Gifts of the latter variety were commonly made by landowners in return for masses being said for the salvation of their souls. *Morte meyn* or 'dead hand', whereby a donor would tie up his lands in perpetuity by gifting them to the Church, was a gift for pious uses and recognized as a charitable gift in the years prior to the Reformation.[2] From the perspective of the rulers, this practice posed a significant threat to the feudal system.

Once property passed into the 'dead hand of the Church' it remained there as the latter prohibited any alienation of its property. A variation of this was 'tenure by frankalmoign' whereby a gift of property to the Church was made subject to a condition that it be held for the use of specified persons, usually the donor and/or his family. By means of mortmain and frankalmoign, the Church and particularly the religious orders came to acquire considerable power, land and political influence. Feudal rulers came to regard a grant of land to the Church by a subject as incompatible with the latter's feudal duties and from the Magna Carta in 1215[3] sought to curtail this practice through successive statutes.[4]

The Court of Chancery, however, was prepared to give recognition to an equitable holding in land. The eventual evolution of the feudal concept of the 'use'[5] into its modern manifestation as a 'trust' was hastened by the Statute of

Uses 1535[6] which gave statutory authority to the approach developed in the Court of Chancery where the transaction involved freehold land.

Trusts and charitable trusts

The law of trusts provides the means whereby property may be held by one person for the benefit of another. As was explained a century ago 'if I give an estate to A upon condition that he shall apply the rents for the benefit of B, that is a gift in trust to all intents and purposes'.[7] This was a conceptual division of property into two components – legal ownership and beneficial ownership. The law of trusts, developed by the courts of equity, provided recognition and enforcement for such a separation. This artificial legal device has become extremely important and is now extensively used in many different forms.[8]

A charitable trust is a species of trust. There are a number of different species within that genre. Each, therefore, is to a greater or lesser extent governed by characteristics common to all. Only charitable trusts are primarily intended to confer a public benefit. Primarily, it is the fact that charitable trusts are established for purposes rather than for persons which sets them apart from other forms of trust. As has been observed:[9]

> . . . trusts for purposes rather than for human beings are rarely valid. They are regarded as difficult, perhaps impossible, to enforce, uncertain in their ambit and generally beyond the capacity of the court to control. In addition, they will very often contravene legal rules against creating perpetuities and inalienability . . . To this general doctrine the great exception is *charitable trusts* . . . the distinctive feature of the charitable trust is that it is *for the public benefit.*

This form of trust must not only be established for a recognized charitable purpose but also vice versa; as the ruling of Macnaghten L.J. in the iconic *Pemsel* case clearly illustrates, the purpose intended must be expressed in the legal form of a trust (see, further, p. 79).[10] The purposes must be exclusively charitable. In addition, the requirement that it be for the public benefit prevents a charitable trust, unlike other forms, from being made in favour of named or specific beneficiaries or those linked by a nexus of relationship (e.g. employees of a particular company).[11] Charitable trusts have also been traditionally entitled to the protection of the Attorney General. Finally, in circumstances where other trusts would fail, a charitable trust may be saved through application of the *cy-près* doctrine.

From at least the fifteenth century, the law of trusts provided the vehicle for giving effect to charitable gifts. All attempts to introduce the charitable corporation failed due to an established policy that viewed any such initiative as a legal device to reintroduce measures providing for the inalienability of property and therefore subversive of the State's interests. The dominance of the trust as the preferred legal form for charities thus became a primary characteristic in the development of charity law in the UK, notwithstanding the introduction in 1862 of companies limited by guarantee and the resulting incorporation of some trusts.[12] As McGregor-Lowndes has noted:[13] 'Over 900 years were to pass before the corporation's original and unfettered capacity to purchase and hold land was restored and during this period the development of the charitable corporation was stunted and the charitable trust ascended.'

The rule against perpetuities

The crucial characteristics of a charitable trust, distinguishing it from other forms of trust, are that it is for purposes rather than for persons and also that it may be perpetual in nature. The latter, an ancient principle, provides that charitable trusts are not time-limited and their resources cannot be lost to charity. The rule dates from the Statute of *Quia Emptores*[14] in 1290 when the judiciary and legislature set limits on the ability of persons to impose alienation constraints on their property to take effect after their death. It requires ownership to vest within the 'perpetuity period'; fixed at life or lives in being plus 21 years or just 21 years where there is no life in being. Once vested a charitable trust enjoys the considerable legal privilege that it may continue in perpetuity. It was this feature, in the context of mortmain, which made the charitable trust such a threat to the rulers of mediaeval England.

The cy-près rule[15]

The fact that a charity may exist in perpetuity can present problems. The courts are bound to give effect to a valid charitable gift in the terms as expressed by the donor but as time passes this may become increasingly difficult. As Sir John Romilly MR stated in *Philpott* v. *St George's Hospital*:[16]

> If the testator has, by his will, pointed out clearly what he intends to be done, and his directions are not contrary to the law, this Court is bound to carry that intention into effect, and has no right, and is not at liberty to speculate upon whether it would have been more expedient or beneficial for the community that a different mode of application of the funds in charity should have occurred to the mind of the testator, or that he should have directed some different scheme for carrying his charitable intentions into effect. Accordingly instances of charities of the most useless description have come before the Court, but which it has considered itself bound to carry into effect.

To cope with the fact that particular purposes or charitable organizations may cease to be valid or viable, the principle of *cy-près* has traditionally allowed the objects to be varied and the resources of a defunct charity or purpose to be transferred to a comparable charity or purpose; to achieve a result as close as possible to the donor's original intention. For the rule to apply a clear charitable intention must be evident, the objects of the gift must be exclusively charitable, the subject must be certain and a '*cy-près* occasion' must have arisen. The traditional constraint, requiring proof of 'impossibility' or 'impracticability' in giving effect to the original charitable intention, has been significantly relaxed by modern legislation. A charitable trust will not be allowed to fail for uncertainty of object if there is firm evidence of a general charitable intent.

The Reformation

The tension between Church and State culminated eventually in the Reformation, which saw Henry VIII taking vigorous action to suppress the Church, dissolve the monasteries and confiscate their property. By mid-sixteenth century a large number of abbeys and monasteries had been dissolved and their lands appropriated by the Crown.

Dissolution of the monasteries had several important consequences for charities. First, it had the immediate effect of removing the single most important source of housing, care and education for the poor; the homeless and destitute were left to roam the towns in search of alms and shelter (see, also, chapter 1). Second, it ended the possibility of making grants of property to the Church in exchange for spiritual benefits. Third, breaking the Church's hold on charities led to the secularization of the objects of charity as the majority of Englishmen 'reflected less on their souls and became more concerned with the worldly needs of their fellow men'.[17]

By the end of the sixteenth century much of its power, land and monasteries had been stripped from the Catholic Church. The Elizabethan era began with the attempt to establish a new and comprehensive national Protestant religion protected by statute. Other religions were not to be tolerated. This in turn led directly to the statute of fundamental importance for charity law, the Statute of Charitable Uses 1601, which modified its predecessor, the Statute of Uses 1597.[18]

Historical background: the Statute of Charitable Uses 1601 [19]

This statute and its Preamble constituted the key statement of the common law tradition and provided a foundation for the development of charity law in the UK and thereafter throughout the common law world. It formed a part of the legislative reforms carried out at the end of the reign of Elizabeth I, the most notable being the Poor Law of the same year.

The Statute of Charitable Uses 1601

Entitled '*An Acte to redresse the Misemployment of Landes, Goodes and Stockes of Money heretofore given to Charitable Uses*' the Statute of Charitable Uses 1601 was a reforming statute with a twofold legislative intent. First, in order to fill the social care gap left by the dissolution of the monasteries and solicit the funds necessary to repair the damage caused by the ravages of war, it sought to channel philanthropic gifts towards identified priorities. Second, it aimed to reform the abuse of property donated to charities by listing the type of purposes which would thereafter be recognized as charitable.

The Preamble

The declaration of purposes to be construed as charitable is in the Preamble rather than the main body of the statute. The following specific charitable purposes are listed:

> Releife of aged impotent and poore people, some for Maintenance of sicke and maymed Souldiers and Marriners, Schooles of Learninge, Free Schooles and Schollers in Universities, some for Repaire of Bridges Portes Havens Causwaies Churches Seabankes and Highwaies, some for Educacion and prefermente of Orphans, some for or towards Reliefe Stocke or Maintenance of Howses of Correccion, some for Mariages of poore Maides, some for Supportacion Ayde and Helpe of younge tradesmen Handicraftesmen and persons decayed, and others for reliefe or redemption of Prisoners or Captives, and for aide or ease of any poore Inhabitantes concerninge paymente of Fifteenes, setting out of Souldiers and other Taxes. . . .

These purposes were treated from the outset as being illustrative rather than definitive; though judicial uncertainty initially prevailed as to whether they could be construed disjunctively or conjunctively.[20] Thereafter the courts would not regard a purpose as charitable unless it could be defined as coming within 'the spirit and intendment' of the Preamble and disclosed an element of 'public benefit'.

The list of charitable purposes

The statute does not purport to address all charitable purposes; it is confined to listing and dealing with those which have given rise to fraud and abuse and is indicative rather than definitive. However, the list constrained judicial recognition of new charitable purposes; wholly new categories were not possible, a link had to be made with the type of purposes listed or since recognized as charitable.

Distinction between public service and poverty relief   The listed purposes fall into two broad categories: for the poor and for public works; these being the areas in which most fraud and abuse had been perpetrated. The fault-line running between the two endured for four centuries and continues to attract controversy[21] (see, further, chapters 5 and 6).

Religion   The Preamble makes no reference to religion or to religious organizations. Although recognition is given to the repair of churches as a charitable purpose, this occurs in the context of a list of public utilities and may simply be an acknowledgement that remedying the wear and tear suffered by all such social infrastructure facilities was equally deserving of charitable status. The absence of an explicit reference to religion serves as a reminder that the 1601 Act did not set out to encode a definitive list of charitable purposes. It also reflects the political wariness of legislators who were mindful of the turbulent relationship between religion and royalty; property donated to religious purposes during the reign of one monarch could be confiscated during the next if the change in reign coincided with a change in the religious affiliation of the monarch.

Social control   In addition to several of the 'service' type public utilities found to be deserving of charitable status, there are also some of a 'social control' nature. The maintenance of houses of correction, assisting poor maids into marriage and the rehabilitation of prisoners are purposes which indicate a legislative intent to promote a congruity between the agendas of charities and government on the assumption that both share a common interest in activities which conform with and tend to preserve the values of contemporary society.

Regulating charities and charitable activity

The Preamble explains that gifts to charitable purposes have been the subject of fraud and abuse:

> Landes Tenementes Rents Annuities Profitts Hereditaments Goodes Chattells Money and Stockes of Money nevertheles have not byn imployed accordinge to the charitable intente of the givers and founders thereof, by reason of Fraudes breaches of Truste and Negligence in those that shoulde pay delyver and imploy the same . . .

The Statute of Charitable Uses 1601 then sets out provisions intended to restrict these abuses. It establishes a body of Commissioners with powers to supervise and inspect charitable trusts. The overriding legislative intent to assert the right and duty to hold to account those who have been entrusted with gifts to be used for charitable purposes is very clear:

> Be it enacted, That the saide Commissioners, or any Fower of more of them, shall an may make Decrees and Orders for recompense to be made by any person or persons whoe, beinge put in Truste or havynge notice of the charitable Uses above mentioned, hathe or shall breake the same Truste, or defraude the same Uses, by any Conveiance Gifte Graunte Lease Demise Release or Conversion whatsoever, and againste the Heires Executors and Admynistrators of hym them or any of them, havynge Assettes in Law or Equitie, soe farre as the same Assettes will extende.

Concern is focused on: protection for donors; prevention of deliberate abuse, careless inefficiency and misuse of status by charities; and providing for the removal of charitable status from bodies found by Commissioners to be in breach of stated standards. The statutory terms of reference of the present Charity Commissioners for England and Wales, though more extensive and sophisticated, clearly originate from this bare outline of regulatory powers.

The 1601 Act and the courts

The legislative intent informing this foundation statute, as Lord Morton noted in *Royal College of Surgeons of England* v. *National Provincial Bank Ltd*[22] was to reform abuses in the application of property devoted to charitable uses rather than to define the concept of a charity. However, in the following years the judiciary repeatedly reaffirmed that only charitable purposes corresponding to those listed in the 1601 Statute would be recognized in law. For four centuries it remained the case that for a purpose to be charitable it had to correspond to one mentioned in the Preamble or broadly come within its 'spirit and intendment'.

Chancery and the common law courts and parens patriae

The *parens patriae* responsibilities of the Crown, as exercised by the Lord Chancellor, came to be administered by the Court of Chancery and were used to determine issues relating to trusts, charitable and otherwise, long before the introduction of the 1601 Act.

Parens patriae   It seems probable that the ancient *parens patriae* powers originated as an incident of the feudal system of tenure. From perhaps the fourteenth century, the monarch – as ultimate landlord to whom all lords, yeomen, serfs and others owed allegiance and paid fealty – was responsible for those declared *sui juris* and who because they lacked the necessary capacity could neither protect their own interests nor fulfil their feudal duties and therefore 'belonged to the King as *Pater patriae*, and fell under the direction of this court, as charities, infants, idiots, lunatics, etc'.[23] In practice it was the property rights of those within such groups that attracted an exercise of the *parens patriae* powers: protecting property from abuse or misuse by officials entrusted to safeguard it was the main concern.

The extent of the *parens patriae* powers, like its origins, are uncertain, but it is clear that they extend beyond the parental duty of care and protection to warrant the taking of positive steps to safeguard the interests at risk. Inherently vested in the monarch, exercised by the Chancellor, delegated to the Court of Chancery and then administered by the High Court and the Attorney General, these powers have been described as 'theoretically limitless'[24] because they 'spring from the direct responsibility of the Crown for those who cannot look after themselves'.[25]

Chancery and the common law courts   The approach adopted by the court in Chancery was very different from that of the common law courts. A petitioner's plea was settled on the basis of principle and good conscience. A defendant could be summoned to appear by the issue of a *sub poena*. If successful, the plea could be enforced by utilizing the prerogative powers, such as the power of injunction or of specific performance, which characterized the traditional authority of the Crown. A paternalistic use of judicial discretion coupled with access to prerogative powers gave this court considerable flexibility and real authority.

The common law courts, on the other hand, exercised the sovereign authority of the Crown. The court of King's Bench, or Queen's Bench, was the more important and powerful of the common law courts. It dealt with criminal and civil matters and supervised the lower courts. In common law no writ meant no action. A petitioner could only succeed in lodging a plea in court if he could fit his complaint within the narrowly defined terms of a particular writ; the range of standard form writs available was limited. On conclusion of the hearing, the range of judicial disposal options was again tightly constrained. Should the plea succeed and the court find in favour of the plaintiff, it quite often lacked the authority necessary to ensure that his rights were enforced.

Chancery, therefore, came to offer an alternative route to justice for petitioners whose cause did not find a remedy in the common law courts. This equitable approach was manifested most clearly in Chancery's treatment of the trust and led to the development of the modern law of charitable trusts.

Chancery and the 1601 Act

The judiciary never fully shared the concern of the Crown that the law should be used solely to prevent abuse. Instead of viewing their role as constrained by the 1601 Act, limited in effect to implementing its provisions, the Court of Chancery took the approach that the authority of the court in respect of charities was inherent and preceded the Statute of Charitable Uses. For example, in *AG* v. *Tancred*[26] Lord Northington acknowledged that even before the 1601 Act the Court of Chancery would have given aid to a defective conveyance in favour of a charity. In *Attorney General* v. *Skinners Company*[27] the court then formed the view that its jurisdiction over charities was inherent, and that the said statute was only declaratory of the existing law. As was subsequently explained in *Moggridge* v. *Thackwell*,[28] 'where money is given to charity generally and indefinitely, without trustees or objects selected, the King as *parens patriae* is the constitutional trustee'.[29] Finally, in *Williams' Trustees* v. *IRC*,[30] the House of Lords indicated that as regards the legal limits of charity, it should be borne in mind that a trust would not be charitable unless it came within the spirit and intendment of the Statute of Elizabeth 1.

The use of judicial discretion, a hallmark of this jurisdiction, allowed the judiciary to formulate a body of principles to guide its determination of matters affecting trusts and charitable trusts. This was quietly developed and consolidated during and following the protracted struggle between Church and State.

Judicial classification of charitable purposes

During the next two centuries and more, as neither statute nor judiciary inter-vened to classify the charitable purposes listed in the Elizabethan statute, the Court of Chancery developed its own separate body of charitable trust juris-prudence. When such classification came it ordered the judicial approach to charities and to charitable activity thereafter.

A first judicial attempt to classify charitable purposes was undertaken by

Sir William Grant MR in *Morice* v. *The Bishop of Durham*.[31] He then stated that a fixed principle existed in the law of England that purposes deemed to be charitable are those 'which that Statute enumerates' and those 'which by analogies are deemed within its spirit and intendment'.[32] He suggested four heads: the relief of the indigent; advancement of learning; advancement of religion; and the advancement of 'objects of general public utility'.

Sir Samuel Romilly's classification was subsequently accepted by Lord Macnaghten in *Commissioners for Special Purposes of Income Tax* v. *Pemsel*[33] with some significant refinements. He classified all recognized charitable purposes under four heads and added that to be charitable, a gift must be 'beneficial to the community'.[34] He ruled as follows:[35]

> 'Charity' in its legal sense comprises four principal divisions: trusts for the relief of poverty; trusts for the advancement of education; trusts for the advancement of religion; and trusts beneficial to the community not falling under any of the preceding heads. The trusts last referred to are not any the less charitable in the eye of the law, because incidentally they benefit the rich as well as the poor, as indeed, every charity that deserves the name must do directly or indirectly.

To be considered charitable in law a trust must fall into one of these four separate but not necessarily mutually exclusive categories. The Macnaghten ruling has been habitually followed not only in England but in all common law jurisdictions.

Then, in *Williams' Trustees* v. *IRC*[36] the House of Lords indicated that two propositions must be borne in mind: a trust is not charitable unless it is within the spirit and intendment of the Statute of Elizabeth 1; and the classification of charity in its legal sense into four principal divisions in *Pemsel* must be read subject to the qualification that every object of public general utility is not necessarily charitable: 'If the purposes are not charitable *per se*, the localisation of them will not make them charitable.'

Fusion of equity and common law

In the centuries following the introduction of the 1601 Statute, judicial discretion was employed to interpret gifts as coming within the 'spirit and intendment' of the Preamble. This served to broaden the range of charitable purposes in an empirical rather than logical fashion; by a process of precedent and analogy the Court of Chancery greatly extended the Preamble list.

Legislative intervention eventually ended the continuation of two parallel judicial systems. In England and Wales, the Supreme Court of Judicature Act 1873 unified the court systems of equity and the common law. This statutory fusion of equitable and common law principles included a directive that, in the event of a conflict between them, the principles of equity should prevail.

Emergence of the modern administrative system in relation to charities

From its common law origins and growth in the courts of equity, its statutory recognition in the Statute of Charitable Uses 1601 and subsequent judicial classification in *Pemsel*, the law relating to charities and their activities has developed in accordance with much the same body of principles across all common law nations. Subject to some important qualifications with regard to the significance of trusts and administrative structures, the lead set in England and Wales by the judiciary and to a lesser extent by the legislators transferred, with the armies of the Crown, to the nations that formerly constituted the British Empire and now largely comprise the Commonwealth.

The courts

The Judicature Acts of 1873 and 1875 abolished the separate courts of equity and common law, establishing in their place a High Court consisting of five divisions: Chancery, Queen's Bench, Common Pleas, Exchequer and Probate. The Chancery Division initially bore responsibility for charities.

Jurisdiction of the High Court

The traditional, inherent or equitable, jurisdiction of the High Court has always been available to allow it to determine issues relating to the validity of dispositions and the administration of trusts for charitable purposes. Under the Judicature Acts statutory jurisdiction in respect of charitable trusts was assigned to the High Court. Initially this jurisdiction depended upon the existence of a trust but this has since been extended to accommodate issues affecting all charities. In addition to hearing proceedings arising under the charities legislation, the High Court also has an appellate jurisdiction. The role and powers of this court in relation to charities is broadly similar in all common law nations (see, further, Part IV).

The Chancery Division of the High Court in England and Wales now exercises a broad jurisdiction in respect of charities and ultimate legal accountability for the proper management of a charity's affairs lies to it. The court provides final authority for decisions taken within an administrative system consisting of the Charity Commissioners, the Inland Revenue and the Customs and Excise. The fact that the jurisdiction of the High Court is geographically limited necessitates charities being located, or otherwise substantially based, within the UK to be subject to its authority.[37]

The Attorney General

The traditional function of the Attorney General is to represent the public interest in litigation. This may be necessary, for example, in situations where an individual has no *locus standi* in a particular matter such as in public nuisance,[38] a criminal act affecting the general public,[39] a statutory authority acting beyond its powers[40] or when enforcing the execution of charitable trusts.[41] Whereas in England and Wales the Charity Commission has been statutorily assigned much of the responsibility previously vested in the Attorney General, the traditional powers of this office continue in theory to be available within a charity law context throughout the common law nations[42] (see, further, Part IV).

Jurisdiction of the Attorney General

The ancient *parens patriae* jurisdiction of the Crown in relation to charities, and the right to bring proceedings in respect of them, devolved from the Lord Chancellor to become vested in the Attorney General:[43]

> . . . the King is to be considered as the *parens patriae*; that is he is the protector of every part of his subjects, and that, therefore, it is the duty of his officer, the Attorney General, to see that justice is done to every part of those subjects.

Indeed a distinguishing characteristic of charitable trusts is that because such a trust is by definition for the public benefit, it thereby acquires an entitlement to protection and enforcement by the Attorney General while a non-charitable trust is void because it is without any enforcement mechanism. The definitional matters, or legal attributes of a charity, are thus of considerable importance as they determine which set of consequences will follow. When so acting, the Attorney General must be advised separately from the State so as to avoid any possible conflict between the interests of the State and the specific interests of the charity.

Proceedings brought by the Attorney General

In keeping with the inherent powers of the *parens patriae* jurisdiction, the Attorney General will initiate proceedings in circumstances where the interests of a particular charity need protection. This may be necessary, for example, where there is evidence that trustees have failed in their duties.[44] It is most likely to be activated where direct intervention is urgently required to prevent or remedy damage to a particular charity. As noted in Tudor:[45]

> Such proceedings are likely to be brought in the Chancery Division of the High Court and the relief sought may include, *inter alia*, the restitution of charity property, the award of damages[46] and interest for breach of trust, injunctive relief[47] to prevent a breach of trust or its repetition, the appointment or removal of trustees or officers, the appointment of a receiver and manager,[48] the establishment of a scheme or the determination, by means of a declaration or otherwise, of questions arising in the administration of the charity or the application of its property.

The public interest in charities requires notice of proceedings affecting a charity, or charities in general, to be served on the Attorney General. The rule is that where proceedings involving a charity are commenced then, if not already a party, the Attorney General should be joined. In many instances, however, the issues that arise do not become the subject of proceedings and therefore do not require the involvement of the Attorney General.

The Probate Office

The Probate Office is of ancient lineage, being a descendant of the common law court of Probate with its jurisdiction in matters relating to wills. Until the Chancery Amendment Act 1858 ('Lord Cairn's Act') and other mid-nineteenth-century legislative reforms to the courts of Chancery and common law, the granting of probate in respect of wills and letters of administration of the estates of intestates remained the prerogative of the ecclesiastical courts. In 1857 the Prerogative Court was abolished and in 1958 the Court of Probate replaced it.

Administrative agencies

Charity law is largely administrative law exercised by government bodies employing the well-established rules and precedents of the common law tradition that remain rooted in the Preamble and the ruling in *Pemsel*. Reserved for the courts are matters referred by the Attorney General and/or by the Charity Commissioners where the issues are complex, involve a fine point of law, require interpretation or where a *cy-près* scheme concerning property above a certain value is needed. Most issues affecting charities never reach the courts. They are filtered out and determined by one of the relevant administrative bodies. While the substance and judicial precedents of English charity law formed the basis of the inheritance passed on to its colonies, the administrative structure (notably the role of the Charity Commission) did not form part of this legacy.

In England and Wales the range of non-judicial agencies now available to settle issues relating to donors, charities and charitable activities apply the *Pemsel* classification to determine charitable status.

The Charity Commissioners

The role and powers of Charity Commissioners for England and Wales can be seen as having devolved from the *parens patriae* authority of the Crown as subsequently exercised by the Chancellor and then by the Attorney General. This responsibility for protecting charitable trusts was first statutorily assigned to a non-judicial body in 1601: 45 decrees were issued in the first year and over 1,000 were sealed before the death of King James;[49] the last commission was held in the reign of Queen Anne and ended in 1803.[50] The Charity Commission ultimately inherited this responsibility, but only after many failed government efforts to introduce measures for registering and regulating charities.

In the late eighteenth century the first registry of charities was introduced and Parliament passed the Returns of Charitable Donations Act 1786[51] which decreed that charities benefiting the poor were to lodge returns sworn on oath to Parliament but, as has been noted, this was 'honoured more in breach than in observance'.[52] Sir Samuel Romilly sponsored legislation to address the problems of delay and expense associated with use of the judicial process to control abuse of charitable trusts.[53] However, this measure met with considerable judicial resistance and fell into disuse.[54] The Charitable Donations Act 1812 required the registration of charitable trusts with the Chancery Inrolement Office and although there were some 400 registrations in the first year these dwindled due to lack of enforcement. These early legislative initiatives to reform the law relating to charities failed mainly because of the lack of supporting administrative and enforcement procedures.

It was not until the Brougham Inquiry of 1819–37, resulting in the prosecution of some 400 charities and thereby demonstrating the value of independent scrutiny, that the modern form of the Commission emerged.[55] The proactive approach of the Inquiry proved much more effective than relying wholly on the traditional role of Attorney General and the courts in detecting the misuse of charitable funds. Consequently this approach was legislatively endorsed by the Charitable Trusts Act 1853, as amended in 1855 and 1860 and consolidated in the Charitable Trusts Act 1858, to establish a permanent Commission to supervise charitable activity.

The powers of the Commissioners were extended first by the Charities Act 1960 and then by the Charities Acts of 1992 and 1993,[56] which in effect transferred to the Commission much of the authority previously vested in the office of Attorney General. The overall statutory duty of the Commission is that of 'promoting the effective use of charitable resources by encouraging the development of better methods of administration, by giving charity trustees information or advice on any matter affecting the charity and by investigating and checking abuses'.[57]

The Commission maintains a national register of charities and monitors, supervises and supports those registered. Being vested with the powers of the High Court, from which their authority initially devolved, the Commissioners can make cy-près schemes, appoint and dismiss trustees and transfer property. In the main the Commission uses its powers to give advice or make decisions upon the many issues affecting the running of charities and it carries out regular inspections. In exercising its powers in relation to registration, the Commission is credited with broadening the interpretation of charitable purposes, particularly under the fourth Pemsel head, to permit a more elastic application of common law principles. Decisions of the Commission are subject to review by the courts but are binding, in particular on the Inland Revenue.

A growing proportion of the proceedings mentioned above in Tudor are now likely to be instituted by the Commission (see, further, chapters 5 and 8). The role played by this body is a distinguishing feature of English charity law, differentiating it from the development and contemporary practice of charity law in all other common law nations (see, further, Part IV).

The Inland Revenue

Primarily, this agency (now called Her Majesty's Revenue and Customs (HMRC)) following the April 2005 merger with Customs and Excise but, for ease of reference, referred to hereafter as the Inland Revenue) continues to give effect to its traditional role of maximizing the revenues payable to the State by way of taxes from which charities, since the Income Tax Act 1799 and the decision a century later in *Pemsel*, have been exempted. It has no special brief for charities but merely responds to applications from all organizations claiming tax exemption on grounds of charitable status. In the UK, since so empowered by the Finance Act 1986, the Inland Revenue has been working closely with the Charity Commissioners by referring cases where it has reason to believe that a charity is engaging in non-charitable activities or is applying income for non-charitable purposes. The Inland Revenue refers to the register of charities maintained by the Commission. The fact that this agency applies established common law principles but is statutorily required to follow the case law precedents set by the Commission marks an important point of difference between its role and that of equivalent bodies in other common law jurisdictions.

Other agencies

The Rates Office and, where appropriate, the Rating Tribunal will determine eligibility for rates exemption on charitable grounds. The powers of the Commissioners of Customs and Excise are exercised to ensure that charities comply with the rules relating to VAT exemption.

Other non-judicial bodies exist to register the existence of certain types of charities and thereafter to set standards for good practice and require a degree of accountability. For example, the many charities with company status must satisfy the requirements of the Registrar of Companies. Other charities with the status of either an Industrial and Provident Society or a Friendly Society must do so in relation to their respective Registrars.

There are no statutory duties placed upon the police specifically in relation to charities nor are their any organizational arrangements for specific police teams to be assigned responsibility for offences relating to charities.

Charity law: emergence of governing principles

The law relating to charities is not a unified coherent body of jurisprudence: the concept of a charity has eluded legislative and judicial definition for four centuries; few absolute and comprehensive rules exist to govern and distinguish their activities. For all common law countries, establishing and expanding the content and boundaries of contemporary charity law has required a return to the founding statutes and to a shared pool of related case law.

However, from the outset a number of principles were available to guide recognition of charities as such in law. First, a charity must have purposes which fit under one of the four *Pemsel* heads or come within the spirit and intendment of the Preamble to the founding legislation. Second, it must be provided for the benefit of the public. Third, unless exempted by statute, it must be exclusively charitable. Subsequently, further refinements emerged to augment these basic principles (see, further, chapter 7).

Charitable purposes

Purposes recognized in law as charitable largely remain as first identified and listed in the 1601 Act and as classified in *Pemsel* (see p. 79). This list has always been treated as indicative rather than prescriptive and its extension within the common law has been guided by analogy rather than by principle. Because a charitable purpose is interpreted relative to the prevailing social context, a trust may lose its charitable status as circumstances change.

The result can be seen in the endless lists and categories of purposes that came to be recognized as charitable, particularly under the fourth head. The recent reviews in common law nations have tended to see this case law legacy of charitable purposes as an obstacle to developing a modern coherent body of law, built around definitional statements and governed by clear principles.

The 'spirit and intendment' rule

Broadly speaking, this rule holds that even if a purpose cannot be defined as coming under one of the established heads of charity, it will nonetheless be construed as charitable if it can be interpreted as falling within the 'spirit or intendment' of the Preamble to the 1601 Act.[58] If it could be shown that the new purpose sufficiently approximated an established charitable purpose, so that it could be viewed as an extension of it or as analogous to it, then the court would hold the new purpose to be charitable on the grounds that it lay within the broad intention of the initial legislation. This rule has underpinned the development of charity law giving the judiciary some discretion to adjust the law to fit contemporary social circumstances.

Most often determining the fact and nature of a charitable purpose is accomplished by reference to the objects stated in the relevant governing instrument. However, occasionally the objects are not specified or are inadequately described. Determining charitable purpose then rests on ascertaining charitable intention.

Charitable intent[59]

Where the terms of a gift are expressed unambiguously in favour of a specified charity then the charitable intent is clearly stamped on the face of the gift but otherwise the court may need to determine the donor's intention. As an aid to discerning charitable intent the courts developed a principle of 'benignant construction' whereby, as stated in Tudor, 'the courts seek to save gifts where there is a charitable intention, although there are no clearly defined objects'.[60] For example, in *Re White*[61] a testator left a gift 'to the following religious societies viz. _____ to be divided in equal shares among them'. No societies were named. The court was able to save the gift by effectuating the donor's charitable intention. It was clear that his intent was charitable; he had merely failed to name the actual objects of charity. In upholding the gift as charitable, Lindley J explained that 'a charitable bequest never fails for uncertainty . . . the nomination of particular objects is only the mode and not the substance of a gift to charity'.[62] This was reiterated by Lord Eldon in *Mills* v. *Farmer*[63] who noted that

> in all cases where the testator has expressed an intention to give to charitable purposes, if that intention is declared absolutely, and nothing is left uncertain but the mode in which it is to be carried into effect, the intention will be carried into execution by this court.

The rule will also be applied if property is left for dispersal among charities selected at the discretion of a specified person.[64]

If the wording of a charitable gift permits an interpretation that may save it, that construction will be adopted. In *Weir* v. *Crum-Brown*[65] the difficulty was how to construe a trust for the benefit of aged and indigent bachelors who had 'shown practical sympathies either as amateurs or professionals in the pursuits of science in any of its branches'. It was argued that such a phrase was so uncertain that the whole gift must be void for uncertainty. The House of Lords adopted the benignant approach and held that the trustees would be able to identify beneficiaries using a common-sense approach.

No charitable intent

The principle of 'benignant construction' was not always sufficient to save a gift. In a line of cases from *In re Harwood; Coleman* v. *Innes*[66] to *In re Spence dec'd; Ogden* v. *Shackleton*[67] the UK courts have held that no charitable intent could be inferred from a testator's will.

Public benefit

Marrying a concept of public benefit broad enough to remain responsive to pressures from an ever-changing social context, with philanthropic intent, and with administrative systems and procedures,[68] to produce an integrated and distinctive body of jurisprudence has always been a central challenge for charity law. This problem was alluded to in *Cross* v. *The London Anti-Vivisection Society*:[69]

> Charity in law is a highly technical term. The method employed by the Court is to consider the enumeration of charities in the statute, bearing in mind that the enumeration is not exhaustive. Institutions whose objects are analogous to those mentioned in the statute are admitted to be charities; and again, institutions which are analogous to those already admitted by reported decisions are

held to be charities. The pursuit of these analogies obviously requires caution and circumspection. After all the best that can be done is to consider each case as it arises, upon its own special circumstances. To be a charity there must be some public purpose – something tending to the benefit of the community.

Private and public benefit

The Macnaghten classification, as has been noted, failed to make clear that for a trust to meet the legal requirements of a charity it must be both of a public character and contain some element of benefit to the public generally. In effect it must first disclose an element of benefit (e.g. the relief of poverty) and secondly, an element of public benefit. The burden of proof in relation to the latter element has varied across the four *Pemsel* heads.

A great deal of charity law jurisprudence has accumulated around the criteria for differentiating between private and charitable trusts. As Jenkins L.J. explained in *Re Scarisbrick*,[70] 'it is a general rule that a trust or gift in order to be charitable in the legal sense must be for the benefit of the public or some section of the public . . .'. This became a statutory rule in England and Wales.[71]

Applying the rule

Two requirements are imposed. First, the rule is not that all persons in the relevant class of the public should derive a benefit but only that they should all be eligible to do so. The number constituting a sufficient proportion of 'the public' has never been determined. This may be affected by whether or not the charity charges a fee for accessing its service. The fact of doing so will not itself affect charitable status,[72] but where the level of fee is such as to discriminate against those who cannot afford to pay and limit the numbers who may avail of the service then the public benefit test will not be satisfied.[73]

The public benefit test will be met, and the trust in question will have charitable status, when, in the words of Lord Wrenbury in *Verge v. Somerville*,[74] the gift is made:

> for the benefit of the community or of an appreciably important class of the community. The inhabitants of a parish or town, or any particular class of such inhabitants may, for instance, be the objects of such a gift, but private individuals, or a fluctuating body of private individuals, cannot.

So, the class of persons who might benefit may be either a section of the public,[75] or a class of the community,[76] or a section of the community.[77] Conversely, it will not be met and the trust will not be charitable if those who might benefit are merely 'a fluctuating body of private individuals'.[78] The basis for this distinction between public and private classes is unsatisfactory because in practice fluctuating membership can be a characteristic of both types.

Second, the rule does not impose an absolute bar on any private benefit accruing from a charitable gift. It does, however, require that any private benefit conferred must be incidental.

Applying the rule: private classes

Where a class is defined so that its membership is fixed then it is necessarily private; a 'closed' class cannot be a public one. The courts have established that in certain instances a class can be defined as private rather than public, although this approach cannot be applied uniformly across all categories of charitable purpose.

A class of specified individuals can never be construed as a public class.[79] Nor can a class which derives from a personal relationship with specified individuals.[80] A subsection of the public or 'a class within a class', and a section of the public as defined by means other than locality, are both outside the definition of public.[81]

Applying the rule: public classes

The courts have come to recognize that certain restrictively defined classes will nonetheless be sufficiently 'public' for the purposes of acquiring charitable status. Where the class is defined by locality, the intended recipients living in the same place, this will be deemed to meet the requirement of being 'public'.[82] Where the class is defined by its faith then the courts construe this as a non-personal relationship nexus and therefore intrinsically public in nature.[83] Where it is defined by membership of a group in a particular locality then even if small in number it may be sufficiently 'public' to qualify as charitable.[84] A class is often defined by the common relationship of its members as descendants of a named person or as descendants of particular group. The former is open to challenge on the grounds of the personal nexus test.[85] The latter may well satisfy the 'public' requirement.[86]

The 'poor relations' exception   Creative judicial interpretation of public benefit in the context of 'poor relations' trusts, where the donor or testator intends to make a gift for the benefit of poor relatives, has been responsible for extending charitable status to a class of beneficiaries who clearly do not satisfy the 'public' requirement. Such trusts have long been recognized as forming an anomalous exception to the general rule that gifts where the beneficiaries are identified by a purely personal relationship to the would-be donor cannot be charitable gifts. As was explained by Evershed MR in *Re Scarisbrick*:[87]

> The 'poor relations' cases may be justified on the basis that the relief of poverty is so altruistic a character that the public element may necessarily be inferred thereby; or they may be accepted as a hallowed, if illogical, exception.

The so-called 'poor relations' or 'poor employees' trusts were recognized in a line of decisions which stretches back to the eighteenth century.[88] In *Issac* v. *Defriez*[89] the court upheld gifts to beneficiaries required to be a poor relation of the testator and a poor relation of his wife selected by the trustees. In *White* v. *White*[90] Grant MR upheld as charitable a trust established for the purpose of providing apprenticeships for the poor relations in two specified families despite the obvious absence of any possible public benefit to the poor in general. The case law was further extended in the nineteenth century to include the descendants of a named uncle,[91] members of a theatrical society,[92] members of a mutual benefit society[93] and the employees of a banking firm.[94] Nowadays, the modification of the public benefit requirement in relation to this category of charitable trust is well established[95] and shows every sign of being relaxed further.[96]

If the class is defined by membership of a particular profession then it is likely to be considered too closed[97] though common nationality may be sufficient to meet the 'public' requirement[98] (see, also, chapter 4).

The rule in relation to charitable purpose

The courts have inferred that trusts falling within the first three of the *Pemsel* categories will be 'assumed to be for the benefit of the community and therefore charitable, unless the contrary is shown'.[99] In fact, although this holds good for the first and third categories, trusts for the advancement of education have quite often not qualified as charitable trusts because of a failure to satisfy the public benefit requirement. No such presumption applies in respect of gifts within the fourth category which has attracted the most stringent application of the public benefit test.[100]

The test never had much viability in application to trusts for the relief of poverty. While gifts to classes of specified individuals will certainly be private, the court is unlikely in this context to rule that gifts to any other class will fail because of a failure to meet the public benefit test. The test is applied in a similarly relaxed fashion to trusts for the advancement of education. In relation to trusts for the promotion of health, however, the test is applied most rigorously.[101] The court will rule that gifts not only to classes of specified individuals but also to those coming within either the 'personal nexus' or the 'narrow *Baddeley*' rule[102] will fail the public benefit test (see, further, chapter 5).

Public benefit: the objective test

In the UK the focus of the judiciary is firmly on deducing the nature of the gift from an objective appraisal of the facts. In *Re Fouveaux*[103] Chitty J held that the abolition of vivisection was a charitable purpose because the testator's intention was to benefit the community; he ruled that it was not for the court to consider whether the community would in fact benefit. However, the House of Lords in *National Anti-Vivisection Society* v. *IRC*[104] expressly overruled the approach taken by Chitty J. The House declared that it was wrong to treat the intention of the testator as decisive; the public benefit test was to be applied by the court. This is quite different from the approach adopted in Ireland. There the judiciary adopt a subjective test in determining whether or not a gift satisfies the public benefit test.[105] That is the courts will pose the question 'Did the donor believe that the purpose to which he or she was directing a gift was of a charitable nature?' If so, then the gift will be charitable in law.[106]

In England, the factors which will prevent the public benefit test being satisfied in the context of trusts for the advancement of education have extended beyond blood ties or a personal nexus to a 'nexus of contract' and trusts for the education of persons, or relatives of persons, in common employment have been found not to be charitable in nature.[107] This approach was in line with the recommendations of the Goodman Committee report on *Charity Law and Voluntary Organisations*.[108]

Exclusiveness

The courts look for an exclusive charitable intent and have resolutely declined to save gifts as charitable where the donor had failed to unequivocally and unambiguously state such intent or had expressed mixed intentions, some charitable and some not. If uncertain language is used as where a purpose or object has been described as 'philanthropic', 'benevolent' or 'for a worthy cause', etc., it will be denied charitable status. If a donor's gift included both charitable and non-charitable purposes, and allowed for the possibility of trustees using at their discretion some or all of the gift for non-charitable purposes, then the courts would refuse to recognize it as charitable. As Wylie explains:[109]

> So long as the objects within the scope of the gift were all charitable, it did not matter that a selection had to be made[110] and the courts even went so far as to uphold gifts requiring an apportionment between charitable and non-charitable purposes.[111] In the latter case, the part of the gift to be devoted to the non-charitable purpose usually failed for want of certainty or as infringing the rule against inalienability. This led to the general impression that there cannot be a trust for a non-charitable purpose.

The exclusivity of charitable purposes continues to be a necessary component of charitable status in the law of England and Wales which requires that 'a trust must not only be declared in favour of objects of a charitable nature, but it must also be expressed that in its application it is confined to such objects'.[112]

Distinction between charities and other not-for-profit organizations

Charities may be differentiated from other types of not-for-profit organizations on the basis of certain principles and the legal form or structure chosen to give effect to their activities.

Types of organization

The most distinctive characteristic of charities, distinguishing them from the range of not-for-profit bodies, is their adherence to the public benefit principle. Other principles (see pp. 147–8) are also distinctive.

A charity

This is a public benefit, non-government organization which in the UK is established exclusively for a charitable purpose and is required to ensure that gifts received are used exclusively for the benefit of those defined by that purpose. Charitable purposes are purposes for: the relief of poverty; the advancement of education; the advancement of religion; and such other purposes, beneficial to the community, which are not accommodated under the previous headings. A charitable trust is uniquely constituted in that it is governed by an independent board of trustees upon whom rests the responsibility to protect the donor's gift, give effect to the charity's objects and ensure that the benefit reaches the beneficiaries. It is also unique in that its status is accompanied by a public recognition of virtue which attracts the commitment of volunteers, financial donations, tax exemption privileges and other resources.

Charitable status confers eligibility for tax exemption, it allows for existence in perpetuity and it attracts the protection of the Attorney General. There are, however, legal restrictions on trading and advocacy activities by charities.

An Industrial and Provident Society

This is a member benefit type of non-government organization, usually a commercial organization, and is required, under the Industrial and Provident Societies Acts 1893–1978, to be registered in the Industrial and Provident Societies Register. It must be formed 'for carrying on any industries, businesses or trades', which includes agricultural producers, group water schemes and housing co-operatives.

A Friendly Society

This is a member benefit type of non-government organization, a mutual assurance association, established under the Friendly Societies Act 1896. These include mutual insurance and assurance bodies, benevolent societies and other societies formed for purposes such as the promotion of science, literature and education. There are three types of Friendly Society, as identified in the 1896 Act: the friendly society; the cattle insurance society and the benevolent society, which is the type relevant to non-government organizations.

Although an Industrial and Provident Society and a Friendly Society are quite different, both were established under the Friendly Societies Acts 1875 and 1896 (as amended), and the Registrar of Friendly Societies must register both.

Structures

The evolution of charities within a common law context has been shaped by their purposes. The starting point has always been: to what legally recognized charitable purpose is this organization seeking to give effect? While the *Pemsel* classification for the most part defines the range of possible purposes, judicial precedent and legislative provision have permitted a degree of variation between the common law nations. Consequently, charitable activity is now housed in a range of different structures. Government bodies, religious organizations and foundations as well as the more traditional trusts, unincorporated associations, incorporated charities and eleemosynary corporations are now all likely to be claiming tax exemption on the grounds of their charitable activities. Industrial and Provident Societies, Friendly Societies and corporations may also, though infrequently, provide structures for charitable activity.

Charities are required to be properly constituted with appropriate governing instruments but this can take a variety of different forms: some may be informal having no legal status separate and distinct from the relationship between its members; others can adopt quite formal, legal structures which provide clearly for such a distinction. Charities are public benefit organizations as distinct from mutual benefit bodies such as Industrial and Provident Societies (occasionally an Industrial and Provident Society will also be a charity), Friendly Societies and co-operatives and other bodies such as trade unions and political parties. In the UK this differentiation between charitable structures is particularly important and determines the jurisdiction of the Charity Commission, which is restricted to the affairs of charitable trusts.

The following are structures for charities with no legal personality or juridical status.

A trust

This is an arrangement whereby one or more persons operating under the authority of a 'deed of trust' hold(s) funds or property on behalf of other persons. The three essential components of a valid trust are: certainty of words; certainty of subject; and certainty of objects or beneficiaries.[113] The governing instrument is a trust deed or will and its executive power rests with trustees appointed under the terms of the trust. It has no legal personality and it is the trustees rather than the body, which must enter into legal relations and accept personal liability. It is to be noted that Lord Macnaghten when classifying charitable purposes in *Pemsel* referred only to trusts – 'Charity in its legal sense comprises four principal divisions: trusts for ... etc.' – the implication perhaps being that he considered this legal structure as having attributes uniquely suited to give effect to charitable purposes.

In England and Wales, unlike some other countries, there is no legal difference between a charitable trust and a charitable foundation. Although the word 'foundation' is more likely to imply permanent endowment, the legal structure is usually still a trust.

An unincorporated association

This is not a legal entity and its creation rests on an agreement, oral or written, between identified members; usually its governing instrument is its constitution or rules.[114] An unincorporated association has no legal personality and therefore no capacity, independent of its members, to enter into legal relations with other bodies. It is usually the structure of choice for small charities. As explained in Tudor: 'The use of unincorporated associations as a legal structure for charities gained popularity in the 18th century with the rise of voluntary societies and reflected the change from individual to associated philanthropy.'[115]

Other structures

Charities may, alternatively, assume one of the following incorporated structures and thereby acquire a legal personality.

A company limited by guarantee   A limited company is a body, incorporated under the legislative provisions regulating companies, the memorandum and articles of association of which are registered in the designated registry office for companies. Many charities, as they grow in size and complexity, become incorporated and must then comply with statutory registration requirements and have their names entered in the appropriate registry. This has become an increasingly popular structure.

An incorporated foundation   The term 'foundation' most usually refers to a body established by an initial endowment which may or may not be dedicated to charitable purposes (see, also, chapter 2). A charitable foundation acquires legal personality on incorporation although the charitable purpose to which the endowment is addressed will always remain as stated by the founder in the governing instrument. The endowed charitable foundation has traditionally been established by a successful business and most often served as a grant making body providing financial assistance to projects that came within its designated purposes (e.g. Ford, Rowntree, Nuffield, Carnegie and Rockefeller).

Advantages of legal personality

For charities the advantages of adopting a formal legal structure include:

- separation of members' responsibilities from those of the organization, including protection for members from liability for any debts incurred by the organization;
- the organization can own property, enter into contracts and employ people in its own name;
- the organization can bring and defend court proceedings in its own name; and
- the organization can apply for charitable recognition in its own name.

Conclusion

The current common law foundations for the charity law of many nations lie in the Statute of Charitable Uses 1601, particularly in the Preamble, and in the judicial principles and precedents established before and after that date.

The overarching requirement that above all else a charity must be for the public benefit still provides the governing and distinguishing principle for charity law. These and other characteristics underpinned the development of charity law for many centuries and across many diverse common law jurisdictions. They also, however, contributed significantly to contemporary difficulties in fitting the law to meet patterns of social need. These difficulties will be explored in the following chapter.

Chapter 4

Alienation, philanthropy and the common law

Introduction

The common law heritage, underpinning the statutory infrastructure of many modern western nations, has proved enduring. Some of its characteristic components have been very serviceable. The public benefit test, for example, has lent itself as a means for the flexible reinterpretation of what in law can be defined as charitable in the light of changing social and economic circumstances. The protective nature of the *parens patriae* jurisdiction,[1] coupled with the prerogative powers of the High Court, for centuries provided a supportive framework for sustaining charities and their activities. However, for common law nations the charity law framework may now provide an inadequate and in some respects even an obstructive means for addressing the social inclusion issues.

The four heads of charity as classified by Macnaghten in *Pemsel*[2] (relief of poverty, advancement of education, advancement of religion and other purposes beneficial to the community not included under the previous three heads) together with the 'spirit and intendment' rule[3] provided the basic common law toolkit for determining charitable status. Unsurprisingly, this now very dated toolkit has developed problems. One area of difficulty is that it carried with it vestiges of the era for which it was assembled; these basic common law characteristics are often no longer appropriate. Then there are problems associated with the *Pemsel* heads of charity: some of a technical nature, others to do with relevance and sufficiency. Finally, from the perspective of the modern social inclusion agenda, charity law lacks the capacity to authorize the range of possible methods of intervention most likely to leverage positive change to the circumstances of the chronically socially disadvantaged.

Cumulatively, these deficiencies give rise to the question, Is the common law toolkit now fit for the purpose of facilitating appropriate, sufficient and effective philanthropic intervention in contemporary western society?

This chapter briefly considers the growing alienation of minority groups in modern common law nations and the threat this presents to the consolidation of civil society (see, also, chapter 2). It then examines the four *Pemsel* heads of charity before considering the implications of the above constraining aspects of the common law legacy for philanthropic intervention in respect of social inclusion issues.

Forestalling alienation

Facilitating the social inclusion of marginalized groups is now perhaps the most important challenge facing all democratic governments. In its most acute form, this challenge is very evident in national and international responses – appropriate/inappropriate or lack thereof – to the alienation experienced by minority culture-specific groups. This is set to become increasingly significant as population displacement, driven mainly by factors of economics and conflict, continues to impact upon all modern western nations. It must now also be viewed in the uncertain unfolding politics of the post-9/11 world and with particular reference to the pressing need to build a new rapprochement between those nations and the culture of Islam.

Alienation: indigenous people

The record of philanthropic intervention on behalf of indigenous people in Australia, Canada and elsewhere demonstrates the failings of the related legal framework that authorized the nature and extent of the related charitable activity (see, further, chapter 2 and Part IV). Their experience has been not unlike that of some minority cultures in other countries.

Recent history provides many examples of countries experiencing debilitating and at times destructive tensions because of the inability of government to respond in an appropriate and timely fashion to the needs of a minority culture which is then left to perceive itself as increasingly alienated from mainstream society. When the need for a level of separate recognition and affirmation by and within the prevailing social infrastructure is not accommodated by government then – as demonstrated for example in Northern Ireland, the Balkans, parts of Africa and the Middle East – there is every possibility of a drift from alienation to confrontation. Governments often cannot intervene effectively: their continuation in power rests on satisfying the wishes of the majority; they have complex interests to protect; are distanced from and usually mistrusted by the marginalized; have only blunt, heavy-handed methods at their disposal; and cannot respond swiftly, with the sensitivity and discretion appropriate to the particular circumstances. Philanthropists, facilitated by an appropriate legal framework, would be much freer to develop an acceptable, appropriate and flexible contribution that could make the crucial difference in forestalling any such a drift. For philanthropic intervention to be effective, however, the charity law framework must fit contemporary social need and facilitate the mediation of organizations able to strategically address the needs of marginalized minority groups on a community, national and international basis.

International law

The principles and provisions of international law, particularly the European Convention for the Protection of Human Rights and Fundamental Freedoms 1950 and the Declaration of Indigenous Peoples 1993, have a bearing on the issues facing such communities. The Preamble to the former, for example, includes a reference to 'the importance of the traditions and cultural values of each people'. Article 4 of the latter, for example, emphasizes the right of indigenous peoples to maintain and strengthen their political, economic, social and cultural characteristics as well as their legal systems (see, further, chapter 7).

Alienation: the domestic agenda

Arguably, from a charity law perspective, the issues and possible solutions in relation to minority, culture-specific communities such as the Indigenous people of Australia apply also to a large extent in respect of the marginalized groups that typically appear on the domestic social inclusion agenda of modern western nations. The risk and possible consequences of a similar drift towards alienation should not be underestimated simply because it is unlikely to lead to civil unrest. The dangers posed to civil society by disaffected youth, for example, are real enough. Again, an appropriate legal framework is crucial if effective philanthropic intervention is to facilitate the meaningful and authentic social inclusion of groups that perceive themselves as marginalized and forestall their possible alienation (see, further, chapters 2 and 6).

Characteristics of the common law

The seventeenth-century legacy remains very evident in a number of distinctive characteristics that uniformly colour the contemporary regulatory frameworks for charities in the common law nations. Some of these characteristics have inhibited effective philanthropic intervention.

Judge-made law

The common law was referred to as 'judge-made law' in recognition of the fact that when travelling on 'assizes' and dealing in the main with law and order issues, the judiciary often had to administer justice in an ad hoc fashion. This distinguished it from the prescriptive approach required by statutory law and applied more fastidiously when cases could be listed and given a full hearing in the main courts. The expression also refers to the weight placed on the value of precedent, the hallmark of the judiciary in the courts of equity. Following the amalgamation of equity and the common law, with the requirement that the principles of the former should have priority, the judicial approach thereafter was firmly confined to developing the law in accordance with established cases. In the absence of specific legislative provisions, any progressive development to ensure that the law was adjusted to fit the circumstances of the presenting case, relied entirely on judicial decision-making. This was perhaps particularly true in relation to charity law where legislation avoided definitional matters, restricting itself to dealing with powers and processes, and the judiciary was largely left to exercise their discretion as guided by precedent.

Emphasis on rights and duties of the individual

The common law has always placed an emphasis on the rights and duties of the individual. Perhaps the single most distinctive common law characteristic found expression in the catch phrase 'no writ no action'. A petitioner could only succeed in lodging a plea in court if he could fit his complaint within the narrowly defined terms of a particular writ; the range of standard form writs available was limited. On conclusion of the hearing, the range of judicial disposal options was again tightly constrained. Should the plea succeed and the court find in his favour, it quite often lacked the authority necessary to ensure that the plaintiff's rights were enforced.

This approach, coupled with a fixed reliance on precedent has, in some parts of the common law world, resulted in a bar on class actions; rights and duties fall to be determined by the courts on a case by case basis.

Extension of status by analogy rather than principle

In the common law any extension of status is by analogy rather than by principle. The Preamble to the Statute of Charitable Uses 1601, the legislative progenitor of charity law in all common law nations, consisted largely of a list of activities which were then considered charitable. This common law approach of listing subjects for legal redress, permitting subsequent empirical extension by analogy, has itself proved to be problematic. A grindingly logical approach led to the law being constrained by the rigidity of the specified where case law developments could only be accommodated by painstakingly distinguishing the facts of new cases from the old. Most importantly, it prevented the emergence of unifying principles which could have brought more coherence to charity law. The result can be seen in the endless lists and categories of purposes recognized as charitable, rather than in a coherent body of law, built around definitional statements and governed by clear principles. The evolution of charity law in a common law context is a victory of form over substance.[4]

Respect for social institutions

The common law would seem to be predicated on maintaining the status quo in society: most particularly it embodies a respect for social institutions by giving protection to the government of the day, the place of religion, the role of the Church and the authority of the judiciary. It is not concerned with matters of public policy or contemporary politics but requires an almost feudal respect for king and country and for the institutions of the land. This tends to induce a complicit relationship between charities and social institutions.

Freedom of association

The place of voluntary organizations, including charities, within the social infra-structure alongside government bodies and business enterprises owes a great deal to the very basic common law principle that people have a right to form associ-ations. This right to gather together as a body, for lawful purposes in order to better represent and advance collective interests found early recognition in law and rapidly became a crucial strategic building block in the relationship between government and the governed as well as a cornerstone in the development of commerce and in such other areas as the pursuit of philanthropy. The very existence and consequent growth of the voluntary sector is essentially attributable to this right. Such associations do not need permission to exist nor to assume any particular legal form and are free to maintain their independence from government bodies

Particular respect for religion

There is a common law presumption that religious organizations are for the public benefit and therefore should have charitable status. In the increasingly secular societies of the modern common law world there has been considerable debate regarding the continued merits of such a presumption. Where religion no longer functions as a 'pillar of society', and perhaps particularly in those societies where it is a divisive force then, arguably, activities of religious organizations should be subject to a more stringent and broadly based public benefit test before qualifying for charitable status.

Respect for government, policy and law

The respect for king and country and the institutions of the land continues to find expression in the specific prohibition on political activity by charities. This requires a fine distinction to be drawn between political purposes and charit-able purposes. The distinction is not easily made: deprivation, homelessness, unemployment, civil liberties, animal rights, conservation, etc., are all matters which in practice are often the business of both politicians and charities. The hallmark advocacy role of charities on behalf of the disadvantaged can often shade into political lobbying – the former being permitted, the latter not.

Role mutuality of charity and government

The common law carries an assumption that the purposes of public service bodies and charities are coterminous; that a complementarity naturally lies between the roles of government and charities in maintaining social values and ensuring social service provision.

Maintaining contemporary social values

The Preamble includes in its list of charitable purposes references to the maintenance of houses of correction, assisting poor maids into marriage and the rehabilitation of prisoners. These now appear to us as measures of social control. It
would seem the government of the day was then implying that it was the business
of charities to assist it in maintaining order. This approach continues to be evident
in the current policy to promote a congruity between the agendas of charities and
government on the basis that both share a common interest in ensuring the
provision of facilities that conform with and preserve contemporary social values
and promote civil society.[5]

The in-built assumption, that defending the contemporary social policy status
quo is appropriately treated as a priority for both government and charity, clearly
has its roots in the founding charity law statute. This, again, resonates with the
legislative intent behind current charity law and is evident in provisions such as
those which uphold the charitable status of religious purposes, deny this status to
organizations pursuing political aims and prohibit any trading activity which
might compete with commercial bodies.

Providing social services

The Preamble also clearly indicated that public utility provision was a charitable
purpose and thereby laid the foundations for a partnership between government
and charities in providing services for those in need. However, the retreat of the
public sector and the devolving of responsibility for service provision to the voluntary sector has become a widespread phenomenon in the common law world.
There is now a growing concern to clarify the distinction between the remit of
government and charity in relation to public utility and the attendant respective
responsibilities of government bodies and voluntary organizations[6] (see, further,
chapter 5).

A fiscal regulatory environment

The common law was always a law based on rules accompanied by a complex
system for levying and collecting fines. This led to an emphasis on administration
rather than adjudication and to a fundamental concern with financial matters. In
many ways the development of charity law has been driven by a concern to
improve control of charity finances.

The Revenue authorities

Charity law has its origins in legislative and judicial attempts to maximize tax
revenues by establishing agencies and processes designed to regulate practice,
detect abuse and restrain the availability of exemption on grounds of charitable
status, as clearly illustrated by both the 1601 Act and the *Pemsel* case. The

deep-rooted preoccupation of charity law with tax, rates, trading and more recently with the contract culture and the intricacies of profit distribution illustrates this aspect of its common law heritage. The present-day role of the Inland Revenue in the UK in relation to charities, and of other such government bodies in all common law countries, grows from this very basic traditional concern.

The taxation statutes, granting considerable exemption to those fulfilling the eligibility criteria for charitable tax exemption, are also a source of judicial precedent for the definition of 'charity'. In England and Wales, where registration with the Charity Commission is recognized by the Inland Revenue as satisfying such criteria and determining entitlement to tax exemption, there have been calls to separate the definitions.[7]

Pemsel and the four 'heads' of charitable purposes

The common law heritage, consisting of the Macnaghten classification of charitable purposes as subsequently enlarged under the 'spirit and intendment' rule, continues to provide the basic legal framework for charities and their activities. The relief of poverty, advancement of education, advancement of religion and other purposes beneficial to the community not included under the previous three heads still constitute the principal heads of charitable purposes across the common law world. Their judicial interpretation over the centuries has resulted in charity law acquiring certain features, some limiting and others liberating, that now constrain its capacity to respond to poverty and issues of social inclusion.

The relief of poverty

Charity law has its origins in trusts for the relief of poverty. As was explained in *Pemsel* 'the popular conception of a charitable purpose covers the relief of any form of necessity, destitution or helplessness'.[8] Poverty, however, and the means of providing for its relief, is not as readily susceptible to definition, classification and regulation as was the case when the foundations of charity law were first laid down;[9] the 'poor relations' case law, for example, has introduced some uncertainty (see, further, chapter 3). There is also a view that in this context the law in the UK has become curiously ossified:[10] that it has taken little account of the emergence of the Welfare State and the nationalization of education, health and welfare. This is illustrated by the example of educational charities which gained their charitable status at a time when they provided the only means available for educating the poor. The advent of State education for all led to the transformation of such schools to exclusive fee-paying establishments but they nevertheless retained their charitable status.[11] Medical care raises similar problems. Following the nationalization of health services, private insurance schemes were declared charitable as they relieve the burden on State facilities, but membership fees effectively exclude the poor from their benefits.[12] Again, although access to justice is facilitated by statutory schemes for legal aid and assistance, in practice charities find it prohibitively expensive to seek judicial guidance.

The poor

Poverty is not an absolute concept but is relative to the circumstances of each individual poor person. When *Re Coulthurst*[13] was appealed to the Court of Appeal, Evershed MR attempted a partial definition: 'it may not unfairly be paraphrased for present purposes as meaning persons who have to "go short" in the ordinary expectation of that term, due regard being had to their status in life and so forth'.[14] As explained by Viscount Simonds in *IRC* v. *Baddeley*,[15] 'there may be a good charity for the relief of persons who are not in grinding need or utter destitution' and a trust to provide for persons of limited or reduced means may come within the ambit of this category. The relative nature of poverty is illustrated by the wide range of cases associated with persons of professional standing such as out-of-work actors as in *In Re Lacy*[16] and *Re de Carteret*.[17]

Being poor will not itself be sufficient to justify intervention that is charitable in law. Moreover, the definition of 'poor' has also carried with it some connotations of 'the deserving poor'. For example, in 1904 ladies in reduced circumstances (defined as having an income of not less than £25 nor more than £55) were objects of poverty relief[18] while in 1914 employees (earning £39) were not.[19] Also, for the purposes of charity, 'poverty' does not include an object to relieve unemployment unless the unemployed person is additionally both poor and in need.[20]

Implied poverty

A gift need not expressly state that it is for the poor, 'such intention on the part of the donor may be implied from the nature of the gift looked at as a whole'.[21] In *Re Dudgeon* it was stated that 'it is not absolutely necessary to find poverty expressed in so many words',[22] which conforms with the view in *Re Lucas* that 'the court will look at the whole gift, and it if comes to the conclusion that the relief of poverty was meant, will give effect to it, although the word poverty is not to be found in it'.[23] The court will look at the identity of the intended beneficiaries to see if it can imply poverty into their circumstances as in *Re Coulthurst* where 'the status of "widows and orphaned children" suggests the possibility, or perhaps the probability of impecuniosity'.[24]

Gifts to the poor

The 'public' dimension to the 'public benefit' test has always had little relevance when applied to determine eligibility of the poor or impotent. The class of poor may be appropriately defined by reference to a locality, to members of a particular religious faith/profession/nationality or to a particular line of descendants.

Specific class of poor   Gifts made to the poor of a specified town[25] or city[26] or of a particular religious denomination[27] have been upheld in the courts. So also have gifts to the poor in a particular parish;[28] a gift to a parish itself, the poor of the parish being intended;[29] and a gift to the poor maintained in a hospital.[30]

Similarly, gifts made to the poor of a specified town[31] or city[32] or of a particular religious denomination[33] have been upheld in the courts. Gifts which are gender- or status-specific such as for the benefit of spinsters,[34] widows,[35] working-men[36] or debtors[37] have all been upheld as charitable trusts. The poverty component, however, must be satisfied unless the identified class can be construed as coming within the alternative category in the 1601 Act of 'impotent' rather than 'poor'.[38] In *A-G for Northern Ireland* v. *Ford*,[39] for example, a gift to widows who were not necessarily poor was found not to be charitable while in *Re Lewis*[40] a gift in similar terms to blind girls and boys was charitable because the latter were classed as 'impotent'.

A gift will not fail to be construed as charitable solely because the intended recipients were identified only in very general terms[41] or by reference to a personal nexus.[42]

Charitable intent

In common with all charitable trusts, a gift to provide for the relief of poverty must be made with a charitable intent if it is to come within the definition of charity.[43] Usually the purpose is stated with such clarity that there can be no doubt about the donor's charitable intent.[44] Where problems arise this is often due to an ambiguous or non-explicit use of language.[45] As Picarda explains:[46]

> The word 'deserving' on the other hand does not necessarily connote poverty so that, whatever else it is, a trust to provide dowries for deserving Jewish girls is not for the relief of poverty.[47] Nor is a trust to advance deserving journalists a trust to relieve poverty.[48]

The advancement of education

As explained by Buckley LJ[49] 'educational' entails an 'improvement of a useful branch of human knowledge'. The usefulness, or possible prospective usefulness, and to whom, of particular knowledge can be difficult to determine.

General educational purposes

A gift for the advancement of education in a general manner will usually be recognized as charitable. So, for example, a bequest for 'educational . . . purposes'[50] or a gift 'for the benefit, and advancement, and propagation of education and learning in every part of the world'[51] or to finance 'a body of persons established for the purpose of raising the artistic state of the country'[52] will be upheld. Similarly, a gift to schools,[53] or to colleges, either generally, or to found a scholarship[54] will be recognized as charitable under this heading. But if the purpose is expressed too generally then charitable status will be denied.

Specific educational purposes

The list of judicially approved charitable purposes in the context of trusts for the advancement of education is extensive. There has never been any doubt, for example, that a charitable trust would be for educational purposes if it provided for the study of subjects such as languages,[55] law,[56] medicine,[57] natural history,[58] archaeology,[59] economics,[60] theology,[61] religious instruction,[62] comparative religions,[63] agriculture,[64] mechanical sciences and engineering[65] or shorthand typewriting and book-keeping.[66]

However, the less vocational the subject the greater the judicial scepticism regarding its intrinsic educational value. So, for example, literature of no literary merit will not be viewed as educational and a trust to protect a testator's manuscripts will not be upheld as charitable;[67] though a biographical study may be viewed more positively.[68]

Aesthetic educational purposes

Providing aesthetic education is charitable. No firm definition has been given of what precisely constitutes aesthetic education. It would seem to encompass the appreciation, promotion and development of art of a certain calibre, the cultivation of skills such as play and the imparting of civilized values. It has been stated that 'the education of artistic taste is one of the most important things in the development of a civilised human being'.[69]

A gift to provide for the upkeep of ancient cottages so that modern craftsmen could learn from them is charitable.[70] Establishing art galleries and museums is charitable.[71] Exhibiting a collection of arms and antiques can be charitable.[72] Advancing or promoting literature is charitable.[73] A choral society can be charitable[74] as can music generally.[75] Gifts to promote the training of singers of 'serious music' have been held charitable,[76] as has a gift to promote interest in a particular composer (Delius).[77] Theatres can be valid educational charities,[78] but it will depend upon the quality of their productions. In most cases concerning aesthetic education, the courts will need to be satisfied of the artistic content of a particular purpose.

The advancement of religion

Religion has been defined as 'the promotion of spiritual teaching in a wide sense, and the maintenance of the doctrines on which it rests, and the observances that serve to promote and manifest it'.[79] Judicial defence of religion and religious organizations is embedded in the common law.

It is clear from the cases that an essential prerequisite is a belief in the existence of a god. The view that the legal definition of religion could be satisfied by a system of belief not involving faith in a god was explicitly rejected by Dillon J in *Re South Place Ethical Society*.[80] English case law stresses that the 'two essential attributes of religion are faith and worship: faith in a god and worship of that god'.[81] Worship is defined as 'conduct indicative of reverence or veneration for that supreme being'.[82] Worship is not regarded as merely any lawful means for formally observing the tenets of a cult.[83]

The exclusivity rule applies and a trust will fail if it contains a mix of both charitable and other purposes.[84] The basic rule was set out by Sir William Grant nearly two centuries ago: 'the question is not whether the trustee may not apply it upon purposes strictly charitable, but whether he is bound so to apply it'.[85] Gifts to ministers are charitable as being for the advancement of religion[86] as are gifts for building and maintaining churches, the maintenance of tombs and for missionary purposes.

Equality of religions

The law holds that all religions are to be treated equally. It will not inquire into the inherent validity of any particular religion nor will it examine the relative merits of different religions.[87] Even if the gift deliberately discriminates against particular religions it may still be charitable.[88] As has been said, 'although this court might consider the opinions sought to be propagated foolish or even devoid of foundation, it would not, on that account declare it void'.[89] The Church of Scientology was refused charitable status by the Charity Commissioners because its core practices of training and auditing (counselling) did not constitute worship of a supreme being,[90] even though it had been deemed charitable in the USA and in Australia.[91]

In *R* v. *Registrar General ex parte Segerdal*,[92] it was held that Buddhism was a religion despite a lack of belief in a supreme being. The judicial view is that for a religion to be charitable it must be founded on a belief in and reverence for a god or gods. In line with a progressive and evolving approach to religion, faith healing has also been deemed to be charitable where it was open to members of the public.[93]

Beneficial to the community, not falling under any of the preceding heads

This fourth *Pemsel* head is a residual one, of charitable objects that cannot be conveniently fitted under the other heads. In order to qualify for charitable status under this heading it is not necessary that a gift should be directed solely towards relief of the poor (see, further, chapter 5).

Charitable purposes under the fourth head

It is becoming increasingly anomalous to refer to this body of case law as a category when often the only factor the cases have in common is that they do not readily fit under any of the other three headings. Some of the case law groupings, such as those within the broad umbrella of 'health', are coalescing and growing at such a rate as to warrant recognition as separate and distinct areas of charity law.

The flexibility permitted by this *Pemsel* head has also, however, allowed the judiciary across the common law world some room for manoeuvre in the struggle to align charity law with contemporary and local manifestations of social need. By creatively interpreting the public benefit principle in accordance with current circumstances and within the parameters of the 'spirit and intendment' rule, the courts have been able to expand the application of charity.[94] In this way it has proved possible to extend charitable status to organizations established for purposes such as the relief of unemployment, the promotion of urban and rural regeneration, rehabilitation and for the benefit of particular localities.

Pemsel and the four 'heads' of charitable purposes; the public benefit constraints

Four centuries of relatively ad hoc decision-making on issues of charitable status resulted in certain anomalies being accommodated within the body of common law precedents. That these now constitute technical constraints on the effective application of charity law is particularly evident in the application of the public benefit test under each of the four heads.

Relief of poverty

Although there is a presumption that the public benefit test is now virtually automatically satisfied in relation to gifts for the relief of poverty, nonetheless practice in this context has led to some curious idiosyncrasies becoming part of charity law.

Poor

The assumption that to be charitable a gift or an organization should, if not dedicated to public utility, be for the benefit of the poor has proved contentious. A great deal of case law has revolved around whether dedication to education, training, religious purposes, etc., is sufficient to acquire charitable status or whether this must be accompanied by a requirement that the end-user also be poor.[95] This fundamental issue, stemming from some uncertainty as to how the opening words of the Preamble should be construed, exercised considerable influence on the development of charity law within the common law tradition (see, further, chapter 5).

Benefit

The fact that not all gifts directed towards poor people necessarily assist in the alleviation of their poverty has often been judicially noted. For example, Harman J in *Baddeley* v. *IRC*[96] commented that a gift to amuse the poor would not relieve them and would therefore not be considered charitable. In *Re Hadji Daeing Tahira binte Daeing Tedelleh's Estate*[97] it was held that the donor's gift, establishing a fund for the purpose of admitting the poor to dog races, would not relieve their poverty and so would not be charitable.

The link between 'impoverished circumstances', the nature of the gift and the capacity of that gift to actually ameliorate the poverty of the defined class of persons in those circumstances can be difficult to determine. In *Re Sanders' Will Trusts*[98] Harman J held that a bequest to provide housing for the 'working classes' and their families resident in a certain district did not qualify as a charitable trust. However, in *Re Niyazi's Will Trusts*,[99] Megarry VC upheld as a valid charitable trust a gift 'for the construction of or as a contribution towards the cost of a working men's hostel' in the town of Famagusta in Cyprus. Peter Gibson J in *Joseph Rowntree Memorial Trust Housing Association Ltd. v. Attorney General*[100] stressed that the need, to be relieved by the charitable gift, must be attributable to the condition of the intended recipient.

The public benefit test

In *Re Scarisbrick* the court held that 'the relief of poverty is of so altruistic a character that the public benefit may necessarily inferred'.[101] In recent years the judiciary have greatly extended their recognition of the range of exceptions to the 'public benefit' principle in the context of gifts for the relief of poverty. Any organization established for the relief of poverty, or indeed for the purpose of advancing either religion or education, is presumed to satisfy the public benefit test; though this presumption is rebuttable.[102] The public benefit test has now lost any intrinsic viability in application to trusts for the relief of poverty.

The recognition of charitable status, given originally by the courts in England to the 'poor relations' class, has since been extended by analogy to such other classes as 'poor employees' and 'poor members'. The precedent value of this jurisprudence has been accepted and followed throughout the common law world, reducing the relevance of the public benefit test considerably. Judicial recognition of a range of exceptions to the public benefit principle has now reached the point where the public benefit test has virtually disappeared in the context of trusts for the relief of poverty. This development results also from a traditional judicial practice that leant towards saving trusts under the heading of poverty where it seemed likely that they would otherwise fail. If a trust was in danger of not satisfying the more stringent public benefit test under the other *Pemsel* headings then, where feasible, it would be saved under the poverty heading. Inevitably this has resulted in an overall more relaxed judicial approach towards public benefit in a poverty context.

Moreover, in England and Wales the judicial test of whether or not a gift confers a benefit[103] is an objective one. In Ireland the subjective view of the donor is decisive, provided that the gift is neither improper nor illegal and is intended to contribute in some manner or degree to relieve or lessen the poverty of the recipient.

The advancement of education

The public benefit test is more difficult to satisfy in application to trusts for the advancement of education than to trusts for the relief of poverty or for the advancement of religion. The difficulties are evident in both the 'public' and the 'benefit' strands of the test.

The 'public' requirement

As in relation to other charitable purposes, the rules for determining when the 'public' component is satisfied, allowing a trust for the advancement of education to be deemed charitable, are neither precise nor readily applied. It is essential that the size of the class can be ascertained. This leads to problems in relation to both minimum and maximum numbers.

Determining the minimum number necessary to meet an acceptable definition of 'public' has proved difficult. In *Re Compton*[104] the Court of Appeal ruled that too few beneficiaries would invalidate a charitable trust when it found that a trust established to provide for the education of the descendants of three named individuals was too restrictive. Determining maximum numbers, fixing the point at which a class will be regarded as closed, has also proved problematic. Normally, the rule is that membership of a class should be treated as having closed at the death of the donor. However, case law reveals a difference in judicial approach depending on whether the gift is expressed in imperative terms (declaring with certainty the class of persons to benefit) or discretionary (conferring on trustees a power to determine extent of the beneficiaries).[105]

The poor relations exception   The difficulties inherent in defining the parameters of 'class' derive also from further judicial development of the 'poor relations' or 'founder's kin' jurisprudence (see, also, chapter 3). Initially, the rationale for denying charitable status to gifts made by a donor for the benefit of relatives was on the grounds that such recipients formed an essentially private and closed group. In the words of Lord Greene MR, 'a gift under which the beneficiaries are defined by reference to a purely personal relationship to a named *propositus*, cannot on principle be a valid charitable gift'.[106] However, his lordship then went on to acknowledge that in certain circumstances the 'founder's kin' class could be eligible for exemption from this principle. He ruled that where a donor made a gift clearly intended for the advancement of education, attaching a stipulation that preference be given to the donor's kin, this would be a valid charitable gift provided the preference was 'merely a method of giving effect to this intention'. So, for example, a gift to a college coupled with a direction that the donor's kin be given preference in availing of the benefit of the gift, constitutes a valid exemption to the traditional ban on charitable status being awarded in respect of gifts to relatives.[107] This class of exemption has since been judicially broadened by the decision in *Re Koettgen's Will Trusts*[108] where charitable status was awarded in respect of a trust established to advance the education of British-born persons subject to a direction that preference be given to employees of a particular company.

The dissemination requirement   The public benefit test is also difficult to satisfy in relation to trusts for the advancement of education because of the significance of 'dissemination' which is an essential and distinguishing characteristic of a charitable trust in this context. In *Re Shaw*,[109] Harman J stressed that 'if the object be merely the increase of knowledge that is not in itself a charitable object unless it be combined with teaching or education'. This view was subsequently endorsed by the Court of Appeal in a ruling which stressed the importance of sharing or publication, rather than the simple accumulation of knowledge.[110]

The 'public schools' controversy   In England the fact that schools such as Eton, established for the children of rich parents, should attract charitable status, has long been a matter of contention. However, it has never been a requirement that educational purposes should be for the benefit of the poor. A private school may permit fees to be paid but the trustees must not make a profit from the enterprise.[111] Within those constraints, it is of no significance that the educational facility restricts access either through levying fees or by offering specialist tuition.

Gifts to schools 'for the sons of gentlemen' have long been recognized as charitable trusts. As was explained by Leach V-C:[112] 'The institution of a school for the sons of gentlemen is not, in proper language, a charity; but in the view of the Statute of Elizabeth, all schools of learning are to be considered.' While the law accepts the charitable nature of gifts to prestigious schools catering largely for fee-paying privileged minorities, it must be acknowledged that the general public has a difficulty in sharing that view. Any application of the public benefit test which can result in affirming the charitable nature of elite institutions does give rise to scepticism and serves to emphasize a difference in perception between judiciary and the general public in what constitutes a charity. Gifts to such schools for the purpose of providing for organized games have also been assured a sympathetic judicial hearing.[113]

The 'benefit' requirement

The authorities are clear that to be charitable a trust for the advancement of education must have a purpose which meets criteria of 'usefulness'. The courts in the United Kingdom have had little difficulty in ruling that some donor intentions do not comply with usefulness criteria. For example, the compilation of lists of Derby winners[114] and the public exhibition of junk[115] have failed this test.

The advancement of religion

A religious charity must not only be so constituted as to satisfy the legal definition of religion, including having objects or purposes of a religious nature, but its activities must also advance religion. The courts will require evidence that a gift to a religious organization satisfies the public benefit test.[116] That it will not do so when given to a closed contemplative order was demonstrated by the ruling of MacDermott LCJ in *Trustees of the Congregation of Poor Clares* v. *Commissioner of Valuation*,[117] where charitable status was denied. The requisite evidence may, for example, take the form of proof that masses will take place in public. The decision in *Gilmour* v. *Coats*[118] quite decisively established that in the UK acts of worship by private contemplative orders confer no public benefit; it is necessary to prove tangible and direct public benefit. In Ireland, the judiciary take the opposite view (see, further, chapter 9).

Beneficial to the community, not falling under any of the preceding heads

Trusts for 'other purposes beneficial to the community' form the category of charitable gifts to be found under the fourth of the *Pemsel* headings. It has been held that it may seem anomalous to speak in terms of a public benefit in relation to this category as it is defined in terms of trusts for the benefit of the community.[119] Nevertheless, it is to this category that the public benefit test has been applied with most rigour.[120]

'Public'

As with all charitable trusts it is vital that a gift for other charitable purposes is potentially available to a significant number of beneficiaries, who are not linked in a private relationship nexus with the donor, if it is to be upheld as a charity.[121] This was emphasized by the House of Lords in *I.R.C.* v. *Baddeley*,[122] where it was held that 'if a charity falls within the fourth class, it must be for the benefit of the whole community or at least of all the inhabitants of a sufficient area'.[123]

'Benefit'

While the 'benefit' quotient necessary to meet charitable status requirements is different under each of the four *Pemsel* heads it is most difficult to satisfy in the residual category 'other charitable purposes'. As has been explained:[124]

> The essence of the charitable nature [of trusts within Lord Macnaghten's fourth category] is that the beneficiaries should not be a private class, nor should any limitations be placed upon the gift which would prevent the public as a whole from enjoying the advantage which the donor intends to provide for the benefit of all the public. It would be quite consonant with this concept that it should be more difficult for a trust under the fourth head to satisfy the requirements of public benefit, and that a bridge to be used only by Methodists should fail to qualify where a gift for the education of the children of members of that church might be a valid charity.

Trusts for promoting recreational facilities   In England and Wales the Recreational Charities Act 1958 was introduced to establish that it is charitable 'to provide or assist in the provision of facilities for recreation or other leisure time occupation if the facilities are provided in the interest of social welfare',[125] and this legislation was then replicated in Australia. While recreation in itself is not charitable,[126] it will acquire that status if its provision is ancillary to a recognized charitable purpose, is for the benefit of a locality or is open-air public recreation.

There is no equivalent to this legislation in the Republic of Ireland. Instead, where a gift is for the purpose of providing social or recreational facilities, charitable status will normally be withheld. Only if the intended beneficiaries are the elderly, youth, handicapped and disadvantaged, or where the gift fails to be determined under one of the other *Pemsel* headings, will it qualify as charitable. In Ireland, whether the recreational facility is provided indoors or outdoors is of no relevance to the issue of charitable status.[127] In Northern Ireland, however, the position is different. As MacDermott LCJ declared in *Commissioner of Valuation* v. *Lurgan Borough Council*,[128] 'the law does not regard the mere provision of recreational facilities charitable unless they are provided in the open air on land dedicated to the use and enjoyment of the public'. Moreover in Ireland, unlike the UK, a subjective judicial approach will be employed to ascertain the donor's intention.[129]

Gifts for the benefit of animals   A gift for the benefit of a particular type of animal or for animals will generally be charitable. In Ireland, the subjective approach to the public benefit test has been evident in decisions grounded on a belief that the donor's intention to safeguard the welfare of animals was sufficient in itself to attract charitable status under this heading.[130] This interpretation has tended to be viewed as insufficient in the courts of England and Wales.[131] For example, in *Re Grove Grady*,[132] Russell L.J. expressed the opinion that the charitable status of gifts to animals depended upon whether or not they were of benefit to mankind; broadly speaking, domesticated or farm animals would satisfy this test but wild animals would not.

Trusts for the promotion of health   In the UK the public benefit test is applied most rigorously in relation to trusts for the promotion of health.[133] Until the ruling in *Re Worth*,[134] the same could have been said of the judicial approach in Ireland. Keane J then formed the view that a gift, having the effect of providing 'a haven of quiet intellectual relaxation' for certain staff, thereby benefited a hospital and consequently met the definition of a charity. This interpretation significantly broadens the grounds in a way unlikely to be followed outside Ireland.

The public benefit test and the European Convention

The fact that charitable status under the fourth *Pemsel* head, unlike the other three, is conditional upon this test being satisfied may not be wholly compliant with the non-discrimination principle of the ECHR.

Common law constraints on charities; implications for addressing contemporary social inclusion issues and forestalling alienation

The complex nature of much contemporary social need can no longer be adequately addressed through a law that in the main is constructed from – and still requires to be applied with regard to – case law principles and precedents that relate to an earlier and wholly different social context. This is particularly true in relation to the extreme and embedded nature of social disadvantage suffered by indigenous people. In many modern western societies the reasons for the current failure of charity law to address contemporary social inclusion issues can be traced directly or indirectly to the legacy of the common law.

Outside the spirit and intendment of the Statute of Elizabeth

The 'spirit and intendment' rule has been a crucial to the development of the public benefit test for charitable activity (see, further, chapter 4). Those organizations with purposes that did not fit within the *Pemsel* classification, or were not analogous to those listed there, could only acquire charitable status on the grounds that their purposes could instead be construed as coming broadly within the legislative intent of the Preamble to the 1601 Act. Four hundred years later it can require some ingenuity, and more importantly a willingness, to interpret the public benefit of a modern activity (such as Internet access) to correspond with a Preamble activity (such as repair of highways) and so qualify for charitable status.[135]

In England and Wales the ingenuity and willingness to provide a modern interpretation of activities constituting public benefit is provided by the rulings of the Charity Commissioners. This agency acts as a foil for the more defensive approach of the Inland Revenue, the primary concern of which is to maximize tax revenues by minimizing opportunities for organizations to evade tax liability through claiming charitable status. The Inland Revenue approach is typical of that adopted by equivalent agencies in other common law nations, notably by the ATO (Australian Tax Office) in Australia (see, further, chapter 10), where it is not counterbalanced by any equivalent to the Commission.

A particular achievement of the Commission has been its ability to gradually broaden the interpretation of public benefit within the confines of the spirit and intendment rule. Unlike other common law jurisdictions, including both on the island of Ireland, the non-legislative development of charity law in England and Wales has in recent years been a consequence of a deliberate strategy to constructively stretch the boundaries of this traditional rule. As it has forthrightly declared:[136]

> The Commission will take a constructive approach in adapting the concept of charity to meet constantly evolving social needs . . . In considering new purposes as charitable we will look closely at those purposes which have

already been recognised as charitable either under the Preamble or in subsequent decisions of the court or the Commission . . . While in most cases a sufficiently close analogy may be found, in others an analogy may be found by following the broad principles which may be derived from the scope of the Preamble or from decided cases of the court or the Commission.

In pursuing its intention to further develop the spirit and intendment rule the Commission has increased the capacity of charity law to address contemporary social inclusion issues (see, further, chapters 5 and 8).

The absence of a forum for adjusting the law

The common law has always been wholly dependent upon a continuous case flow to permit judicial review of principles in the light of practice. The fact that in most common law nations no mechanism exists to permit an ongoing review and adjustment of the law to ensure an appropriate fit with new or embedded forms of social disadvantage, amounts to a structural flaw in their charity law frameworks. In countries such as Ireland and Australia, a judicial review of principles and precedents occurs so seldom and randomly as to provide little capacity for effectively addressing changes in social need or, as in Canada, the court may simply decline to respond when the opportunity arises.[137] When they do occur then, as in Ireland, they are very likely to concern a relatively peripheral aspect of charity law; in that jurisdiction the case law for generations has been mostly to do with rates related issues. This is partially because the traditional role of the judiciary has been displaced by a variety of administrative bodies each concerned with their own necessarily narrow terms of reference. These bodies filter out issues amenable to administrative decision-making thereby depriving the courts of the opportunity to consider their more strategic significance. It is also a natural consequence of the division of powers between courts and parliament, indeed

> it would run counter to the strongest traditions of our judiciary for the courts to consciously assume the responsibility of charting the areas of social need into which private benefaction might usefully be channeled and thus, to act as arbiters of social policy at any given time.[138]

In England and Wales, however, the rulings of the Charity Commission to a large extent provide not only a substitute for the judicial role but also permit an ongoing review of the law in relation to emerging practice requirements. By referring issues of principle and policy to court or government respectively, it also serves as a proactive channel for furthering the development of the law.

Reliance upon outmoded legal structures

Emerging from the law of equity, the trust became the legal vehicle for carrying a donor's gift and giving effect to their charitable intentions in the common law of

England and Wales. This transferred to the common law nations, although not to the same extent, and continued to provide the mainstay of the law and practice of charity until well into the latter half of the twentieth century.

Corporate structures

The mid-nineteenth-century introduction of companies limited by guarantee acted as a significant catalyst for generating growth in trade and manufacturing in England and Wales. This development extended to the incorporation of some charities but insufficiently to affect the world of charity as it did the world of commerce. By the twentieth century other common law nations, particularly the US, had adopted the corporate structure to a much larger extent than in England and Wales. In the US, the corporate form triggered the rise of large endowed foundations, many of which came into being in the first half of the twentieth century as part of the social reconstruction in the immediate aftermath of the Second World War. A similar surge of interest occurred in England and Wales towards the end of the twentieth century but failed to translate into as significant a commitment to incorporation and the trust continues to provide the main legal structure for charities. Experimentation with corporate structures for charities is only now acquiring some respectability and momentum in England and Wales (see, further, chapters 2 and 8).

Causes rather than effects of poverty

Poverty, admittedly a relative concept in any western society, continues to resist government assurances that the rising tide of affluence will lift all boats. Social deprivation maintains a persistent presence even in the most affluent of contemporary western societies, most often affecting the groups that appear on the domestic social inclusion agenda and falling particularly heavily on the minority, culture-specific communities within such societies. It may be that the concept will have to be legally redefined in order to facilitate new methods of philanthropic intervention designed to deal with its structural causes.

Established case law confirms that it is the effects rather than the causes of poverty which must be the focus of a charity's purpose and activity. The reasons for this are associated with the status of the poor within common law society.

A hierarchically structured society

The common law is primarily a creature of English society. Its origins, and its evolution over several centuries, occurred within what was a very hierarchically structured social order. From feudal times until at least the end of the Victorian era and the hesitant rise of the meritocracy, this was a society firmly divided according to class. The common law was administered within and served to reinforce this context. Avoidance of revolution, such as had disrupted mainland Europe, required the law to maintain respect for the established social order. The poor had to accept their place and in return they would receive alms from the rich, from philanthropists and indeed from the State in terms of workhouse provision. Alleviating the effects of poverty was philanthropic but to question its cause was sedition.

The benefactor/supplicant relationship

The persistence of attitudes formerly associated with this traditional relationship (see, also, chapter 1) threatens to foreclose any possibility of a more functional and strategic approach, developed in partnership with those in need, intended to tackle structural and embedded causes of social deprivation. Knight, for example, has protested that: 'Charity is a medieval concept that has no place in the modern world. It can reinforce the boundaries between "haves" and "have-nots" finding itself on the cusp between greed and guilt.'[139]

Alms

Charity is irredeemably associated with 'handouts'. Gifts, gratuitously bestowed to provide relief from immediate need, have long been accepted as a sufficient definition of charitable action; though this is now open to challenge on the grounds that it perpetuates dependency (see, further, chapter 1). Providing food, shelter and comfort (but not too much) to 'the deserving poor' (applied with some equivocation to persons such as prostitutes, child criminals, etc.) ensured charitable status for the donor. Only in very recent years has the law been able to accommodate other approaches such as projects for overcoming unemployment or stimulating rural regeneration within the definition of charitable activity.

Training

While the advancement of education is a charitable purpose not all training schemes will necessarily fit under this umbrella. There are various legal pitfalls to be overcome if a scheme is to satisfy the 'public benefit' test.

Public access

The training must allow for sufficient public access: the more tightly drawn the criteria for accessing the training, the greater the probability that the scheme will be insufficiently 'public' to qualify for charitable status. Limitations that restrict access to those of a certain age, to family, relatives or a particular locality will probably prevent the training scheme from being charitable.

Benefit

Not all training schemes will in law meet the 'benefit' test: the benefit quotient involved may be construed as bearing relatively little relationship to poverty. For example, funding the education of and assisting a person to be established in self-employment in a profession does not constitute the relief of poverty.

Profit

A training scheme must be wary of falling foul of the rule regarding profits (see p. 147). Many commercial and professional bodies establish training schemes as entry routes to their organizations. Regardless of how wide the public access or how modest the benefit to the participants, however, such schemes will be denied charitable status if it can be shown that they would also benefit the providers.

Pure research

Again, while the advancement of education is a charitable purpose, an organization that restricts itself to conducting pure research in relation to a subject will be denied charitable status. Activities must do more than simply increase the quantum of knowledge; they must also disseminate it through teaching. Researching the nature and extent of the disadvantage suffered by a group, profiling the causes and gathering the data necessary to identify the resources required to remedy the situation, will not be sufficient for an organization to gain charitable status.

Advocacy/political lobbying

The restraints within charity law on the advocacy activities of disadvantaged groups is a particular obstacle for the organizers of such groups, who are often impelled to draw public attention to their grievances as a method of leveraging change.

Political lobbying

An organization, the main purposes of which are stated to be the pursuit of political lobbying and promotional activities, will be denied charitable status.[140] These activities are allowed, even encouraged in some jurisdictions, when they are 'merely incidental' to a purpose that is otherwise charitable. To establish an organization for the purpose of assertively campaigning on behalf of the needs of a minority group would, however, be to forego charitable status.

Advocating change in law or government policy

An organization set up to challenge government policy or to campaign for change in the law is not a charity.[141] The fact that by pursuing such purposes an organization intends to improve the social circumstances of a disadvantaged group will not prevent it from being denied charitable status in law.

The promotion of justice

As Slade J said in *Mc Govern* v. *Attorney General*, 'the elimination of injustice has not as such ever been held to be a trust purpose which qualifies for the privileges afforded to charities by English law'.[142]

Community development

In theory an organization established for the benefit of a community, a part of a community or a particular locality should have little difficulty in acquiring charitable status. In practice, however, the application of this principle to community development projects has not proved to be so straightforward; although in recent years the Charity Commission has taken steps in this area (see, further, chapter 8).

Self-help groups

Many community-based projects are initiated by small groups whose members share the same vision and organize the necessary resources to engage in an activity or create a facility for their collective benefit. Subject to the 'poor relations' exception (see chapter 3), such groups will not qualify for charitable status, even if some external access is allowed, because they are limited by the nexus of common employment and the necessary 'public' element cannot therefore be met and the activity or facility will be construed as being essentially for member benefit[143] or as being too vague or imprecise.[144]

Cultural affirmation

Where a group belonging to a minority culture sets up an organization to preserve and promote its cultural heritage it will probably not qualify for charitable status because in law such activities may be regarded as essentially social and therefore of insufficient 'benefit' to the community.[145] Such initiatives may also fall foul of the rule that purposes must not be vague or ambiguous.

Businesses

Community development schemes very often have a business component, as disadvantaged communities usually place a priority on projects that may serve to bring in capital and help lift its members out of poverty. Such schemes may not be overtly run for profit but they may have a commercial dimension, involve a private financial contribution and/or generate a surplus. They are often set up solely for the purpose of training the unemployed in skills appropriate to the needs of local industries. This can involve buying land to let to small businesses, advising small businesses and providing paid consultancy services. As in *Inland Revenue Commissioners* v. *Oldham Training and Enterprise Council*[146] such activities will constitute a commercial undertaking with private benefit and will be denied charitable exemption from rates. This is a particular area of vulnerability for organizations engaged in schemes to reduce pockets of unemployment. Not only is there a danger of breaching the public benefit test by focusing on a closely defined number of people and thus being more 'private' than 'public', but also such schemes tend to involve investments, small businesses and a degree of individual gain. Such activities can be fatal to charitable status.

Conclusion

The role of philanthropy is governed by law, specifically by charity law, but this no longer provides an appropriate or sufficient means for channelling philanthropic resources in a way that effectively addresses issues of social inclusion and forestalls alienation. The reasons for this are largely to be found in certain aspects of the common law heritage that continues to underpin much of charity law in many modern western societies. The chronically disadvantaged circumstances of some minority culture groups such as the Indigenous people of Australia, who remain impervious to generations of philanthropic intervention, graphically illustrate the consequences of a misfit between law and social need. The same issues are in play in respect of such socially marginalized groups as the mentally ill, the disabled, disaffected youth, etc. in all modern western nations. The extent to which responsibility for addressing these issues falls to government in the form of public service provision and the degree to which this may be supplemented by the contribution of charities will be explored in the following chapter.

Chapter 5

The 'public benefit' test and social inclusion

The roles of government and charity in a common law context

Introduction

'Public benefit' is the hallmark of a charity within a common law context. In practice, however, applying the 'public benefit test' has never been sufficient to clearly distinguish the activities of charities from those of other non-government organizations or from government bodies. The business of providing services for the benefit of the public has traditionally been shared, pretty much on an ad hoc basis, between government and charity, although the common law has placed constraints on the latter. This has implications for how common law nations now respond to the social inclusion agenda.

This chapter begins by examining the common law origins of the public benefit test in the Preamble, its enduring but equivocal association with poverty and public utility and its resulting usefulness as a means of differentiating between the roles of charity and government. It does so from the perspective of developments in the UK, or, more accurately, as these have unfolded in England and Wales. The chapter then considers the record of charities and government as service providers in relation to the socially disadvantaged, analysing the impact of the Welfare State and the consequent adjustment to their respective roles. It outlines the emergence of the modern relationship between government, charities and the public benefit, noting the importance of the 'contract culture' phenomenon. The chapter concludes by considering a crucial component for the future development of this relationship: the role of the Charity Commissioners as determinant of partnership arrangements in practice between government and charity in public service provision.

The common law, poverty and public utility

The public/private distinction, as represented by the roles of government and charity in relation to the provision of public utility facilities, is uncertain. The reasons for this are deeply rooted in the common law and may be traced back to the Preamble.[1] There, charitable purposes are simply listed as being either for the poor or for public works. The subsequent classification by Macnaghten in *Pemsel*[2] failed to demarcate between public responsibilities and private benevolence in respect of these charitable purposes (see, further, chapter 3). The 'spirit and intendment' rule[3] (see, also, chapter 3) has further complicated matters by licensing a proliferation of analogous charitable activity in relation to the provision of public utilities. Clarifying the basis of the distinction is crucial to the formulation of successful social inclusion policies.

The Preamble and poverty

In its opening line the Preamble recognizes the 'releife of aged impotent and poore people' as a charitable purpose. In fact trusts established to provide succour for the poor or to relieve the destitute of a parish had been acknowledged even earlier as charitable in English law. The form of recognition provided by the Preamble, however, brought with it the seeds of controversy that grew to become fundamental issues in the interpretation of charity as understood in a common law context.

Charity and the causes of poverty

The roots of charity are to be found in addressing the effects of poverty by providing alms, shelter for the homeless, food for the hungry and care for the sick. There is no suggestion in the Preamble, in the activities of charities before the early nineteenth century, in the Poor Law legislation or in case law that purposes directed towards removing the causes of poverty would be recognized as charitable. The formative centuries for charity law in England occurred within the grip of a feudal or rigidly class-structured society and a Christian value system that combined to instil an acceptance of conditions as they were. This was coupled with an expectation that 'the deserving poor' would receive assistance from private charitable sources (individuals and organizations, usually the Church) and from the public purse. Administration of parish relief and workhouse provision was very localized, reflecting the fact that while communities were willing to assist those known to be 'deserving' they would not pay for 'idle or badly behaved people or for outsiders'.[4] Only comparatively recently has our understanding of poverty developed to accommodate a focus on its causes, its relativity and the needs of 'outsiders' in addition to the traditional focus on its effects.

Charity, the poor and the Preamble

Charity has its roots in providing relief for the poor but is 'relief' only charitable if the recipient is poor?

The problem stems partly from the wording of the Preamble. One interpretation is that the use of 'and' requires the above opening line to be read 'conjunctively', i.e. the 'aged' and/or 'impotent' must also be 'poor'. 'Impotent'[5] in this context indicates a form of disability has come to encompass an indefinite range of separate and distinct areas of need not necessarily associated with poverty.[6] An alternative or 'disjunctive' approach maintains that the wording can only be sensibly interpreted by construing the categories as quite separate, i.e. the 'aged' or 'impotent' do not also have to be 'poor'. In *Re Glyn*,[7] for example, which concerned a gift of cottages to 'old working women', the court was able to imply poverty into the gift, but nevertheless took the disjunctive approach. In *Re Robinson*[8] the gift was to people of pensionable age living in a certain area. Vaisey J stated that 'the gift is to the old people . . . as a group of people who are within the Statute of Elizabeth, qualified not by poverty, sickness or impotence, but by age'.[9] In *Re Lewis*[10] a gift to ten blind boys and ten blind girls, without any accompanying condition of poverty, was considered charitable. By 1983, it was judicially accepted that 'the words "aged, impotent and poor" must be read disjunctively'.[11] In *Joseph Rowntree*,[12] Gibson J held that 'it would be as absurd to require that the aged must be impotent or poor as to require the impotent to be aged or poor, or the poor to be aged or impotent'. In Ireland this problem never arose because the equivalent wording of the Statute of Pious Uses 1634[13] was clearly disjunctive (see, further, chapter 9).

Relief

While it is true that the 'aged' need not also be 'poor' it is certain that the gift must actually address and ameliorate their needs as aged people if it is to be charitable. Similarly so with gifts to persons whose circumstances otherwise bring them within the umbrella definition of 'impotent' by being, for example, blind, alcoholic, drug abusers, etc. As has been said, 'there must be a need to be relieved by the charitable gift, such need being attributable to the age or impotent condition of the person to be benefited'.[14]

Charity, the poor and Pemsel

The conjunctive/disjunctive issue was compounded by Macnaghten's treatment of poverty in the *Pemsel* case. His fourfold classification did not require a poverty component in charitable trusts for the advancement of education or religion nor in respect of trusts in the fourth category for public utility purposes. As Lord Wrenbury later observed:[15]

> His [Lord Macnaghten's] fourth head does not contain the word 'poor'. He does not say 'beneficial to the poorer members of the community'; he says, 'beneficial to the community'. Did he mean his words to be confined to the poor? Education and religion, two of the heads which he had just mentioned, do not require any qualification of poverty to be introduced to give them validity. If he was going by general words to add a fourth class in which poverty must be an ingredient, he would surely have said so.

From its earliest beginnings, then, charity in a common law context was not necessarily concerned with the poor and, when it was, it focused on the effects rather than the causes of their poverty. This equivocal relationship between charity and poverty was responsible for considerable subsequent uncertainty in the law until all that could be said with any confidence was that a gift exclusively to the rich would not be charitable.[16]

As the law in the UK now stands, poverty is not a necessary condition for a purpose to be deemed charitable. In fact a gift benefiting the rich may nonetheless be charitable, although the advantage conferred must benefit them incider ally.[17] Public schools and private hospitals, for example, qualify for charitable sta us as do concert halls, art galleries and opera houses; all of which cater prin arily for those with the high income necessary to access such facilities. In Aust ralia, however, the concept 'public benevolent institution' which was introduced into charity/tax law in 1928, has developed to require evidence that an organization is engaged in the direct relief of poverty or some other form of need if it is to attract tax exemption (see, further, chapter 10).

The Preamble and public utility

References in the Preamble to such forms of civic provision as the 'Repaire of Bridges Portes Havens Causwaies Churches Seabankes and Highwaibuilding' clearly indicate that public utility was then recognized as worthy of charitable status. Such a range of municipal utilities would today be regarded as core public services and thus more properly the responsibility of government than charity. The fact that these activities carry an entitlement to charitable status has built into charity law an assumption that government and charity are jointly and similarly engaged in public benefit work. Then as now this is undoubtedly the case if only because charitable provision of public utilities enables government to divert equivalent tax revenues into other public services. Again, the reference in the Preamble to 'paymente of Fifteenes . . . and other Taxes' implies that a gift that contributes to the provision of a public amenity will be charitable simply because, if nothing else, the gift relieves the general public of the liability to pay for that amenity through taxes and rates.

This blurring of the distinction between private gifts and public responsibilities is of fundamental importance and is at the conceptual heart of many of our problems in modernizing charity law.

Charity and public utility

In *Morice* v. *Bishop of Durham*[18] charitable purposes that did not relieve poverty, nor advance religion or education were classified under the fourth head of *Pemsel* as 'objects of general public utility'. In *Incorporated Council for Law Reporting for England and Wales* v. *Attorney General*[19] it was accepted that 'if a purpose is shown to be beneficial or of such utility it is prima facie charitable in law'.

Range of public utility [20]

The type of activity and facility of a public utility nature found to be charitable under the fourth head includes, for example, trusts for recreation, the improvement of cities, the protection of animals and the benefit of a locality. While most of these have no particular significance for social inclusion they indicate the extent of an overlap between public services and private philanthropy.

In *Commissioners of Inland Revenue* v. *Yorkshire Agricultural Society* [21] the advancement of agriculture was found to be charitable while in *Crystal Palace* v. *Minister of Town Planning* [22] so also was the promotion of industry, commerce and art. The fact that charity could include commerce was demonstrated by the enthusiasm with which it was extolled in the founding charter of the Philanthropic Society established in 1788 to 'unite the spirit of society with the principles of trade, and to erect a temple to philanthropy on the foundations of virtuous industry'. [23]

By analogy with references in the Preamble to the maintenance of 'maimed soldiers' and the 'setting out of soldiers', gifts for the defence of the realm have since been held to be charitable. [24] As Lord Normand explained in *Inland Revenue Commissioners* v. *City of Glasgow Police Athletic Association*: [25] 'gifts exclusively for the purpose of promoting the efficiency of the armed forces are good charitable gifts'. [26] In *Re Corbyn* [27] a trust for the Mercantile Marine was held charitable, since a merchant navy was essential to a realm unable to produce enough food and the essentials of life. Gifts promoting the efficiency of the police, encouraging their recruitment and preserving public order have all been held charitable. In *Inland Revenue Commissioners* v. *City of Glasgow Police Athletic Association*, [28] for example, the Glasgow police association applied for exemption from income tax for their annual sports meeting. The House of Lords held that 'gifts or contributions exclusively for the purpose of promoting the efficiency of the police forces and the preservation of public order are by analogy charitable gifts'. [29]

Public utility, impotence, and social inclusion; helplessness

The reference to 'impotent' in 'Releife of aged impotent and poore people', the opening line of the Preamble, has long been judicially accepted as an umbrella definition of eligibility for charitable status in the context of health and welfare. It is a term that has to some extent retained its original meaning of helplessness, complete incapacity and total lack of any power or influence with, perhaps, accompanying connotations of awareness and frustration.

The category of impotent has been extended by case law under the fourth head of *Pemsel* and by the 'spirit and intendment' rule to include not only persons suffering from a wide range of different illnesses, disability and impairment, but also the related types of specialized facilities, hospitals, housing and other forms of public service provision. Extension by analogy has largely been confined to recognizing as charitable, gifts to assist those suffering from such modern permutations of incapacity as drug addiction and the provision of such facilities as rehabilitation centres. That is, the range has been enlarged but essentially the category of 'impotent' has continued to be for the most part diagnostically defined and characterized by an incapacitating debility. Judicial creativity in this area, however, provides evidence of potential to address a contemporary social inclusion agenda.

In the Irish case of *Mahony v. Duggan*,[30] for example, the philanthropic intervention was on behalf of prostitutes, a distinctly socially marginalized group. The case concerned a bequest 'for the purpose of reclaiming fallen women in the city of Cork'. As the Master of the Rolls did not attempt to place this purpose within any particular head it must be assumed he had public utility in mind when he explained, in language now viewed as perhaps not wholly politically correct, that 'there may be as high, but there cannot be higher, purposes of charity than the reclamation of fallen women'.[31] In *Re Cohen*[32] the bequest was for deserving Jewish girls on their marriage. Petersen J held that 'deserving' did not mean 'poor', but nevertheless as 'it tended to encourage marriage among Jews, and it was for the benefit of the Jewish religion', it was a valid charitable bequest.[33] Indeed, both are perhaps derived from the Preamble reference to 'Mariages of poore Maides', a provision which seems to recognize a vulnerable social group or 'good cause' and where the intent is to facilitate appropriate social inclusion.

Public utility, impotence, and social inclusion; alienation

As might be expected, the common law has not shown a similar willingness to accommodate as charitable gifts on behalf of those 'impotent' who are not helpless and whose plight does not mostly invoke sentiments of compassion. The doors of charity would seem to be closed in situations where the social circumstances of possible beneficiaries are such as to raise issues of social policy or could imply a political motive on the part of the donor. While admittedly speculative, the absence of any relevant case law would support such an interpretation.

For example, reference in the Preamble to 'repaire of bridges ... and highwaies' has by analogy been extended to include civic institutions such as courthouses[34] and such ancillary services as court reports[35] for assisting the administration of justice and even to family conciliation services.[36] This thread of logic, embracing civic infrastructure designed to reinforce social cohesion, could conceivably have been extended to include other forms of philanthropic mediation and community development initiatives that would similarly serve to generate social capital and promote civil society. But the evidence is to the contrary: purposes such as the promotion of justice or the promotion of peace and reconciliation were repeatedly refused charitable status.

Again, the reference to the 'repaire ... of seabankes' in the Preamble, by allowing subsequent gifts for the protection of human life and property to be charitable by analogy, has implications for social inclusion. The circumstances of the socially marginalized, in all respects impotent within the context of civil society, pose a challenge to the values of the latter which in time may grow to have a destabilizing effect upon it. Arguably, gifts to facilitate philanthropic intervention on behalf of the socially marginalized to forestall their alienation and possible drift into violence would be sufficiently analogous to the repair of sea-banks to warrant recognition as a charitable purpose. Whether the potential threat to mainstream society arises in the form of anti-social behaviour from groups such as disaffected youth or from the civil unrest generated by an alienated minority culture group such as Catholic nationalists in Northern Ireland[37] or the Tamils in Sri Lanka, in theory charitable status could be extended by analogy to gifts, activities and organizations the purpose of which is intended to facilitate mediation, address grievances, forestall alienation and possible violence and promote inclusion. However, the common law views the circumstances of such groups as being the business of government rather than charity and attempts at philanthropic intervention by the latter as unwarranted interference in the policies of the former.

Public utility, impotence, and social inclusion; overseas aid

The fact that a charity registered with the Commission operates wholly outside the jurisdiction is no obstacle to its recognition as a UK charity unless its activities are contrary to public policy.[38] A number of organizations committed to providing disaster relief, development aid or relief from poverty are so registered. In that respect their purposes are often similar or identical to particular government bodies.

Social inclusion and prevention of 'impotence'

Charitable intervention on behalf of the 'impotent', as defined in case law and as may be included by analogy, has not been limited to treating the effects of their impotence. In contrast to its treatment of gifts in respect of poverty, charity law has an established track record of approving those intended to address the causes of 'impotence'. So, in England and Wales, the court in *Re Hood*[39] approved as charitable a gift to prevent alcoholism by promoting temperance through the preparation and distribution of educational leaflets and a similar approach has been taken in Ireland.[40] However, in keeping with the general rule against political purposes, any gift intended to support advocacy or a lobbying campaign to change the law relating to impotence (e.g. imposing prohibition or legalizing the use of cannabis) is not charitable. This contrasts with the law in the US and Canada where political lobbying for such a purpose has been recognized as charitable.[41]

Charities, the State, service provision and social inclusion: a brief historical background

The role of charities has traditionally been associated most strongly with activities that addressed the effects of poverty including the provision of such public utilities as hospitals and homes for the aged, disabled or destitute. To that extent, the history of philanthropy within a common law context records that the social inclusion agenda has long been more the business of charity than government.

The traditional role of charities; primary social services provider

In the UK, from at least the time of the Reformation until local authorities were established in 1929, the responsibility for meeting the needs of the poor, the ill and disabled and those otherwise disadvantaged fell mainly to charities – a responsibility gradually and increasingly shared with the State under the Poor Laws. The present social and health care infrastructure, particularly hospital provision, owes a great deal to the earlier contribution of the Church, the philanthropic endeavours of individuals and to religious groups such as the Quakers. Together they provided a charitable foundation for the modern State system of health, education and welfare services.

Health care

In mediaeval England a parish-based system of residential provision for the ill, wounded soldiers and those otherwise destitute was most usually maintained by the Church as distributor of alms and pastoral care. At that time 'hospitals' were more a form of hostel in which some in need of food and shelter, including those requiring medical treatment, could take refuge. In London and other urban centres these facilities might be provided by the State from tax revenues but most often they were built and staffed by religious organizations as the latter had the wealth, the geographic spread and perhaps most importantly the capacity to organize their members.

Subsequently, provision was extended to include more specialized health care facilities such as asylums, homes for the poor, the elderly and orphans. Gifts for the 'sick and wounded',[42] for a home of rest for persons in a condition of strain,[43] and for the maintenance of aged persons in a nursing home have all since been held to be charitable. The range of providers of charitable relief also broadened as individual philanthropists and charitable societies emerged to initiate intervention on behalf of abandoned children and others in need.[44] One such was Thomas Coram who in 1739 established a hospital for foundling children. This example of a philanthropic initiative to address a significant aspect of social inclusion in the early eighteenth century survived into modern times. By the end of the nineteenth century a number of organizations such as Dr Barnardo's[45] and the National Society for the Prevention of Cruelty to Children[46] had begun their current child care services by rescuing children who were orphaned, abandoned or abused.

Education

The history of the development of education in England is one in which the separate provision made by Church and the wealthy initially prevailed at the expense of a State system. Public secular education for young children in England was not universally available until the latter half of the nineteenth century. Private education had been available to those who could afford it at least a century earlier and the Church maintained a patchwork of schools for poor children.

For most of the nineteenth century, the State contribution took the form of grants aiding the education provided by Church-based and nonconformist schools. The 'public school' system, educating the children of a wealthy elite, was established during this period and consolidated in the early decades of the twentieth century. Until the latter half of the nineteenth century, such schooling as existed for all others was provided by the Church and other charitable organizations. The education and preferment of orphans, being within the terms of the Statute of Elizabeth, allowed the care of orphans in Ireland[47] and children's homes in England[48] to be charitable. In 1856 a Department of Education was established and the Education Act 1870 finally laid the foundations for a system of mandatory primary education which was to be secular and freely available to poor children.

The emergence of new forms and functions for charities

Eighteenth-century England saw trade and commerce flourishing and an empire expanding, bringing prosperity and a degree of enlightened social awareness. However, as has been said:[49]

> Essentially, the institutions of early eighteenth-century charity were still those first set in place after the sixteenth-century Reformation. The structures established then and the functions they performed were based on locality; and inherited from the medieval parish system.

By the end of the nineteenth century, as with so many other social institutions, the role of charities in a newly industrialized and urbanized England had changed quite radically.

Charitable associations

The traditional legal vehicle for giving effect to a charitable gift, usually in the form of a bequest, was the charitable trust, which required a named trustee or trustees to carry out the instructions of the donor, honour the terms of the trust and do so without taking any personal advantage from their appointment. Although to be charitable a trust had to have a public benefit dimension, the process of appointing a trustee made its implementation mainly a matter of private law.

The eighteenth century saw the emergence of innovative legal structures for organizing collective enterprises which were to provide a new basis for philanthropy. The introduction of joint stock companies for furthering commerce offered a model for channelling philanthropic effort. Entrepreneurial philanthropists, such as Thomas Coram in 1739 and the founders of the Philanthropic Society in 1788, established charitable associations that adopted the form, the management systems and the funding mechanisms of the new trading companies. Charitable associations,[50] like joint stock companies, were collective social entities that relied upon public subscription, required professional systems of governance and whose functions were similarly subject to public law.

Advocacy

Charities did not necessarily confine their activities to poverty relief and the provision of public utilities. It is unlikely that there was any government pressure on them to do so. In the Victorian era, many important initiatives resulting in policy changes by government were led by charities. The protests against the conditions suffered by children employed in factories or as chimney sweeps etc were led by charities such as Dr Barnardo's and the NSPCC. The Infant Life Protection Society, founded in 1870, provided such support as was then available for the protection of newly born babies in workhouses and campaigned for the introduction of the Infant Life Protection Act 1872. The Charity Organization Society, established in 1869, was a good example of reflective philanthropy at work, mixing provision for the poor with a sociological analysis of the causes of poverty.

Then as now it was not necessary to be poor to be socially disadvantaged and this was reflected in the activities of charities. They were to the fore in the rallies against the slave trade, the lobbying to halt the practice of 'baby-farming' and in support of the suffragette movement.

Overseas aid

In the late nineteenth and early twentieth centuries UK-based religious organizations established their practice of distributing charitable aid alongside the dissemination of Christianity in the underdeveloped countries of Africa and elsewhere. It was a requirement of charitable status that such missionary bodies should have the advancement of religion as their primary purpose.[51]

Leaders of voluntary action

By the end of the nineteenth century charities were the primary providers of health, social care and education services for the socially disadvantaged. The State provided facilities such as workhouses in the towns and funds and officials to manage care facilities such as hospitals. However, the role of charities was diminishing. Partly this was due to the State gradually assuming more responsibility but it was also due to the emergence in England of voluntary action in a myriad of forms that were to flower prolifically in the early decades of the twentieth century.

Following revolution in France and America, socialist principles had begun to mix with philanthropy in England, giving rise to both theoretical and very practical expressions of a new liberal activism. Collectivism as a basis for organized mutual support became evident in initiatives such as those that launched the Friendly Societies. Prominent liberal activists, such as Mary Wollstonecraft[52] and Mary Carpenter,[53] generated public awareness of issues then constituting a contemporary social inclusion agenda. Leadership for a new approach was provided by 'chocolate philanthropists' from the Quaker families of Fry, Cadbury and Rowntree. Their construction of model villages enabling whole communities to be self-sufficient but mutually supportive offered a new challenging interpretation of philanthropy that contrasted sharply with the previous centuries of alms, the workhouse and ignominious dependency (an approach that may well be applicable in a contemporary context with indigenous communities). It was an ethos that saw the birth of organizations formed to provide sustained economic security for its members such as co-operatives, mutual benefit associations and the Credit Union movement.[54] This was the era that first saw the emergence of 'social economy' a concept developed by writers such as Herbert Spencer,[55] Kirkman Gray[56] and the Fabian socialism of the Webbs.[57]

The turn of the century was a period in which the traditional role of charity came to be viewed by some as unsatisfactory, as a pernicious corollary to persisting structural divisions in society, complicit with and ultimately serving to reinforce the position of the wealthy.[58] However, not until this perception firmed up into a new political frame of reference with the advent of the first 'labour' government in the UK did the role of charity become redefined. Two world wars later, the value system that had for generations supported the class divisions in English society was no longer accepted unquestioningly. A new willingness to consider responsibilities for addressing the needs of the poor and for the provision of public utilities found expression in the creation of the Welfare State, which reset the roles of government and charity in respect of such matters.

The Recreational Charities Act 1958 and social welfare

Following the House of Lords decision in *IRC* v. *Baddeley*,[59] the 1958 Act was introduced (and subsequently replicated in other common law nations) to confirm the charitable status of 'facilities for recreation or other leisure-time occupation, if the facilities are provided in the interests of social welfare'.[60] As explained in Tudor:[61]

> Facilities which are likely to meet such an objective test are those whose dominant feature is that they reduce social exclusion and encourage public participation or improve education or health where previously no, or no adequate, facilities existed.

The beneficiaries must be young, old, infirm, disabled or otherwise socially marginalized and be unable to provide such facilities for themselves. For example, in *Springhill Housing Action Committee* v. *Commissioner of Valuation*[62] a community centre serving a housing estate qualified and community associations or recreational organizations for specific minority groups would similarly do so where it can be shown that the group has a need for that type of facility. The concept of 'social welfare' clearly has potential to be developed further in this context by the Charity Commissioners and applied to the circumstances of the socially disadvantaged.

The traditional role of the State; provider of last resort

The traditional *parens patriae* responsibilities of the King – requiring that he use his powers of guardianship to protect wards, lunatics and charities (or more accurately, to protect their property) – eventually broadened to include a care responsibility for other vulnerable groups of subjects and then devolved via Parliament to the relevant institutions of the State.

The Poor Laws and service provision

In the UK, State provision for the destitute can probably be safely traced back to the Reformation. Certainly by 1572 a parish-based system of poverty relief was in existence. This was extended by the Elizabethan legislation of 1597–1601, which secularized Church facilities, provided for the appointment of parish overseers to work with local churchwardens and raise the funds to assist all classes of destitute persons. The Act for the Relief of the Poor 1601 was perhaps the first legislative indication of State commitment to a social inclusion agenda. It has been claimed that the Statute of Charitable Uses 1601 'set the course for the evolution of philanthropy as a voluntary partnership between the citizen and the State to fund and achieve social objectives'.[63]

However, the care of the needy was viewed by both State and Church as primarily the responsibility of the families concerned and government provision under the Poor Laws for the ill, the destitute and those otherwise in dire need was rudimentary and coupled with a regime intended to discourage malingering. It was left to charities to provide the hospitals, the care services of nurses and almoners and the long-term support needed by the impoverished ill, unmarried mothers, abandoned children, etc. This arrangement of shared responsibility, resting on locally based public service utilities manned and often provided by charities but managed by State officials, was developed in the Poor Law legislation of the eighteenth century and ultimately regulated by the Poor Law Amendment Act 1834 which defined the roles of government and charity until the introduction of the Welfare State. The fact that in the UK the authority of the State had survived intact since 1689 was perhaps both cause and effect of a pervasive and enduring acceptance of the balance between government, charity and the poor/impotent in relation to the nature and extent of public benefit service provision.

The Welfare State: a new partnership between government and charity

The Welfare State was launched in 1948 when the National Health Service Act 1946 came into effect. Beveridge, its chief engineer, concluded in his eight-point plan that for reasons of principle as well as expediency the government should make room for the continued involvement of voluntary organizations in public service provision, where leading charities were well established, and should support that role through a programme of grant aid.[64] To some this partnership policy was merely formalizing an arrangement first recognized in the Preamble when, as was noted in the Nathan Report,[65] 'a partnership was established in which the State filled in gaps left by charity rather than charity filling in gaps left by the State; and this has continued down to the changed situation of our own day'. The relationship between the government and the voluntary sector in relation to public benefit provision has endured throughout the lifetime of the Welfare State.[66]

Charity, the Welfare State and public utility: a new role for charities

Nothing could more graphically demonstrate the mutuality of purpose of government and charity in public benefit provision, and the balance of power in that relationship, than the building of the Welfare State. The network of hospitals and many of the schools, established and maintained for generations by charities, were abruptly nationalized. As the Charity Commissioners subsequently commented: 'the NHS and other statutory services provide for many needs which in the past, used to be met by charities established for the relief of sickness or for the general benefit of the sick poor'.[67] Arguably, as the process is now gradually reversed, the same mutuality of purpose and imbalance of power are equally apparent as the government colonizes the charitable sector in a strategic withdrawal from comprehensive service provision that will leave charities as its proxy service provider.

As the State assumed comprehensive responsibility for ensuring that basic levels of social care were met, charitable activity focused on supplementing State service provision for the socially disadvantaged. Health care facilities, particularly those hospitals that retained their independence, played an important role in augmenting State provision but such public utilities had to satisfy the 'public benefit test' to acquire charitable status.

Public   The requirement that a hospital be open to the public, or a sufficient section of it, is a condition of charitable status. While it is not necessary that a hospital be used exclusively by the poor it cannot be charitable if used exclusively by the rich. Where public access is restricted by the imposition of admission fees then the degree to which this affects the balance between public and private patients will be a key factor in determining a hospital's claim to be a charity. In *Re Resch's Will Trusts*[68] the non-profit factor proved to be determinative when Lord Wilberforce came to consider the status of a gift to a hospital which admitted only 'persons of means'. He upheld the charitable status of the gift but conceded that he would be unable to do so where the functions of such a hospital were 'carried on commercially, i.e. with a view to making profits for private individuals, or where the benefit provided was not for the public, or a sufficiently large section of the public to satisfy the necessary tests of public character'.[69] Where, however, the hospital does make a profit but this is then re-invested in the facility, perhaps to refurbish wards or buy additional medical equipment etc., then its charitable nature remains uncompromised.

A gift to a hospital is *prima facie* a charitable gift. In England and Wales valid charitable gifts have included a bequest for patients in named hospitals,[70] gifts for the endowment of hospital beds[71] and the endowing of ancillary hospital facilities.[72] Moreover, the status of the hospital does not affect the validity of a charitable gift: the public benefit test in relation to the donor's gift is equally satisfied whether the hospital is a government or non-government facility,[73] provided, as in *Re Resch's Will Trusts*,[74] the non-profit requirement is met.

Benefit In addition to providing for a certain breadth of access, a gift must also satisfy the 'benefit' requirement if it is to be recognized as charitable. In *Re Dunlop*,[75] for example, Carswell J commented that in a trust established to found a home for 'Old Presbyterian persons' it would be insufficient to merely 'admit as beneficiaries any aged persons, whatever may be the amount of their resources and irrespective of their needs arising from their condition of advancing years'.[76] His finding in favour of charitable status was grounded on evidence that the trust would be providing a form of sheltered accommodation appropriate to the needs of such elderly persons. Sheltered accommodation for the elderly, disabled, mentally ill and other such groups often attract charitable gifts.

With the increasing hegemony of the public sector in providing health care, the opportunities diminished for charities to engage in public service provision that did not merely duplicate State provision. Charities during this period were able to consolidate their identification with specific groups (Help the Aged, MENCAP, Save the Children, etc.) but were unable to extend their brief to assist others not traditionally regarded as 'impotent'. Their traditional role as principal service provider had been displaced by the State while their capacity to develop new roles in relation to the needs of the socially excluded was restricted by the common law. This was a time when charities were valued for their capacity to supplement State provision and to pioneer new models of intervention that if successful could then be subsumed into such provision.[77]

A framework for partnership

In England and Wales, following the Nathan Report,[78] the regulation of charities was substantially overhauled by the Charities Act 1960 which provided a template for similar legislation in the neighbouring jurisdictions[79] and was widely studied and emulated throughout the common law world. England and Wales remained unique, however, in its strategic approach to addressing and representing the concerns of charities: the Charity Commission was positioned to counterbalance the Inland Revenue and become a key instrument in the government policy of delivering public services in partnership with charities. Over the following several decades this body used its new powers under the Charities Act 1960 to compile a register of all charities while continuing its monitoring, preventative, remedial and investigative work. It also became more actively engaged in the issues facing the sector and in adjusting the interpretation of public benefit to induce a better fit between charities and the pattern of contemporary social need.

Partnership for the public benefit: emerging characteristics of the modern relationship between government and charities

In the closing decades of the twentieth century there was no doubting that Thatcherite policies in the UK had succeeded in rolling back the public sector and much debate ensued as to how a partnership might be formalized between the public, the private and the voluntary sectors to better share responsibility for future public service provision while maintaining social progress. The key to building any such new relationship lay in policy negotiations between government and charities, the two parties legally committed to advancing the public benefit.

Charities, the waning of the Welfare State and growth of the 'contract culture'

In the UK, as elsewhere in the common law world, the last decades of the twentieth century witnessed the retreat of the State accompanied by a steady increase in the devolving of public service responsibilities, mainly to the voluntary sector. While the State withdrew from direct service provision it did not relinquish control as the services franchised out were subject to statutory regulations that specified benchmarks for standards of quality etc. and to government powers of monitoring and inspection. Moreover, the concept of 'social economy' had taken hold bringing with it an awareness of the broad responsibility for building and maintaining the infrastructure for civil society to be shared between government, non-government and for-profit bodies (see, further, chapter 7).

Shaping the modern role of charities

Government policy in the UK to withdraw from much direct public service provision was planned to ensure that voluntary organizations provided substitute services, often then acting as agents of government bodies. In community care, health and education the organizations concerned were invariably charities and their close working relationships with government enabled many to become repositioned as major service providers, but in the process their traditional role in relation to social inclusion, as independent advocates for the disadvantaged, robustly challenging government policies, diminished. Other charities such as Law Centres and the Citizens Advice Bureau, retaining greater autonomy, were more critically aware of the effects of government action or inaction and developed a role as 'pressure groups' working to shape social, economic and environmental policies. Some provided forums for the coherent expression of such general fundamental rights as freedom of assembly and speech. Others became champions for the cause of particular socially disadvantaged groups or focused on disaster relief and overseas aid. A small number of charities diversified into research and concentrated their resources on assembling sophisticated data banks profiling the needs of the socially excluded. Among the latter were charities such as the Rowntree Trust,[80] which spearheaded the modern evidence-based approach to challenging government policies that cause or fail to deal with poverty, inequity and social exclusion.

Public services and non-government bodies

In the UK, the retraction of the State occurred across many areas until then regarded as core public services. Transport, housing, education, social and health care and prisons were among those areas where responsibility for future provision was to be devolved to or shared with non-government bodies. Some of the latter were entrepreneurial commercial organizations, concerned with exploiting opportunities for growth and increasing profit margins, the participation of which was by way of private finance initiatives often induced by government grants.

It was government policy to manage the strategy for achieving the necessary partnership arrangements, determine the nature and extent of the responsibilities borne by for-profit and not-for-profit bodies and to retain some degree of control over the services provided. Paradoxically, this was a process of increased central-ization, in terms of government strategic management and in terms of reducing the authority and resources available at local authority/county council level, while imposing procedural and regulatory mechanisms to monitor and control the quality and cost-effectiveness of service provision.[81] As well as increasing its central control, government simultaneously sought to strengthen transparency and accountability mechanisms for those on the receiving end of public service provision. After 1997, the New Labour government continued and reinforced the Conservative Party policy of putting in place the means for recognizing and protecting the rights of service users through 'citizens' charters', consumer complaints procedures, etc.

Finding itself squeezed from both ends, local government in the UK set about building new allegiances within the voluntary and community sector to assist first in the delivery of public services and gradually also in the identification of social need and in the planning of appropriate services. This development, encouraged by central government for reasons to do with furthering its policy of generating social capital and community capacity while embedding a broader sense of civic responsibility, led to a more confident voluntary sector and to the growth of umbrella bodies that were increasingly able to articulate and negotiate on behalf of the sector's interests.[82]

The contract culture

The process of delegating responsibility for public service provision to non-government bodies was and continues to be managed by government contract.

Across the UK, in the closing decades of the twentieth century, government departments at local, regional and national levels increasingly sought to devolve responsibilities to charities, other voluntary organizations, commercial enterprises and to various combinations of such bodies. A mixed economy of provision emerged. All contracts were to be governed by the public benefit principle and benchmarked against standards of value for money, effectiveness, transparency and accountability, etc. However, as the contract culture phenomenon became established certain characteristics of the newly developing relationship between government and charities emerged, some of which caused disquiet.

Voluntary participation in public benefit activity   The retraction of State social/health care service provision and the corresponding rolling forward of the voluntary sector was accompanied by a new found State enthusiasm for a vigorous, independent voluntary sector with its use of volunteers as a means of promoting civic engagement, building social capital[83] and stimulating a more participative democracy.[84] In the main, the involvement of volunteers in locally based social care activities proved beneficial for such recipients as the house-bound frail elderly, the disabled and other socially disadvantaged groups while also being therapeutic for the volunteers and contributing to the growth of more aware and caring communities. This was balanced by a concern that volunteer involvement was at times a cheap and insufficient substitute for professional care, that active engagement of volunteers in their community was not always a good thing,[85] and that many recipients would have preferred not to endure exposure to neighbours as the price of service provision.

Unacceptable charity   By the end of the twentieth century the voluntary sector in the UK had grown to become confident, extensive and richly diversified, embracing a wide range of not-for-profit bodies of which charities formed a significant but not a numerically dominant part.[86] In fact many organizations did not want charitable status because of the associated restrictions on trading, models of governance or perceptions of paternalism. Others could not acquire it due to their political activism, their involvement in locally based self-help groups, co-operation with business enterprises or because their altruistic activities failed in other ways to satisfy a legal interpretation of 'public benefit'. Many voluntary organizations were single-issue bodies that simply wanted the flexibility and freedom to pursue their objectives without having to comply with the administrative requirements that accompanied charitable status.

Charitable status, however, was also problematic for those service users who did not want to receive, or be seen to be receiving, 'handouts'. Whereas government service provision was acceptable as of right (associated with payment of taxes) charitable provision (associated with paternalism) was not. By contracting with charities to channel the same services to the same recipients, government departments risked lowering service uptake by the socially disadvantaged.

Market competition by and between charities   As the larger charities extended their activities, they engaged and competed in the market place in a manner almost indistinguishable from, and at times in direct competition with, commercial businesses. The convergence between the two became evident in their funding arrangements, activities, use of salaried professional staff, etc. Most familiar in this period was the claim that charities, using the public appeal and exemption from rates associated with their status, were gaining an unfair advantage over other high street traders.

This was also a time when there were many takeovers, mergers and bankruptcies which while inducing a more acute awareness of cost efficiency and the importance of good management, skills not traditionally associated with charities, also resulted in greater hegemony and less diversification in the sector. Revenue being the lifeblood of charities, competition for government contracts led to accusations that some (e.g. those engaged in cancer research or in domiciliary care services) were becoming more concerned with issues of market share and strategic positioning than with the further development of needs-sensitive services.

Government colonization of the voluntary sector   The granting of government contracts, even if on the basis of open and competitive tender, inevitably served to favour some charities at the expense of others. For many the income derived from such contracts constituted the largest or even their sole source of revenue, providing financial security and opportunities for expansion. Those without government contracts were not only relatively less financially secure but they also lacked leverage as the government was able to treat its contracting partner as representing relevant client interests. For smaller charities with a restricted market and range of services the lack of government contracts often meant they were unable to survive. Government patronage, as played out through the contract culture, significantly reshaped the voluntary sector in the UK at the end of the twentieth century.

Independence of charities   Charities, unlike for-profit and other not-for-profit bodies, are legally required to establish and maintain independent governance. Being bound by its objects and purposes as stated in its governing instruments, a charity must resolutely continue to pursue the objectives for which it was established regardless of any external influence. However, charities dependent upon contract renewal were susceptible to developing a compliant relationship with government bodies and, arguably, compliance with the latter's agenda became an implicit criterion for their selection and deselection. The concern that short-term government contracts threatened to compromise the independence of charities was highlighted in two important reports where the authors spoke of their fear that such contracts 'may lead to unhealthy dependencies'[87] and has recently been addressed by the Charity Commission.[88]

There was also cause for concern regarding the flexible interpretation of charitable purposes adopted by some charities as original objectives were redefined to conform with the policy of a government funding body in order to secure contracts: the pragmatic adjustments made were at times open to a challenge of illegality on the grounds of abandoning the trust and/or seeking an unfair trading advantage. The Deakin report drew attention to the fact that 'the distinctive nature of voluntary action in our society is now in danger of being compromised as organisations move away from their original objectives and take on new roles defined for them by others'[89] or, as Knight protested, 'organisations that follow the State into new contracting arrangements can no longer think of themselves as sufficiently independent to warrant the adjective "voluntary" '.[90]

A general muting of dissent   The contracting/partnership strategy pursued by government bodies had the effect of persuading their voluntary partners that 'biting the hand that feeds them' would not be conducive to a renewal of contractual arrangements and consequently the monitoring, lobbying and advocacy roles traditionally pursued by charities and other voluntary organizations in relation to the policies of government bodies became increasingly inhibited. Moreover, the process of competitive tendering for government contracts fragmented the capacity of similar organizations to co-ordinate any lobbying activity.

This general development was noted as a matter of concern in both the Kemp and Deakin reports, which stressed the need for equality in any partnership between the voluntary sector and government while also emphasizing that 'voluntary bodies must be free to be advocates even where they are also partners'.[91] However, it may also be the case that the advocacy role traditionally borne by voluntary organizations was increasingly perceived as the responsibility of other bodies such as the Equality Commission, the Ombudsman or Law Centres, etc.

Politics and partnership

In the UK, the political significance of a balanced relationship between State and voluntary sector had been articulated in the Nathan report: 'The democratic State as we know it could hardly function effectively or teach the exercise of democracy to its members without such channels for and demands on voluntary service.'[92] In recognition of their mutual dependence, the Deakin report sought to formalize the relationship between central government and the voluntary sector in a partnership to be expressed in a concordat or compact.[93] Following the accession of Labour to government in May 1997 four separate compacts (for England, Scotland, Wales and Northern Ireland) were then developed.[94] These 'compacts' set out to clarify the respective roles of government and the voluntary sector in the context of the shared values and principles that underpinned their partnership. While they relate to the wider voluntary and community sector and not only to charities, and while there is always the danger that they will function more as aspirational declarations of intent rather than as an enforceable code of conduct, they do represent a further stage in the development of the centuries-old relationship between government and charities in their mutual commitment to promoting the public benefit.

The public benefit and political activity by charities

The advocacy role of charities has been compromised not only by the contract culture[95] but also by a hardening of the judicial view that charitable status and lobbying for change, in the law and government policy, are incompatible activities. The timing of the latter development strengthened the hand of a government determined to engage the voluntary sector on its terms in a partnership for the future delivery of public services.

The common law rule regarding political activity by charities

In common law jurisdictions it is a long-standing legal rule that a voluntary organization seeking to acquire or retain charitable status, and all the attendant financial benefits, must avoid having political purposes and engaging in most forms of political activity. A legal distinction is drawn between bodies with political purposes and bodies that engage in political activities: the former are not charitable; the latter will be charitable if the activities are ancillary but subordinate to and in furtherance of its non-political purposes.

This rule is a singular characteristic of charity law in common law nations. In a survey of 24 countries, undertaken to establish the nature of such links as might exist between the freedom of voluntary organizations to engage in campaigning and political activity and the prevailing type of civil law regime, a clear distinction was found to exist between countries with a common law legacy and others. As the authors state:[96]

> At some stage in their history, all the charity law countries have followed the general approach which descends from the 1601 English Statute of Charitable Uses ... of the countries to constrain the campaigning activities of non-profit organisations specifically because of their organisational form or status, all were charity law, and ... originally common law, countries. *In other words, only the USA, Northern Ireland, Ireland, Canada, England and Wales, Australia, Scotland and India have specific constraints on campaigning by charities.*

All other non-charity law countries in the survey not only refrained from imposing any restrictions on campaigning by non-profit organizations but many openly encouraged an advocacy role. It would seem that in the common law nations charitable status and political activity are almost mutually exclusive. This is a difficult moral proposition to sustain as was pointed out in the Nathan report:[97]

> Some of the most valuable activities of voluntary societies consist, however, in the fact that they may be able to stand aside from and criticize State action or inaction, in the interests of the inarticulate man in the street.

Political activity or inactivity often provides a rallying point for minority groups, providing the *cause célèbre* that brings them together and a focus for collective action in pursuit of common goals. It is therefore also a necessary focus for charitable activity. In the context of social inclusion the rule is particularly obstructive as it at least inhibits and often prevents campaigning by charities for change in government policy or law in relation to disadvantaged minority groups (e.g. asylum seekers).[98] The rule applies equally to campaigning for such change within the jurisdiction or elsewhere.[99]

The rationale

The accepted rationale for denying charitable status to bodies engaging in political activity rests on several related arguments. They all essentially stem from the view that such activity subverts the established democratic political process. Because a charity has not submitted to the electoral system it is not publicly accountable. Because it is not usually internally organized in a democratic fashion it is seldom in a position to proclaim that other systems are unfair. It is therefore claimed that a charity has no mandate to represent issues before the 'body politic'. It is also suggested that the social value of a charity lies in the latter's independence, which would be compromised if it became politicized – a corollary being that the legitimacy conferred on a charity by virtue of its formal recognition as such would, in the eyes of the general public, be extended to the cause it chose to espouse, with corresponding disadvantages for causes not championed by charities. Allied to this is the argument that it would be illogical for the State to defray the liability of an organization to contribute towards the 'public purse', thereby imposing a duty on others to make good the tax loss, only to find that by so doing it was subsidizing the capacity of the organization to undermine State policies. Again, by granting public monies to charities the State is channelling taxpayers' funds on a preferential basis, but it has no way of knowing which campaigns taxpayers support and which they do not.[100] Moreover, as illustrated by the anti-vivisection cases,[101] a cause may gain or lose public support thereby rendering uncertain the public benefit component which is so crucial to charitable status. The judicial dilemma when faced with policy issues arising from action or inaction by government or Parliament was pithily expressed by Simons L.J.: 'it is not for the court to judge and the court has no means of judging'.[102]

The decision in McGovern v. Attorney General[103]

This case concerned an attempt by Amnesty International to create a trust in order to have some of its work deemed charitable. The purposes of the trust were fourfold:

1   looking after the needy, i.e. prisoners and ex-prisoners;
2   promoting the abolition of capital and corporal punishment;
3   researching and disseminating information on human rights;
4   securing the release of political prisoners.

Slade J held that, although purposes 1 and 3 could be charitable, the other two were political. The political nature of these two contaminated the whole trust and the entire trust was void as being for political purposes. In the course of the hearing Slade J made a finding as to matters that could be construed as political purposes. These were:

- to further the interests of a particular political party;
- to procure changes in the laws of this country;
- to bring about changes in the laws of a foreign country;
- to bring about a reversal of government policy or of particular decisions of governmental authorities in this country;
- to bring about a reversal of government policy or of particular decisions of governmental authorities in a foreign country.

This list was added to in *Re Koeppler's Will Trusts*:[104]

- to oppose a particular change in the law or a change in a particular law.

As pointed out by Dal Pont, it may also have been extended, in New Zealand at least, by the ruling on the corollary in *Molloy* v. *Commissioner of Inland Revenue*[105] that 'advocating or promoting the maintenance of the *present* law is equally a political purpose because the court has no means of judging whether a change in the law would *not* be beneficial to the community'[106] (see, further, chapter 11).

The ruling in the *Amnesty* case, as endorsed by subsequent case law, served to underpin the traditional common law approach to political activity by charities, emphasize the difference between it and the approach taken by other modern western societies and prevent or obstruct future campaigning by charities on behalf of the socially disadvantaged at a time of public service retrenchment.

The Charity Commissioners and a broadening interpretation of public benefit

The potential for broadening the interpretation of matters constituting the 'public benefit' to ensure a better fit between the law and contemporary social need has always rested primarily with developments in charitable activity under the fourth and most extensive *Pemsel* head. While the public benefit test in England and Wales is presumed satisfied in relation to gifts made under the first three heads, the fact that it requires to be proven under the fourth provides considerable opportunity for the scope of charity to expand (and contract – purposes can cease to be charitable, as was the case with gun clubs) incrementally.

As the role of the High Court in developing the common law interpretation of matters constituting the 'public benefit' petered out, due to the decline in litigation (attributable to the associated expense and the negative effect of publicity), it was replaced by the more discrete, systematic and comprehensive probing of the Commission. Initially, as has been pointed out, the outcome was much the same:[107]

fossilisation is virtually institutionalised. The interposition of the Charity Commissioners means that fewer cases now reach the courts, but the Commissioners regard themselves as wholly bound by the decisions of the courts, and so even that slow development of the law which judicial creativity can produce, is to a large extent denied us. This is an area which is truly substantially ruled from the grave.

In the closing years of the twentieth century, however, this body had adopted a more proactive and strategic approach towards broadening the interpretation of 'public benefit' to address issues of contemporary need including those relating to social inclusion.

Pending the Charities Acts 1992/1993

Where new issues arose the Charity Commissioners were often able to rule that the public benefit was satisfied.

Rehabilitation   The Commission reports reveal a number of cases where gifts for the purpose of providing rehabilitation were found to be charitable, including for the benefit of those suffering from a disability[108] and from abuse or deprivation.[109] In *Joseph Rowntree Memorial Trust Housing Assoc. Ltd.* v. *A-G*[110] the court held that it was charitable for a housing association to provide housing for young and old people in need by a method that included selling the tenants a leasehold interest in allocated property.

International and race relations   The established judicial view that trusts for promoting better relations between nations and races are not charitable[111] has been significantly relaxed. As noted in Tudor: 'Since 1983, the Commissioners have accepted as charitable trusts for the promotion of good relations, for endeavouring to eliminate discrimination on the grounds of race and for encouraging equality between persons of different racial groups.'[112]
   For example the Commission registered the Community Security Trust which had, as one of its purposes, the promotion of good relations between the Jewish community and others by seeking the elimination of anti-Semitism, this being a form of racism. Trusts to support equal rights for women and for the gay community have similarly been held to be charitable (see, also, chapter 6).

Research   The Commission found itself able to move beyond some of the restrictions previously associated with pure research (e.g. the requirements regarding dissemination and a pupil – teacher relationship).[113] Consequently, research itself became charitable without the necessity of it having to form part of a recognized educational activity (see, also, chapter 4).

Political awareness   Again, following the decision in *Att-Gen* v. *Ross*[114] which recognized the purpose of encouraging political awareness as charitable, the

Commission has developed a slightly less restrictive interpretation of 'political activities'.

Post the Charities Acts 1992/1993

Following the legislative extension of their powers, permitting closer monitoring and control of charities, the Charity Commissioners initiated a review of the Register of Charities in 1997. The Commission's review, using a checklist of identified principles for screening charitable purposes and activity,[115] proved to be a fruitful mechanism for clarifying the public benefit test[116] and developing the scope of charitable status in relation to matters such as unemployment,[117] rural and urban regeneration,[118] training[119] and co-operation between charities and business. These matters, with significant implications for increasing the capacity of charity law to address issues of social inclusion, were the subject of considerable guidance notes from the Commission which, as noted in Tudor:[120]

> sets out possible activities for charitable regeneration organisations including the provision of housing for those in need, assistance and training to the unemployed, assistance to businesses and the provision of roads and public amenities . . . Linked with urban and rural regeneration is the decision of the Charity Commissioners that the promotion of community capacity building in relation to communities which are socially and economically (or in some cases simply socially) disadvantaged is charitable.[121] Community capacity building here means developing the capacity and skills of members of a community in such a way that they are better able to identify and help meet their needs and to participate more in society. The relevant communities may be geographical or may be a community of interest, for example, membership of a particular ethnic group.

As also noted, care must be taken to ensure that the public benefit test is satisfied, in particular that any private benefit remains incidental.

Instead of being dependent solely upon relevant issues arising to provide opportunities for broadening the interpretation of 'charity' the review process allowed the Commission to systematically filter registered charities, abstract data and issue guidance accordingly. Moreover, it was a process that saw the Commission gradually move away from the constraints of the 'spirit and intendment' rule. During this period it was able to endorse as charitable novel methods of tackling poverty such as the positive discrimination approach adopted by the Fairtrade Foundation to identify products provided in a manner that benefits those involved in the production process[122] and by the Garfield Poverty Trust which provided loans to enable the less well-off to acquire mortgages for accommodation.[123] It issued advice explaining how charities could engage in political activity and exercise influence on government policy without endangering their status.[124] It declared its approval of the promotion of the voluntary sector as a whole[125] as charitable and the promotion of greater effectiveness in the use of resources by bodies within it.[126] Again, the Commission has broadened the approach to poverty relief by advising that instead of one-off grants it may in some circumstances prove more effective to arrange a programme of staged investments.[127] The review process also provided many opportunities for creative *cy-près* schemes to transfer assets from dormant or redundant charities to those capable of applying the resources to alleviate contemporary instances of social need. Moreover, following the introduction of the Human Rights Act 1998, the Commission has recognized the promotion of human rights as charitable[128] and has taken into account ECHR principles when examining charitable purposes (see, further, chapters 6 and 8).

Conclusion

The distinction between the remit of government and charity in relation to public benefit service provision remains, as it has always been, somewhat confused. This was perhaps an inevitable consequence of the initial blurring of boundaries in the Preamble, the subsequent common law approach and the history of an alternating responsibility for certain aspects of public service provision. In recent decades this legacy has come to be viewed as providing a timely political opportunity for advancing a policy that positively promotes shared responsibility for future provision, implemented through the 'contract culture', as a cost-effective means of facilitating the civic engagement of volunteers in – and the corresponding withdrawal of central government from – servicing the social and health care needs of local communities. One outcome of a policy that has succeeded in positioning some charities at the frontline of public service provision, ironically, is a reduction in the overall capacity to address social exclusion issues.

Charities, many of which have existed for centuries, are uniquely placed to know and to address the contemporary social inclusion agenda. The 'poor' and the 'impotent' have always been their core business and are central to a contemporary understanding of social inclusion. The common law however, for reasons outlined above (see, also, chapter 4) restricts their effectiveness and this is now further inhibited by the growth of the 'contract culture'. If charities are to play a full role in partnership with government and meet the challenge presented by the socially disadvantaged to the goal of achieving a sustainable civil society, then they must be freed up to hold an authentic, independent negotiating position within that partnership.

In recent years the Charity Commissioners have significantly ameliorated the common law approach and strengthened the capacity of charities in relation to social exclusion issues. In particular, the review process undertaken by the Commission corrects a very real structural flaw within the common law, namely that it can only progress by judicial decisions taken on a case-by-case basis in response to litigation which necessarily appears on a random and infrequent basis before the courts. The methodical screening of all registered charities has enabled the Commission to identify and map areas where charitable purposes are out of synch with contemporary social need and to plan related strategic adjustments.

However, as the Commission's powers remain constrained by the 'spirit and intendment' rule, any broadening of the interpretation of 'public benefit' is by analogy rather than by paradigm shift.

Given the history of four centuries of uncertainty, it is probable that a legislative initiative is now required to ensure that the future roles of government and charity are appropriately realigned around the central concept of 'public benefit' and their respective areas of responsibility, mandatory and discretionary, are clarified in respect of public service provision. This would enable a government/charity partnership to proceed, and the Commission to hold the ring, in relation to their common goal of ensuring that charitable purposes are appropriately applied to address social inclusion issues (see, further, Part IV for jurisdiction-specific accounts of contemporary relationship between charity law and social inclusion and chapter 8 for developments in respect of England and Wales).

Part III

Legal rights and functions

A framework for philanthropy

Chapter 6

Legal functions relating to social inclusion in a modern regulatory environment for charities

Introduction

This chapter identifies and examines the main functions of the law relating to charity and considers how it and the themes that emerged in Part II impact on social inclusion within a contemporary political context.

It opens by briefly considering the significance of the political context for charity law with particular reference to implications arising from the recent international emphasis on anti-terrorism legislation. This leads into an exploration of the concepts of 'civil society' and 'social capital' and the related broader relevance of the charity law reviews. It examines some shared themes in the current social inclusion agenda of the common law nations engaging in such reviews and considers the potential of an appropriately reformed charity law for promoting civil society.

The chapter then identifies and analyses the core legal functions that comprise contemporary charity law in common law nations and therefore constitute the main ingredients for a template. It notes and explores the concern in all charity law reviews with definitional matters. It focuses on the main mechanical aspects of a regulatory environment: the existence of a statutory or voluntary system for registration; the separation or otherwise of the functions for determining charitable status and tax exemption; the role of the government body with primary responsibility for philanthropic organizations; and the role of various other regulatory bodies etc. It assembles the components for a standard template of such functions that can be applied as a research tool to survey the regulatory framework for philanthropy in a selection of representative common law nations and notes jurisdiction-specific characteristics.

Drawing from themes running through the reviews and evident in the developmental history of the common law (see, further, Part II) the chapter then turns to consider the nature of factors currently inhibiting effective philanthropic activity. It identifies and evaluates the effect of such general operational constraints as: partnership with government; restrictions on advocacy/political activity; human rights and anti-terrorism concerns; fiscal issues, particularly tax orientation; the role of the courts; legal structures; and public benefit issues. This chapter basically identifies and assesses those functions of the law and other inhibitors that act to constrain philanthropic activity in relation to the social inclusion agenda. It thereby prepares the ground for conducting the comparative analysis that follows in Part IV.

Government, charity law and social inclusion: a political frame of reference

The responsibility of good government in relation to social inclusion must be to ensure that the relevant legislative and institutional infrastructure is in place and is functioning within a healthy social capital environment in such a way that the needs of the socially disadvantaged are appropriately addressed. If this is the case it then begs the question as to what, in that context, should be the contribution of charities and other non-government organizations? The answer depends upon where, on a political continuum from liberal democracy to totalitarianism, the society in question wishes to be positioned, or, more accurately, where in fact any particular government has positioned that society. Charity law is among the more significant means whereby a government can orchestrate the public/private balance deemed to be politically appropriate in its management of social need.

Charity, the law and politics

A sense of perspective needs to be kept in mind when considering the capacity of charity law to address issues of social inclusion. The legal functions available to modern western societies to deal with such issues are not confined to those provided by charity law. The extent, for example, to which a government subscribes to international law and to the related policy frameworks for dealing with issues of human rights and social justice while also deploying anti-terrorism measures will be very influential, as will the extent to which it has in place a national institutional infrastructure for addressing issues of equity, equality, non-discrimination, etc (see, further, chapter 7). The legal functions of charity law cannot be viewed in isolation.

Public/private

The public/private balance in modern democratic nations and the resulting distribution of responsibility for social service provision has changed greatly over the past two or three decades. There has been a marked shift from a position that the State should own and maintain its national resources, institutional infrastructure, etc., to one that it should, to some degree, settle for controlling access to services and their standards by regulatory legislation and inspectoral bodies. Across the world, the move towards privatization of social utilities has enabled the State to leave the market to provide, at a price, services such as water, sanitation, transport, housing, electricity, gas, etc., and it is demonstrating an increasing enthusiasm for similarly shedding responsibility for nursing home care, residential care of the elderly, etc. For many in the UK, the privatization of water supply in the late

1980s, followed by the disconnection of thousands of families from running water for failure to pay, provided stark evidence of a new public/private balance being struck in the distribution of responsibility for safeguarding the interests of the socially disadvantaged – a lesson driven home by the policy, currently evident in some hospitals and HSS Trusts, to manage resources and waiting lists by unilaterally ceasing to provide standard public health and social care services. This shift in the balance struck between public and private responsibilities was graphically underlined in the US by the recent dedication of immense private wealth to immunisation programmes; leaving to charity the responsibility for eradicating malaria constitutes an interesting benchmark in government disengagement from its traditional public service role. All modern democracies are now wrestling with the implications arising from privatizing access to such basic necessities for life and working through the considerable challenges for sustaining civil society that flow from the consequent reshaping of relationships between governments, business and charity.

The principles governing the dividing lines between State provision of essential services, State funding of not-for-profit bodies to do so and State transfer of service provision to commercial enterprises are hard to find. In particular, the principle that charity cannot be left to bear responsibilities that more properly fall to the State is less helpful in a context where it is far from certain what it is that remains or should remain with the State. It is a context in which legal rights must assume a greater salience.

Charity law

The extent to which a society, at any point in time, allows or relies upon philanthropic activity to provide for the needs of its disadvantaged reveals a great deal about where it is then located on the political spectrum from democracy to totalitarianism. At both extremes there is an acceptance that social need will always exist and will require a social policy response. However, whereas one values independent discretionary acts of the individual as a means of addressing social need and legislates to protect and encourage the right to do so, the other subordinates or suppresses this in favour of structural intervention by government. Many modern western nations have developed sophisticated systems of charity law to identify and regulate approved philanthropic activity, to ensure that it contributes to meeting contemporary social need and to provide preferential tax status and other financial benefits for the organizations concerned. Totalitarian States have tended to view this hallmark of democracy with suspicion. It is seen as an area of voluntary activity with potential to undermine approved values and policies, established social priorities, strategies for social and economic development and ultimately the authority and control of the State. But there is now no denying the central importance of charity law for democracy, as evidenced by the scale and vigour of philanthropic activity in all modern democratic nations, coupled with the enthusiasm with which it has been embraced by the many east European states newly emerged from under their blanket of totalitarianism.

In the modern world, the law regulating charitable activity has become a significant measure for differentiating not only between totalitarian and democratic States, but also for differentiating between the latter on the basis of their relative values and social policy priorities. The particular such values and concerns of a government will inevitably be reflected in the legislative framework provided by it to define and regulate charitable activity and to justify related tax exemptions and other concessions. The government of the day in any modern western society will shape the statutory basis of charity law to strike the balance between voluntary and statutory sectors, and adjust the relationship between for-profit and not-for-profit economic activity, that it considers most appropriately reflects its position on the socialist/liberal/conservative political continuum. Charity legislation is a useful means of orchestrating the relationship between the voluntary sector and the State (though not the only one: service agreements and contractual relations rather than legislation can achieve the same ends). By providing a mediating mechanism for adjusting the respective remits of the voluntary and statutory sectors, such legislation sets out the rules for managing the interface between the two. The nature and extent of regulations governing the functions of charities provide a revealing indicator of the terms on which a government has chosen to share its social economy responsibilities with non-government organizations. It also structures activities within the voluntary sector: differentiating between informal and formal voluntary organizations and between the latter on the basis of their charitable status; classifying charities by purpose; and providing such authority as there may be for regulating their affairs.

Charities and terrorism

There has been a sudden surge of interest among governments around the world in the regulatory environment for charities. In the aftermath of the events of 11 September 2001 and subsequent related outrages in Bali, India, Spain, England, Egypt and elsewhere, the growing willingness to adjust this environment has a firm emphasis on creating new powers to detect and control the abuse of charities. There is some irony in the timing. Just as the governments of common law nations were slowly finalizing preparations for new legislation to liberalize the interpretation of charitable activity they are now hastily introducing measures that are bound to restrict it. It would be naïve to ignore the fact that, in the post-9/11 world, the charitable sector is now seen by many as a weak link in the fight against global terrorism.

Anti-terrorism legislation

The United Nations Security Council Resolution 1373 has been interpreted as placing a requirement on all governments to pass legislation to prevent the flow of charity money to fund terrorism. There can be no denying the existence of a link between some fundraising bodies, whether or not registered as charities, and the subsequent use of some such funds by terrorists: sending money home for the cause has long been seen as the duty of overseas supporters for the 'freedom fighters' in the 'motherland' and the necessary chain of socially respectable but bogus organizations has existed for this to be accomplished. Equally, there can be no denying the persistence of the shibboleth that soup kitchens are inherently subversive: that the best intentions of good people can nonetheless serve to undermine the prevailing social order; that literally or metaphorically, money for bread may become explosive. The two must not be conflated.

Among the problems now facing the governments of modern western societies, as they calibrate the legislative powers necessary to regulate the supposedly terrorist-related element of the charitable sector, is that of differentiating between victims and those that satisfy the definition of 'wilful' in the Resolution. The common supposition among such governments, that new powers are needed to prevent or detect the flow of overseas money into the bogus national charities that fund terrorism, is not necessarily wholly accurate. That scenario, which presumes the common and culpable intent of both giver and receiver, while undoubtedly to some extent valid is a dangerous oversimplification of the complexities surrounding the role of charities in this matter: dangerous because the resulting legislative powers may be used to close down organizations and their support networks which are largely engaged in bona fide charitable activity but may unwittingly accommodate a terrorist-related element. Various examples come to mind.

Fraud   Organizations established to provide long-term support for the dependent families of prisoners convicted of terrorist offences may find their good work jeopardized by revelations that money donated to defray costs of prison visits has occasionally been diverted for other use by the prisoner's terrorist group. Such a diversion of assets constitutes a straightforward criminal offence of fraud and needs to be dealt with simply on that basis.

Lobbying   An immigrant minority culture group – formed to provide mutual support and to assist other new immigrants – which finds itself rallying around a common grievance (e.g. lobbying for change in the related law and policy) may be faced with the challenge that it has transgressed the boundary of free speech to become an advocate for subversive activity.

Incidental assistance   Again, there are those who innocently give to a fraudulent organization believing that they are providing food and shelter for a bona fide cause. However, by giving terrorists food they may be freeing their funds to be used for buying guns.

Then, of course, there are those who are simply and genuinely giving money to assist victims. In each instance the flow of funds may well be wholly internal to the jurisdiction, rendering the need for new powers to combat the funding of international terrorism as beside the point. A proportionate and discriminating legislative response, that is human rights compliant, to the real but limited threat presented by the link between charities and terrorism, that does not impede the vital link between charities and the socially marginalized, would seem to be all that is necessary.

Social inclusion: the international dimension

Given the largely north/south global economic divide, coupled with the number of unstable societies in Africa, the Caucasus and elsewhere, there are and will continue to be many occasions when modern western societies will be presented with opportunities to practise social inclusion policies with an international dimension. The pressing challenge to do so in response to the deepening alienation experienced by some Islamic groups, communities and nations will test the veracity of the social inclusion agenda currently espoused by western governments. Whether dealing with the exclusion, or perceived exclusion, of countries from the comity of nations, of ethnic groups from the social infrastructure of a State, or of minority groups such as the disabled from within their local communities, the differences in scale should not obscure the fact that the issues and need for mediatory intervention are much the same. The potential role for non-governmental organizations in facilitating social inclusion and the legitimacy of their right to claim charitable status for engaging in such activity, are as relevant on an international as on a domestic level.

External

A need for benign, consensual intervention in the affairs of some underdeveloped nations by modern western society may arise for various reasons. Most obvious and least contentious is the need for emergency relief to be provided promptly, on an international and co-ordinated basis, in the immediate aftermath of a local disaster, usually for a short period. Intervention of a focused nature and again on an international and co-ordinated basis but probably for a more sustained period may also be invited and necessary in circumstances of endemic poverty and/or disease such as in sub-Saharan Africa, or following economic or socio-economic collapse, such as that experienced in Argentina when its currency was sharply devalued. More controversially, intervention in the affairs of an unstable or failing nation may well be necessary even though an invitation by consensus is not forthcoming. This may be the case in countries on the verge of internal fragmentation due to civil strife such as subsequently occurred, for example, in Yugoslavia, Rwanda, Lebanon and, arguably, Northern Ireland. Finally and most controversially, because again an invitation by consensus may not be forthcoming, mediatory intervention could be justified in the affairs of two or more nations in a state of mutual antagonism that are drifting towards, or have become embroiled in, actual conflict. The dynamics of ethnic tensions in the Middle East, sub-Saharan Africa, the Caucasus and elsewhere provide examples of circumstances where such intervention might well be appropriate.

Clearly, in situations where conflict is underway, then third-party intervention in the affairs of sovereign states can only be justified, and in practice may only be possible, within a framework set by international law and diplomacy and conducted under the auspices of the United Nations. Before and after an outbreak of violence, however, in response to an invitation from any one or more of the parties concerned, mediatory third-party intervention such as may be provided by an independent non-government organization established and legally mandated for that purpose would in theory be feasible. Arguably, a modern charity law framework should facilitate the creation of such bodies and positively discriminate in favour of their work (see, also, chapter 7).

Internal

Many common law countries are currently experiencing, along with other modern western nations, a wave of economic migration causing difficult, largely urban, tensions due to fluctuations in the balance between different and sometimes opposing cultures. From Quebec to Bradford, from Paris to Sydney and elsewhere, similar tensions are becoming evident. It is highly probable that this phenomenon will increase as the more stable developed nations struggle to cope with refugees fleeing economic and political turmoil. The influx of sizeable numbers from different ethnic groups is now challenging many western societies. Including but not assimilating new cultures, while preserving those already established and in the process maintaining social equilibrium and promoting opportunities for further growth, will test government capacity to sustain civil society across the western world.

Social inclusion: the domestic dimension

In addition to the above international aspects of social inclusion, all modern western societies are struggling with domestic issues relating to the distinctive needs of socially disadvantaged minority groups such as the disabled, the elderly, the mentally ill, the drug-dependent, disaffected youth and the gay and lesbian community (see, further, Part IV). The domestic social inclusion agenda may well be further complicated by issues relating to post-colonial matters and/or to the circumstances of indigenous, culture-specific, ethnic groups (see, further, chapters 2 and 4). Again, inclusion rather than assimilation, facilitated by appropriate charity law provisions, would seem to be indicated.

Civil society, charity law and the reviews

It is axiomatic that any review designed to improve charity law – currently understood as providing for the relief of poverty, the advancement of education and religion and providing for such other public benefits as better social and health care facilities – must thereby also promote the development of civil society. A major challenge for the future is to ensure that these four *Pemsel*[1] heads of charity – as amended, supplemented or replaced – continue to give effect to the underpinning principle of public benefit by addressing contemporary social circumstances in an effective, appropriate and sufficient manner.

Charities and civil society

Arguably, to meet the challenge presented to the common law nations by the opportunity of charity law reform is to put in place the core components for the future development of civil society. Activities legally defined as charitable are also those that are essential to establishing and sustaining an equitable, inclusive and stable society: to promote a truly contemporary interpretation of the public benefit is to promote civil society.

The role of charities

Even if viewed solely in terms of economics, charities constitute the most significant component of the voluntary and community sector (or third sector). Charities are at the heart of the sector, controlling most of its assets, generating much of its income, contributing longevity and consistency, deploying the majority of its volunteer workforce (which constitutes a significant proportion of the total national workforce) across most sector activities. Particularly in the areas of health and social care service provision, education, culture (and sport/recreation in some jurisdictions), the role of charities within the sector has been expanding rapidly in recent years. However, they are also distinctive among non-government organizations for characteristics that uniquely lend themselves to promoting the growth of civil society. The distinctive underpinning principles of charity require charitable bodies to strive with a 'moral mission' to improve the circumstances of the socially disadvantaged,[2] to maintain independent governance and to neither make nor redistribute any profits for private gain in the process. Through their activities in the areas of poverty, education, religion and in such other areas of benefit to the community as health and social care charities thereby ameliorate hardship, address the issues of fundamental concern and facilitate the growth of civil society.

A rich diversity of organizational form allows charity the flexibility to permeate and grow within the socio-economic fabric of society; from the informality of the small local unincorporated association to the large multinational corporation, including foundations, trusts, etc., charities find the level and space best suited for their particular contribution.[3] Charity also helps to sustain that fabric; it contributes to the alleviation of poverty and to the articulation of grievance and by so doing, it reduces social tensions. It reinforces the standing of religion and education, provides the means for both to become more generally pervasive and to build their institutional infrastructures. As an employer, manager of assets and generator of income it fuels a significant sector of the economy. By mediating at such interfaces, charities contribute towards maintaining balance and equity in society.

Civil society and its limitations

A society may be civil but this provides no guarantee that it is either efficient or right. Social capital, shared values and a common purpose, voluntary activity and community development may each be either cause or effect of an engaged and coherent body politic while together they do not necessarily add up to a civil society.

Clearly a conflicted society such as presently exists among the Balkan nations, the Middle East and elsewhere cannot also be a civil society. It can, nevertheless, display some of the characteristics normally associated with the concept. It may have a strong sense of identity, its citizens may exercise mutual care, share common values and concerns, and a large proportion may be active volunteers demonstrably engaged in the life of that community (as is the case with religious cults). It may also, however, be politically polarized and confrontational in relation to neighbouring communities. Such communities are fundamentally flawed as an expression of civil society because they are totally member-benefit driven and their *raison d'être* is based on opposition to others.

Again, an inert society cannot also be civil. This may occur where a community operates as an integrated, coherent and caring entity but demonstrates a collective denial and lack of engagement in relation to the cause and effect of the conflict surrounding it. Many middle-class communities are often and rightly criticized for continuing to function in their own social bubbles insulated from any association with the problems affecting society as a whole. Such communities cannot claim the status of a civil society because they are member-benefit driven and can only function by denying the needs of their neighbours.

Increasingly in many modern western societies there are those who form affiliation groups which cross-cut the usual geographical and social divides. In societies where locality-based association is problematic, relationships can be quite satisfactorily initiated and maintained despite intervening distances. Most obviously, this is now frequently achieved through use of email. A rich subculture exists of people who do not share the same geographical or even social context but relate through a common interest via the Internet. These communities are very real and self-sustaining and have a claim to be considered as legitimate if narrow and attenuated expressions of civil society.

Civil society and societies in transition

Not all societies are civil and those that achieve that state do not necessarily remain in it. Those that are undemocratic, where there is no freedom to associate and no market economy and where control lies with a dictator or with a socialist collective are most clearly wholly outside the civil society model. This has been well illustrated by the eagerness with which so many nations in middle and eastern Europe, newly emerged from under the blanket of totalitarianism, have sought to build democratic institutions and attain the coveted recognition as a civil society. Others societies are either not coherent entities or not at a point where their development is susceptible to the influence of such a progressive concept. In regions where national boundaries do not coincide with the ethnicity of the population the countries concerned are particularly unstable. The recent experience of nations in the Balkans and the Middle East as earlier in the history of countries such as South Africa, Rwanda and Borneo can be cited as illustrative of the many such countries lacking the preconditions for establishing civil society.

As evidenced above, the status of civil society is largely politically determined. However, some societies may be largely civil in nature but experience fluctuations in whole or in part, which from time to time threatens the sustainability of their civil status. This may have its origins in a context outside the political control of the society in question, as is the case with the current experience in north-west Europe of economic migration from the poorer nations of the south.

Government, charities, charity law and civil society

Charities are viewed by government, for all the reasons noted above, as having significant potential to assist in the goal of achieving civil society. Their proven capacity to harness armies of committed volunteers, reach the socially marginalized and deliver public benefit outcomes provide convincing partnership credentials for a government tied to a policy of generating social capital, increasing community capacity and embedding a broad sense of civic responsibility. For any government seeking to engender and develop a sense of participative as well as representative democracy, charities are well placed to stimulate community involvement in local politics (see, also, chapter 5).

The pressing need to achieve harmony in the face of increasing diversity has recently prompted a number of governments to reflect on the potential bridging role of charities and ensure that by facilitating a better fit between charitable activity and social need, charity law thereby promotes the growth of civil society. The focus has tended to concentrate on the extent to which charity law could be reworked to promote a greater degree of congruity between the purposes of charities and the agenda of government. The central plank to any such happy marriage is the principle of 'public benefit'. Because charitable status is at all times dependent upon an ability to satisfy the 'public benefit' test, a charity law with a contemporary interpretation of this principle at its heart that addresses issues of social inclusion will necessarily be conducive to promoting a civil society.

The capacity of charity law to facilitate or impede the work of charities makes it crucially important to civil society. For all modern western societies this entails at least putting in place a legal framework for philanthropic intervention conducive to facilitating the social inclusion of such marginalized groups as the mentally ill, the disabled, disaffected youth, etc. Arguably, to be fit for the philanthropic challenges of the twenty-first century, any such framework must also extend to addressing the additional domestic and international aspects of social inclusion referred to above.

The charity law reviews

Charity law is largely administrative. Once the statutory framework is in place then, for the most part, it has fallen to government bodies rather than the courts to exercise such regulatory powers as may be available. On the rare occasions when matters of principle are brought before the courts then the common law roots of charity law have allowed the judiciary some leeway in their efforts to keep the law relevant to changing social circumstances. Generally, the governments of those modern western societies with a common law foundation have been slow to resort to legislation in order to realign charity law with its contemporary social context.

Charity, contemporary social need and the common law

Legislation, then, has not been the tool of choice for ensuring that charity law remains appropriately and sensitively attuned to the fluctuating manifestations of social need. By the end of the twentieth century there was increasing dissatisfaction in England and Wales, as elsewhere in the common law world, with a charity law based on a seventeenth-century perception of social conditions. The criticism included charges that it failed to provide either a definition of charity or a body of integrating principles and that the legacy of ancient precedents imposed limitations on the extent to which it could be adapted to meet the challenges of new forms of social need. It was claimed that leaving the law to be extended by analogy with established charitable purposes in response to the vagaries of causes randomly presented by litigants, instead of subjecting it to substantive legislative control, avoided the opportunity to ensure that it developed coherently. This necessarily resulted in the law having to focus on regulating and administering a motley collection of entities and their activities; unable to assert a formative role it was left to struggle with matters of process. The singular strength of the 1601 Act, its elasticity, enabling a responsive if not a directive approach to the activities of charities, had come to be viewed as a constraint. Across the common law world – in Canada,[4] Australia,[5] New Zealand,[6] Ireland[7], the US[8] and the UK[9] – a protracted period of charity law reform ensued.

The coincidence of relatively contemporaneous charity law reviews presents a unique opportunity for the common law world to collectively consider how reform could best contribute to the promotion of civil society within and between the different jurisdictions. At a minimum, the nations concerned might agree common indicators for domestic social inclusion, the wording of related provisions and the functions of tax revenue bodies. At best they could agree to a co-ordinated harmonization of the core legal functions, including definitional matters, that constitute contemporary charity law, so as to maximize future opportunities for their shared common law heritage to address issues of social inclusion and promote civil society on a national and international basis.

Common review themes as a template for comparative analysis

Several distinct themes emerge from the various reviews. These include a focus on definitional matters, a concern to balance the key components in the regulatory environment and an interest in increasing the capacity of charity law to address the contemporary social inclusion agenda. These themes, together with material from Part II, form the key components for constructing a template which is applied in Part IV to conduct a comparative study of contemporary charity law, policy and practice across a number of common law nations.

It has to be acknowledged, however, that constructing and then applying a standard template in a snapshot exercise across such diverse cultures is methodologically imperfect. Clearly all law must be contextualized and therefore appropriate context setting needs to be undertaken when profiling the regulatory environment of charitable activity in each jurisdiction, while allowing also for local developments occurring since this exercise began which may require template adjustments. Some account, for example, needs to be taken of the history of the nation concerned as regards issues of social inclusion and the development of related legislation, particularly charity law. Attention will also need to be given to such contemporary factors as the capacity of the charitable sector, the social circumstances of particular minority culture groups, the domestic social inclusion agenda, the related government policy and the current legislative framework. The blunt effect of categorizing a nation's law, policy and practice to fit template imperatives will need to be balanced as far as possible by a sensitivity to context matters.

Charity law and definitional matters

A particular trend can be detected in the charity law reviews: they all, though in varying degrees, give attention to definitional matters. This is clearly crucial: to define 'charity' and 'charitable purposes' is to define the parameters of the charitable sector; to thereby legally delineate the boundaries between charity and government is to suggest the terms of reference for future partnership arrangements between the sectors.

Charity and charitable purposes

There is widespread acknowledgement among the common law nations that the time has come to change the traditional definitional basis of charity law. They are demonstrating a new willingness to move towards basing the future development of charity law on statutory definitions or at least on a specification of matters that might constitute definitions.[10] Invariably this entails enlarging the existing range of charitable purposes by identifying new charities drawn from the cases currently emerging from within the fourth *Pemsel* head. The type of charitable purposes now listed for incorporation within a prospective new statutory definition provides tangible evidence of how the future common law framework for philanthropy will and will not address social inclusion issues.

Source of current definition

In all common law countries the *Pemsel* classification is the starting point for a definition of purposes deemed to be charitable. The definition will be satisfied if the purpose is exclusively charitable and fits under one of four heads: the relief of poverty, the advancement of education, the advancement of religion, and certain other purposes which cannot be accommodated within the first three. If a purpose cannot be defined as coming under one of the four heads it will nonetheless be construed as charitable if it can be interpreted as falling within the 'spirit or intendment' of the Preamble to the 1601 Act,[11] a rule that has been variously employed in the common law jurisdictions to extend the definition of 'charity' to address social inclusion issues.[12]

An ancillary issue is the nature of the agency that provides the definition. Most often but not always, in common law countries, the definition is tax driven and the agency responsible for determining charitable status is the one for collecting taxes and rates.

Elements of current definition and issues for the future

The essential elements in the common law definition of charity are well established, have subsisted for many years and are recognized as such, with some differences in emphasis, throughout the common law world. It has in particular been the breadth and constancy of their adherence to matters of definition that have enabled the common law nations over the centuries to draw from much the same pool of judicial precedents and develop their present shared understanding of charity law. This unique thread of cross-jurisdictional jurisprudence now offers the possibility of strategic concerted change to address the agenda of contemporary social inclusion issues that face the same nations. The corollary, however, is also true. This is a vulnerable thread and if one or more nations should choose to introduce statutory definitions at variance with established precedents and/or with such definitions introduced by others, then it is hard to see how the common law legacy can survive to provide a shared platform of charity law for the twenty-first century.

Charitable intent   The charitable intent of the donor is an all-important element. The judiciary in most of, but not all, common law jurisdictions applies an objective test to determine whether or not a gift satisfies the public benefit test and thereby qualifies as 'charitable'.[13] Should the objective test prevail?

Exclusively charitable   Case law in the common law jurisdictions has long established that for a trust to be charitable its purposes must be confined exclusively to charitable purposes. The attendant difficulty in distinguishing between a purpose that is merely ancillary to the charitable purpose as opposed to one that is itself a main purpose (e.g. fees for hospitals/schools) has attracted considerable judicial attention. The exclusivity of charitable purposes, however, continues to be a necessary component of charitable status, and in some jurisdictions this rule finds explicit legislative endorsement. Should a trust wholly fail to acquire charitable status because compromised in part?

Public benefit Interpreting this concept sufficiently broadly,[14] so that it remains responsive to pressures from an ever-changing social context, is the central challenge for charity law. In England and Wales, much work has been done in response to this challenge by the Charity Commission, while integrating altruism as a distinct test to be applied alongside public benefit has been usefully articulated in the Australian charity law review report. Should legislation ascribe this crucial test of charitable status a more exact meaning, weighting and uniform application?

Independent A charity is required under common law to be a free-standing, independent entity founded by and bound to fulfil the terms of the donor's gift. The duty resting on trustees to honour the terms of their trust and ensure that the objects of the charity prevail has always been seen as the primary means whereby the integrity of the donor's gift could be protected. Fulfilling this duty has required trustees to be resolutely committed to the charity's objects and free from any influence which may deflect from that focus: this is most clearly represented in the endowed foundation which, with its present and future funding secured and its management legally required to pursue certain charitable objectives, has the capacity to act independently. The rule is most often confined to trust law and can give rise to inflexibility – the dead hand of the donor ruling from the grave. Should the rule be placed firmly on a legislative basis with mandatory and comprehensive effect?

Non-governmental The distinction between the public benefit activities of government and charities in addressing issues of social inclusion is not always clear-cut (see, also, chapter 5). The above rule, regarding the need for charities to maintain their independence does, however, require that they do not become merely 'an arm of government'. Different jurisdictions have developed different methods of managing this interface. The extent to which governments and charities can forge a real partnership, allowing for genuine autonomy and mutual criticism, will be critical for their future capacity to address social inclusion issues. Should any future statutory definition exclude bodies that are not independent from the State?

Non-profit distributing A charity does not compromise its standing by making a profit. Entering fully into the commercial market place by engaging in trading, competitive practices, mergers and management takeovers, etc., has become a modern necessity for many charities. The recent emergence of social entrepreneurs in the field of charitable activity owes much to the available profit-making margins. It is, however, of crucial importance that any profit gained does not accrue to the benefit of individuals but is directed towards the fulfilment of the charity's objects. Is this rule currently treated with sufficient understanding and compliance so as not to require prescriptive legislative provisions?

Non-political A common law characteristic of charities, which has attracted attention in all modern charity law reviews, is the restraint on their freedom to engage in political activity. Initially interpreted as an embargo on party political campaigning by charities, this characteristic has developed to the point where it is now no longer certain to what extent, if any, charities may lobby for change in social conditions and/or government policies without compromising their charitable status. Given that effective intervention on social inclusion issues will always necessarily involve assertive advocacy and lobbying for change in law and policy, it is of considerable importance that charities are in future legally enabled to do so. Does the law require a statutory clarification of the distinction between party political involvement by voluntary organizations, and advocacy for social/political change on behalf of the disadvantaged, and the implications for the charitable status of both?

Structures for charitable activity

In the common law jurisdictions, charitable activity is housed in a range of different structures. Being public benefit organizations, charities are usually readily distinguished, sometimes legislatively, from mutual benefit bodies such as Industrial and Provident Societies, Friendly Societies and co-operatives and other bodies such as trade unions and political parties; though in the UK, some old and large charities such as the older universities and religious organizations are also outside the charity law framework. There are issues arising as to the future basis for and significance of any distinction between charities and other public benefit or not-for-profit entities. There may also be issues regarding the type of charitable vehicle, such as hospital foundations, that are best suited or are to be permitted to convey charitable activity, and issues as to their relative effectiveness in relation to questions of social inclusion.

Perhaps the most significant pressure on modern charities, with implications for appropriate structure, is their need to operate within a competitive commercial environment. Some, such as schools and hospitals, have a pressing need for access to capital; this may, as is often the case in the US, force them to become for-profit organizations in order to access the equity markets. For many commercial pressure means launching their organization from the outset as a company, for others it means changing their legal status from unincorporated association or charitable trust to a limited company. In all common law jurisdictions, charities find themselves being increasingly governed by a weight of company law.

Types of charitable structures

A variety of different types of legal vehicle are usually available to further the work of charities. It is difficult to construe each type of vehicle as being of equal standing in terms of relative capacity to represent the ethos of charity and ability to give full and unqualified effect to charitable purposes. Arguably, there is a distinction to be drawn between those vehicles which derive wholly from a charity and would not exist if it were not for the need to give effect to that charity's purpose; the charitable gift/activity, resulting from a voluntary gesture, came first. The trust, unincorporated association and incorporated company would come into such a category. Then there are a number of secondary vehicles whose activities may well be charitable but may not necessarily be established for such purposes, or be exclusively or indefinitely charitable; the authorizing body, obliged to provide such a vehicle, came first. Into this category fall a range of government public benefit service institutions such as hospitals, universities, leisure centres, etc., and also, perhaps, many religious organizations. Finally, there are new vehicles such as types of foundations and perhaps Incorporated Charitable Organizations (as proposed in Scotland) which differ from both previous categories by being designed specifically and solely to give effect to charitable purposes. All three categories, needless to say, differ from other not-for-profit and mutual benefit vehicles such as an Industrial and Provident Society or Friendly Society (though both may, occasionally, be charities), co-operative or trade union, etc.

Some common law jurisdictions classify charities as either private foundations or public charities. Public charities include schools, hospitals, churches and any other charities that receive their financial support from a broad group of donors or patrons. Private foundations, which have not traditionally conducted direct charitable activities, receive their financial support from the endowment of a single individual or family.

A modern regulatory environment for charities

The Charitable Uses Act 1601 was the first legislative attempt to regulate charities and their activities and this served as a baseline for the creation of a regulatory environment for all common law nations. In the UK, as elsewhere, it was not until the enactment of nineteenth-century statutes that effective regulatory provisions of a general nature began to be introduced. Since then, while the balance struck between support and inspection has varied across the common law jurisdictions, they have mostly moved towards putting in place the same basic institutional components. Where they differ is in the extent to which in constructing a modern regulatory environment they make provision for mechanisms that protect, support and positively reinforce opportunities for the further development of charitable purposes.

Registration functions

Registering charities and regulating their activities are two distinct sets of functions, though they may be legislatively assigned to the same government body. Some countries make no statutory provision for the registration of charities. In most countries there is one government body, usually the agency responsible for collecting tax revenues, that keeps a register of all 'live' charities.

Statutory process

Where a common law jurisdiction, such as England and Wales, has a statutory requirement that a central register be maintained, this duty will be assigned to a specific government body which will then at least list all charities that have their headquarters within that jurisdiction. The classification system used in any system of registration, which can be a significant means of establishing the relevance of charities for social inclusion in that jurisdiction, usually provides minimal information including name, address of headquarters, organizational structure, primary charitable purpose and contact information regarding the executive officers. The government body authorized to maintain such a register is usually also required to first examine an organization's founding documents to establish its charitable status before entering it in the register of charities. Registration may also impose duties on the registered charity such as an obligation to submit annual financial accounts and perhaps an activity report.

In addition, charities will often have to meet registration requirements under such other legislation as company law.

Voluntary process

In some common law jurisdictions, such as Ireland, there is no statutory requirement for the particulars of an organization to be entered in a register of charities, though they may well have to submit to the registration requirements of company law. Instead, as a means of facilitating the voluntary and community sector, an umbrella organization may elect to compile such a register. In such circumstances, where there is no legal onus on a charity to register as such, the database is often incomplete and/or out of date and unreliable in terms of legal status.

Regulatory functions

Charity law, at least within jurisdictions such as Ireland and England and Wales that remain wedded to the trust model (the US, New Zealand and Australia being based more on the corporate model), treads an uneasy path between leaning in favour of recognizing the philanthropic intentions of a donor and seeking to ensure that his or her gift is properly applied. The traditional protective role of the Attorney General as guardian of charities is maintained in most common law jurisdictions. Although this office does maintain an overview of charities and their activities, while retaining a pivotal role in the commencement of any proceedings relating to them, for most practical purposes its functions in this context have become more symbolic than regulatory in nature.

As a means of reinforcing the probity of charitable organizations, legislation is often introduced to provide the powers necessary to regulate those bodies which receive and use charitable donations. At the very least, due to the fact that the law governing charities in the common law jurisdictions is fundamentally tax driven, statutory provision is invariably made for the government agency with tax revenue responsibilities to determine the tax exemption eligibility of organizations claiming charitable status. The further step of establishing an independent body at 'arm's length' from tax collection and introducing the statutory provisions and mechanisms necessary for it to enforce probity, require transparency and accountability, to set and monitor standards in respect of charities and further the development of charitable purposes, is not adopted in all common law jurisdictions.

In some jurisdictions, instead of a specific body being statutorily assigned the duty to determine charitable status, a number of different bodies may be involved without the benefit of one definitive checklist of criteria for determining such status.

Charitable status and fundraising/trading

The common law jurisdictions invariably provide a statutory framework for regulating the fundraising activities of charities. As the accompanying legislative intent is focused on identifying and proscribing fraud and other forms of abuse, the provisions tend to be generally applicable to public donations and simply include charities among all other organizations engaged in eliciting funds from the general public for 'good causes' by such means as raffles, church collections, house-to-house or street collections. These traditional forms of fundraising are now supplemented by more professional and entertaining fundraising techniques including national lotteries and telethons. Laws governing fundraising tend to focus on process and procedures with the issue of permits designating collectors, collecting points and methods of collection. Enforcement, with the exception of national lotteries, tends to be mainly through the normal criminal law proceedings relating to theft, fraud and embezzlement.

Trading, in common law jurisdictions, is not itself a charitable purpose though charities can and do undertake trading activity in furtherance of their primary purposes. In the UK charities will most often set up a subsidiary company to undertake trading on its behalf and to which any after-tax profits will be returned for expenditure on its charitable purposes. The relevant regulatory provisions focus on ensuring that trading is not compromising an organization's charitable status, determining eligibility for tax exemption on trading profits and on the post-tax use of those profits.

National laws regulating fundraising/trading are not usually susceptible to analysis on the basis of a differentiating application to charitable purposes nor as regards whether the latter are domestic or international in nature.

Charitable status and tax/revenue collection

As well as having responsibility for granting or refusing charitable exemption from tax liability in accordance with common law principles and contemporary legislation, the government agency responsible for tax collection may also play a limited regulatory role in checking that income has, in fact, been applied exclusively for charitable purposes (or indeed applied at all rather than left to accumulate).

Revenue agency with sole responsibility for determining charitable status

Where this agency is the sole government body involved in regulating charities then it will in effect determine charitable status and its *raison d'être* of maximizing tax revenue returns will inevitably restrain its discretionary capacity to extend the boundaries of eligibility for charitable status. The onus is then left on any organization seeking registration to challenge that agency, perhaps through the courts, to expand its interpretation of 'charity' to include the objects and activities of that organization. In such circumstances the primary means of adjusting charitable purposes to facilitate their capacity to address the contemporary social inclusion agenda is by legislative manipulation of the exemptions and incentives provided through the tax framework and the rules governing fundraising.

The tax regime is the cutting edge of any government policy governing the relationship between charity law and social inclusion. Whether the goal is to assist charities in general and/or to favour those whose activities comply with its current policy, it will be implemented through the government's explicit or implied tax exemption incentives; not just income tax, but VAT, rates and customs and excise duty. Enabling provisions may be introduced to favour donor's gifts, overseas aid, etc., while disincentives may be applied in other areas. Personal, company and institutional donor tax incentives reveal whether domestic and/or overseas charitable activity is being promoted and sometimes even indicates the intended nature of the activity and/or the circumstances to be addressed. Modern western societies have developed sophisticated tax regimes, intensively managed and often subject to annual legislative revision, in which a government's social inclusion commitment can be thematically tracked over time.

Charities may also be subject to the revenue collection functions and related inspectoral powers of other government bodies such as those responsible for determining the rateable valuation of property and the annual rates payable. Again, the government body exercising powers to collect custom and excise payments on the import and export of goods may well have cause to inspect the bona fides of an organization claiming exemption from liability on the grounds of charitable status.

Charitable status and philanthropic purposes; the courts and the Attorney General

In all common law jurisdictions, the ultimate default mechanism for regulating charities, controlling their activities and broadening the range of charitable purposes is provided by the court system. In addition, judicial capacity in this area has been significantly reinforced by widespread national adherence to the European Convention for the Protection of Human Rights and Fundamental Freedoms 1950 (see, also, chapter 7). However, the accompanying expense, bad publicity and nature of litigated issues results in this forum now having random and infrequent opportunities to exercise a regulatory influence.

Again, in theory, the powers of the ancient *parens patriae* jurisdiction (see, also, chapter 3) vested in the Attorney General, as protector of charities, should provide significant authority for the protection and development of charities and their purposes. Instead, the office of Attorney General has become of marginal significance for charities.

Charitable status and philanthropic purposes; administrative bodies

Some common law jurisdictions have in place a government body (or quasi-government body), alongside but independent of the tax authority, which is vested with statutory powers and duties that balance, to a varying degree, support and regulatory functions. The remit of this agency in relation to the courts and the tax authority is of central importance.

There are those jurisdictions, such as Ireland, in which the functions of such an agency are explicitly supportive rather than supervisory. The tax authority is viewed and empowered to act as gatekeeper to the acquisition of charitable status and accompanying tax exemptions, thereby leaving the support agency free to promote good practice, facilitate good governance, assist organizations to become formally established within an appropriate legal framework and to provide advice and guidance on matters such as trusteeship and *cy-près* schemes. Such services are usually made available on demand, the agency having little or no responsibility to be proactive and usually very little capacity to direct change. As all statutory responsibility relating to charitable status remains with the tax authority, the support agency has virtually no capacity to address newly emerging social inclusion issues.

A distinctively different regulatory model is in place in England and Wales (see, also, chapters 5 and 8). There the Charity Commission – while vested with registration, supervisory and support functions – is also legislatively positioned alongside but independent of the Inland Revenue to determine purposes and activities that constitute or cease to constitute charitable status. This body requires all charities to keep proper accounts and, unless excepted or exempted on the grounds of having an annual income of less than £10,000, they are all subject to accounting and auditing regulations. In jurisdictions without any equivalent to the Charity Commission, where the regulatory framework is applied through the tax/revenue collection agencies, there can be a lack of financial transparency and regulation particularly as regards unincorporated associations.

The Commission is also vested with powers which in other common law nations continue to constitute the jurisdiction traditionally associated with the powers of the High Court in relation to charities. Sufficient powers have been transferred from the latter to permit the Commission to exercise a judicial remit in matters such as arbitrating issues of charitable status, the creation of *cy-près* schemes, etc.

Depending on the legal structure adopted, charities may also be accountable to a professional regulatory body for its standards of practice. In the UK, most obviously, if registered as a company, a charity will be required to file with the Companies Registry an annual certified statement of accounts and its management and governance structures may be open to inspection.

Charitable status and crime

In all jurisdictions the police have a role in regulating the activities of charities. In any case where there is a suspicion that a criminal offence (for example, fraud, theft, obtaining money under false pretences) has been committed by or against a charity or its trustees, or by any body or person falsely claiming to be a charity, this is automatically dealt with by the police under the general criminal law. Similarly, where there may be a violation of standard commercial regulations or anti-trust laws etc., the police will investigate and prosecute as necessary. In addition, the issuing of permits for permission to carry out fundraising collections is most usually the responsibility of this agency. The capacity of the police service to influence the response of charities to the contemporary social inclusion agenda is virtually non-existent as it is confined to the prevention/detection/investigation of abuse wherever this occurs.

Constraints on modern philanthropic activity

Common law countries, in varying degrees, share a common colonial history derived from their having constituted a part of the British Empire. Consequently, while each country has its own unique historical experience they often have a similar legacy of indigenous ethnic groups that require distinctive need-sensitive strategies to facilitate their future inclusion. In addition, the range of contemporary social problems affecting many common law nations is largely similar, with much the same issues appearing on what is a relatively shared social inclusion agenda. The challenge for philanthropy and therefore also for the law is to respond appropriately to the social circumstances of minority culture groups (e.g. the indigenous people of Australia and Canada) and to the contemporary domestic social inclusion agenda (e.g. the disabled, elderly, mentally ill, disaffected youth, etc.). The modern cultural context of each nation may also differ in many respects from the others but the main constraints on the potential capacity of philanthropic activity to address such issues again remain broadly similar.

Policy constraints: partnership with government

The public benefit principle, underpinning charity law in all common law jurisdictions, has become the basis for a widespread contemporary policy whereby government seeks to share with charities the responsibility for public service provision, particularly in the areas of education, social services and health care. This has proved problematic for charities. One consequence of being enticed into such 'partnerships', or becoming ensnared in the 'creeping contract culture' phenomenon, is that charities necessarily have to compromise their independence by accepting government priority setting and directing their resources towards the alleviation of government-defined need (see, further, chapter 5). The option of not co-operating with government can also carry serious risks. Government funding now provides the main source of income for many charities and to avoid that source in today's very competitive environment, as many charities have discovered, is to jeopardize financial viability and be exposed to possible liquidation or a hostile takeover. As the locus for determining public benefit moves more within government control so there is a risk of a proportionate diminution in the probability of charities independently championing the cause of dissident socially marginalized groups.

International charitable activity

The provision of aid to developing countries, or indeed to any country in need, is usually a matter on which government and charities work in tandem. However, this arrangement has arguably undergone a considerable shift in the post-9/11 world of geopolitics. Government aid is now conditional upon the recipient government conforming to an approved democratic model that is judged likely to foster the growth of civil society. The UN Millennium Development project,[15] for example, is increasingly being delivered by western nations on this basis. Charities are coming under increasing government pressure to be similarly discerning in their choice of resource input. The threat posed by international terrorism (see, further, pp. 43–4, 377) is prompting governments to constrain the discretion of international charities.

Common law constraints

In addition to the constraints imposed by its traditional definition (the 'spirit and intendment' rule and the four *Pemsel* heads) as outlined above, the development of philanthropy in common law countries has also tended to be restricted by other aspects of their shared charity law heritage (see, further, chapter 4). Some of these constraints are legal functions, others are rules or presumptions, which form part of the regulatory environment and impact negatively on the capacity of charity law to address the contemporary social inclusion agenda. The following are examples of ways in which residual effects of the common law legacy continue to so influence the application of charity law across the common law world; these are examined in more detail, as they apply to particular jurisdictions, in Part IV.

High Court jurisdiction

The common law is judge-made law and the development of principles and practice in charity law as in all other areas under that jurisprudential umbrella has always been dependent upon the type and frequency of cases appearing in court. The *parens patriae* jurisdiction having devolved to the High Court, it is there rather than in the lower courts that proceedings relating to charity matters are heard, usually after receiving the imprimatur of the Attorney General. The expense, the length of proceedings and the risk of attracting unwelcome publicity have combined to greatly reduce recourse to the High Court on such matters across the common law nations.

Legal structures

Charitable trusts, providing the basic legal structure for giving effect to charitable gifts since well before the 1601 Act, were transferred with the common law to become ubiquitous throughout the common law world. In some jurisdictions, however, this legacy of dependency on trusts has since been legislatively corrected (see, further, Part IV).

Most usually set within unincorporated associations, trusts have over the centuries been supplemented but never wholly replaced by other structures (see, also, chapter 3). The need to minimize personal liability has, in recent decades, resulted in charities seeking the protective shell of incorporation. Similarly, the need to protect a charity's independence and provide for its future financial security (thereby insulating it from the pressures of fundraising, tendering for government contracts and otherwise having to compete in the market place), have boosted the popularity of the endowed foundation (see, further, chapter 3). Otherwise there has not been much experimentation with new legal structures, at least not in the UK, that might offer better ways of delivering resources in accordance with the public benefit principle.

The restrictions on advocacy, political activity, etc.

The traditional common law constraint on advocacy and political activity as a charitable purpose has become a serious obstacle to effective philanthropic intervention in a modern social inclusion context. Modern society has come to rely upon multimedia representation of issues, which makes it particularly difficult when organizations, specifically set up to address some aspect of social disadvantage, cannot use the media to campaign for the changes in policy or law they believe would alleviate that disadvantage.

Fiscal issues

As mentioned above and in earlier chapters, government interest in charity has since at least the Statute of Charitable Uses 1601 been primarily concerned to limit the opportunities available for donors and organizations to use it as a pretext to avoid paying tax.

Revenue driven While policy and legislative intent have focused on identifying and proscribing fraud and other forms of illegal practice occasionally associated with the margins of charitable activity, governments have tended to sidestep any explicit commitment to formulating a basis for the further development of the charities sector as a whole. Instead, almost invariably in common law nations, the gateway to charitable status and accompanying tax exemptions has usually been entrusted to the government body assigned to maximize the return of tax revenues due to the State.

The doctrine of cy-près   Another standard feature of charity law as experienced by common law nations has been the role played by the *cy-près* doctrine (see, also, chapter 3). Again, this power originated essentially in the legislative intent to restrict the common law abuse of charities and the misuse of their assets and it devolved eventually from the courts of equity to the High Court. This default mechanism, allowing the terms of a charitable trust to be varied and the assets of a failed charity or charitable gift to be applied for purposes commensurate with the initial charitable intention, is of considerable importance.

Trading etc.   The capacity of charities to engage in ongoing revenue-raising activities has always attracted considerable government interest (as illustrated above in relation to fundraising, donor-incentive schemes and general eligibility for tax exemption) again with a definite emphasis on reducing opportunities for abuse. This approach would seem to have extended to policing the nature, extent and profits of any trading undertaken by charities (see, further, chapter 4).

Public benefit matters

Leaving aside the definitional aspects of the public benefit test which have so exercised the nations involved in charity law review processes, there are other matters associated with this test which act to constrain the activities of charities. Some of these are generally applicable, such as the uneven application of the public benefit test across the four *Pemsel* heads and the fact that the test excludes matters that would clearly be to the public benefit, such as addressing the causes instead of just the effects of poverty, while others vary from one jurisdiction to the next.

The legal presumption favouring religion   The common law courts were traditionally the enforcing mechanism for the King's decrees and the natural defender of the institutions of the State. For charity law in the UK, this resulted in a legal presumption that gifts to the Church (meaning the Protestant Church following the Reformation) and by extension in due course to other religious organizations were for the public benefit as were any activities they chose to undertake. This presumption has enabled religious organizations to accumulate, over the centuries, vast amounts of property and other forms of wealth. In the present ever more secular society typical of common law nations the fact that a charity is a religious organization, or the nature of that religion, can be an obstacle to accepting assistance. In some common law jurisdictions, notably Northern Ireland, where communities are divided and mutually antagonistic on the basis of differing religious affiliations, it is questionable whether gifts to religious organizations can satisfy the public benefit test. In circumstances where religion is itself a divisive and polarizing influence it manifestly cannot promote social inclusion and at least to that extent the continuation of the presumption may represent a serious constraint on potential philanthropic activity (see, further, chapter 3).

The legal presumption favouring the donor's intent   The common law held that a donor's charitable intent should be interpreted subjectively, the public benefit presumed (i.e. if a charitable intention was expressed or could be inferred then it was a valid charitable gift) and the gift applied in the terms as indicated by the donor. In some common law jurisdictions, such as the UK, this presumption has been displaced by an objective test (i.e. the courts will look to the nature of the gift) and if on rational analysis the gift is incompatible with the public benefit then no expressed or implied intentions of the donor will suffice to make it charitable; as illustrated by the 'anti-vivisection cases'.[16] Arguably, if the social inclusion agenda and charity law are to be aligned along an axis defined by the public benefit principle then the validity of the latter can only be determined in accordance with specified indicators and applied objectively.

Modern law constraints

The fact that philanthropic intervention in relation to social inclusion issues is constrained by aspects of contemporary charity law, in addition to constraints derived from its common law origins, has been explored above and in earlier chapters (see, in particular, chapter 4). The following are some primary examples, drawn from earlier material, of ways in which the functions of modern charity law are currently inhibiting such intervention; again, these are examined in more detail as they apply to particular jurisdictions in Part IV.

Forum for developing charitable purposes

In those common law nations lacking a forum with powers of inquiry and adjudication equivalent to those of the High Court, which for reasons stated above has become less relevant, charity law has failed to respond to the pressures from the contemporary social inclusion agenda. Moreover, in the post-9/11 world, the stringency with which the tax authority customarily views claims for charitable exemption have probably become even more rigorous as the activities of all organizations representing or associated with the grievances of a socially marginalized group fall under increasing government surveillance.

Human rights legislation

In recent years most governments of common law nations have moved to either ratify and incorporate in domestic legislation the provisions of the European Convention for the Protection of Human Rights and Fundamental Freedoms 1950 (see, further, chapter 7) or to largely replicate its main provisions in national legislation. Consequently, certainly in Europe, there is now an onus on all courts and other public bodies to ensure that, in their dealings with charities, the charitable purposes and actual practice of the latter are Convention compliant. For example, the entitlement to charitable status of an organization engaged in activities for the advancement of religion will have to be proofed against Article 9, which deals with the right to freedom of thought, conscience and religion, while if the activities are for the advancement of education then compliance with Article 2 of the First Protocol, dealing with the right to education, will be required. As is pointed out in Tudor, there is also potential for a fundamental difficulty in squaring the public benefit principle of charity law with the Convention's non-discrimination principle in Articles 9, 11 and in particular Article 14:[17]

> future decisions may hold that the public benefit test is only non-discriminatory if it abandons differentiation based on the four heads of charity and moves to a position where there is an assumption that existing charitable purposes are for the public benefit unless the contrary is shown and that all new purposes must prove public benefit.

Arguably, the public benefit principle and indeed the concept of 'charity' itself are both essentially founded on a legal right to positively discriminate in favour of a sector of the public and by so doing the organization concerned becomes eligible for positive discriminatory treatment at the hands of the taxing authority. It remains to be seen to what extent Convention rights, in the new and uncertain world of anti-terrorism legislation, affect the application of charity law to social inclusion issues in the common law jurisdictions.

Anti-terrorism legislation

In response to the United Nations Security Council Resolution 1373, most common law nations and others have in recent years introduced anti-terrorism legislation. New powers requiring the registration of non-government organizations and permitting covert surveillance of their funds, activities and staff have sometimes been accompanied by other new police powers of arrest and deportation. This has contributed to the growth of a climate of insecurity among organizations working with socially marginalized groups. Where these powers are seen to be used mostly in relation to groups of a particular ethnicity/cultural orientation this naturally exacerbates the latter's perception of alienation from the State and greatly increases the gap between philanthropic resources and the needs of the socially marginalized.

Conclusion

Common law nations have for centuries shared substantially the same body of charity law. They now also share some of the same social inclusion issues resulting from their colonial heritage and much the same domestic agenda of issues relating to the needs of disadvantaged groups such as the elderly, the disabled, mentally ill, disaffected youth, etc. Many of these nations are conducting charity law reviews. The outcome of the various review processes is likely to be legislation that will establish the first statutory definitions of 'charity' and 'the public benefit' and form the legal framework for future philanthropic activity. While each of the nations concerned is naturally focused on the quite separate reform of the law in their particular jurisdiction, that law in fact derives and remains conceptually inseparable from the inherited body of common law. To a large extent, the shared experience of the common law nations is now being used to reshape that body of charity law for future generations.

Given the close interrelationship between charity law, philanthropy, social inclusion and civil society, it is possible that these reviews offer a real window of opportunity to identify and co-ordinate the components of a legal framework conducive to consolidating civil society within individual nations and across the common law world. It is certain that it makes this an opportune time to undertake a baseline study of the similarities and differences in relevant aspects of charity law within key representative common law nations. In the post-9/11 world, the rush to man barricades to protect the western world from terrorism must be balanced with measures that address the cause as well as the effects of the alienation that produces the terrorists. Creating the right regulatory environment for the future mediatory intervention of philanthropic organizations could make a significant contribution towards promoting civil society within and between nations.

This chapter has sought to prepare the ground for such a study by drawing from material explored in Part II and from themes evident in the charity law reviews to identify the main functions of the law relating to charity within a common law context and to examine their significance for philanthropic intervention on issues of social inclusion. This sifting process has disclosed and considered a range of characteristics that seem to constitute, in varying degrees, the main elements of charity law within the common law nations. These include key definitional matters and legal structures for charitable activity, registration and regulatory processes, the institutional framework of courts, tax authorities and charity support agencies, etc. It has also identified certain prevailing aspects of the common law and modern law that currently constrain philanthropic intervention on social inclusion issues.

Pulling together this material makes it possible to design a template consisting of the main legal functions in charity law as they relate to social inclusion and as perceived from the heartland of the common law. The template, appropriately customized and contextualized to fit distinctive jurisdiction-specific characteristics, can then be applied to the countries selected for study to establish how each uses charity law to address issues of social inclusion and thereby permit a level of comparative analysis. This is the work undertaken in the following chapters of Part IV.

Chapter 7

International benchmarks for charity law as it relates to social inclusion

Introduction

This chapter looks outside the particular charity law experience of common law nations to identify principles and standards of a more general nature, established on an international basis in recent years, which have acquired the standing of legal 'grundnorms' or benchmarks for law and practice and, arguably, should have a direct bearing on charity law as it relates to social inclusion within those nations. International conventions and related case law are now rapidly promoting a harmonization of principles, policy and practice across many countries. A new jurisprudential floor is being gradually put in place to uniformly strengthen national laws including the law relating to charity in common law nations. The identification of key benchmarks in international law permits an analysis of their application in the context of national charity law and a comparative assessment of national differences in law and practice, insofar as they influence issues of social inclusion. In that way it makes an important contribution to constructing a research template for use in examining and comparing the jurisdictions selected for study in Part IV.

The chapter begins with a review of the different frames of reference that govern State intervention in relation to the circumstances of the socially marginalized. It notes that philanthropy is only one of a number of modes of intervention and may be neither appropriate nor likely to be effective in certain circumstances; much depends on the status of the recipients and the philanthropic model that is used. It then identifies the particular international legal instruments that provide and generate the benchmarks or external reference points for contemporary philanthropy. Of these the European Convention for the Protection of Human Rights and Fundamental Freedoms 1950 (the 'European Convention') is by far the most influential and is reinforced by a swathe of legal mechanisms put in place by the United Nations to monitor and enforce human rights. The chapter, therefore, focuses mainly on relevant principles emerging from the case law of the European Court of Human Rights (ECHR). Consideration is also given to other international conventions and protocols with relevance for specific minority groups. The chapter concludes by reflecting on the broad significance of internationally recognized legal principles, particularly those now being generated by the European Convention, for the future of charity law, policy and practice.

Law, philanthropy and social inclusion: frames of reference

The State can address rights relating to social inclusion within several quite different though often interconnecting legal frames of reference, hierarchically graded and conferring a greater or lesser status upon the subject, that have been in use for centuries. While all other frames of reference have a relevance and importance, which in practice will often usefully supplement the charitable or philanthropic common law model of intervention and may in some circumstances offer a more appropriate alternative, it is this model which is the present focus of interest. Arguably, however, they all ultimately rest on the same basic set of legal requirements.

Public/private law: a juridical entity

Such authority as may be needed to address the circumstances of the socially excluded, however defined, must come from public law through appropriate legal functions and be directed at a specified juridical entity. All frames of reference for such intervention – whether by public body, a State or international body – require much the same set of conditions if they are to be lawfully mandated.

Juridical entity

A prerequisite for authorized consensual intervention in the affairs of the socially excluded, is that the latter falls within a category that is recognized by the law of the intervening State or international body. The lawful use of such authority, in terms of powers, duties and areas of discretionary decision-making, requires as a bare minimum the existence of a juridical entity upon which the law can focus. The frame of reference available will to a large extent be determined by how that entity is defined by the law of the intervening party. If it is recognized as already fully independent and vested with autonomous rights and powers then first party negotiations between sovereign powers is indicated. If it is a recognized entity and further rights and duties can be conferred upon it, then a relationship offering enhanced protection and legal status can be negotiated. If, on the other hand, it is not a recognized entity (e.g. asylum seekers in some jurisdictions) or is, but has no ascribed legal attributes (wards of court and the *parens patriae* role of the King in mediaeval England) then it is left wholly dependent upon the intervening party's acts of discretion. This intervention spectrum may be seen as having treaties at one end, with parity of status for both parties, and the traditional common law model of charity at the other with its characteristic supplicant/benefactor relationship.

Treaties

The State may negotiate a formal treaty with an indigenous ethnic minority in a process which ascribes, or implies, sovereign status to the group concerned. This frame of reference signifies at least a notional parity of legal status between the parties, demonstrates the level of respect and confidence with which the State regards that minority and empowers the latter to negotiate from a position of strength on behalf of the claims, needs and aspirations of their community. The concept of 'internal sovereignty' – by which the State acknowledges that territorial and other rights inherently vest in an indigenous people – is a legal mechanism of uncertain dimensions and burdened with colonial connotations but one that has proved an effective means of recognizing the cultural integrity, autonomy and the rights of a minority group. It has been employed by the State to address, for example, the position of some native Indian tribes in the US and perhaps most convincingly the position of the Maori in New Zealand.

This point is equally well made by its corollary that when a State declines to afford any such recognition to an indigenous ethnic minority then the latter's lack of any legal status enables that State to treat it with impunity. The decision, for example, to treat Australia as *terra nullius*, meaning that it was either uninhabited or occupied only by nomadic people without any organized social systems, allowed the land and its indigenous people to be simply taken into the possession of the Crown.[1] Thereafter the 'Aboriginal people of Australia', devoid of juridical recognition, were left wholly dependent upon the authority, discretionary and gratuitous, exercised by the Crown.

The Maori of New Zealand

New Zealand and Australia, together with their indigenous inhabitants, were 'discovered' by the same intervening authority and at much the same time, but Crown treatment of the former contrasts sharply with its casual disregard of the aboriginal presence in Australia. The established culture, structured society and settled, organized way of life of the Maori earned them recognition as a juridical entity and they were treated as a sovereign power.

The Treaty of Waitangi 1840 is the founding constitutional document in New Zealand and has the status of a compact between the Crown and the Maori. It promised that Maori cultural values would be respected and given effect and that the Maori would participate fully in the new society of New Zealand and its institutions.[2] As a consequence of their status as Treaty signatories, this indigenous group has been able to preserve its cultural identity and coherence while in recent years it has exercised considerable influence over government policy in relation to issues affecting Maori interests.

International, subject-specific, protective legislation

International politics may dictate that the needs of a specific class of socially disadvantaged people are such that it should be singled out for special protection in legislative provisions that offer a form of positive discrimination. Again this frame of reference is evident in relation to indigenous people[3] but is also apparent in respect of such other groups as children.[4]

The United Nations Convention on the Rights of the Child (UNCRC) 1989

One of several conventions that have contributed to the building of an international framework of rights for children,[5] the UNCRC has been signed by nearly 200 countries, lists 42 substantive rights that comprehensively address the needs of children and requires the courts to ensure that decisions broadly comply with the general and specific obligations as set out in it. While the Convention has no specifically designated enforcement mechanism, the UN Committee on the Rights of the Child does make recommendations for improvements in national law and practice on the basis of reports required to be filed with it.

The social justice paradigm

Then there is the social justice paradigm, which requires universal standards of equity, equality and non-discrimination to be entrenched in legislation, applied uniformly across society, largely through the procedures and practice of government agencies with a right of recourse to the courts. This approach is most apparent in national legislation dealing, for example, with civil liberties and freedom of information.

Equal opportunities and non-discrimination legislation

In recent decades, all modern western societies have been putting into place much the same raft of legislation to ensure the provision of equal opportunities for all citizens regardless of factors such as gender and age. The prohibition of discrimination is now to be found in many national laws which apply similar principles in relation specifically to disability, race, religion or belief, sexual orientation, equal pay and fair employment, etc., require more general social legislation to be proofed against those principles and provide for an independent overview by regulatory bodies, commissions or tribunals coupled with power of referral to the court. It is an approach that allows and requires situations of injustice to be remedied.

The legal rights paradigm

In contrast to the blanket safety net of social justice provisions but complementary to it, the legal rights approach provides for assertive action in the courts by individuals for alleged breach of specific rights as established in national legislation and/or in international conventions. Both approaches represent the development of a relatively recent rights-sensitive culture due to a broad recognition of past systemic abuse in the nations concerned and a shared awareness of the need to cultivate the conditions for the growth of civil society.

Human rights

As explained in greater detail below, the rights embodied in the European Convention for the Protection of Human Rights and Fundamental Freedoms 1950, while automatically binding upon all 25 member states of the European Union, are also equally binding upon the many other nations that have elected to endorse the Convention (currently 46 countries have signed). The European Court of Human Rights provides the forum for adjudicating on alleged breaches of an individual's rights and a source of principles to guide practice in member states. The legal rights approach, while providing remedies for individual rather than situational injustice, also, necessarily, contributes to reinforcing the currency of human rights norms and to the building of human rights-compliant practice.

The philanthropic paradigm

Finally, there is the charity or philanthropy paradigm by which the law enables discretionary gifts or activities for public benefit purposes. This feature of democratic societies is now broadly given effect on a structured basis through either the civil code or the common law model of charity law and is usually but by no means exclusively associated with legislative provisions framed to ameliorate the need of those whose social disadvantage has its roots in poverty.

Philanthropy, public law and charitable organizations

Philanthropy, in the common law tradition, has its origins in the charitable trust and retains some of the characteristic features of the private law of trusts. It also continues to carry vestiges of the traditional model of charity which rested on private acts of gratuitous benevolence favouring particular impoverished or otherwise dependent persons. However, charity law has long since placed philanthropy firmly in a public law context. As Mummery LJ has pointed out:[6]

> Under English law, charity has always received special treatment. It often takes the form of a trust, but it is a public trust for the promotion of purposes beneficial to the community, not a trust for private individuals.

Whereas acts of charity may well be, and perhaps most often are, located in the nexus of personal relationships and therefore remain susceptible to private law, charitable purposes and charitable organizations and the broad practice of modern philanthropy are now defined and governed by public law (see, further, below, p. 171).

Philanthropy and social inclusion

Unlike the other models, philanthropy rests on the exercise of a power of discretion. The State does not intend that all should benefit, nor benefit equally, who can fit within the terms of reference of this model but it does require that the benefit satisfies public rather than private interests. The State confines itself to setting down the legal parameters for philanthropic activity and identifying the powers and bodies for regulating it. For many of those suffering from any of the different forms of contemporary social disadvantage this model does not necessarily promote their inclusion and facilitate the growth of civil society. The meritocracy ethos of modern western democracies, after all, rests on an assumption that the aspirations of the poor or otherwise marginalized can itself be a powerful force for reinforcing social conformity and promoting cohesion.

Philanthropy, law and social inclusion

The law not only defines and sets the parameters for philanthropic activity it also provides a medium that offers opportunities for developing methods of philanthropic intervention. Law centres, for example, were once seen as presenting a radical alternative to conventional legal services. The positioning of lawyers in centres of urban deprivation would, it was thought, enable them to work alongside community activists in identifying and tackling the structural issues associated with social disadvantage. By the tactical use of litigation, to further the public interests of a class of persons rather than the interests of an individual, significant strategic change could be achieved in circumstances of endemic deprivation. This vision was never quite realized, being instead absorbed and institutionalized by a powerful legal system and succumbing to the surge of private interest claims in matters such as family breakdown, property disputes and consumer protection. The experiment did, however, serve to make the law more accessible and better understood as a resource for the socially disadvantaged. It at least demonstrated the importance of making relevant advocacy skills available to those groups most in need of them. It also paved the way for the growth of generic advice centres such as the Citizens Advice Bureau and those of a more specialist nature dealing with matters such as tenants' rights, women's rights or entitlement to welfare benefits while encouraging the spread of mediation agencies focused on marriage counselling and the like. The law has proved a fruitful medium for developing and applying skills of advocacy, mediation and reconciliation, all of which have proved to be particularly relevant for philanthropy in the context of social inclusion.

Philanthropy, social inclusion and community development

The community development approach to poverty relief and social inclusion, in contrast to the traditional supplicant/benefactor model of charity, offers a strategic and holistic mode of philanthropic intervention. It addresses not just the presenting problems of the person or persons identified as in need, but takes into account problem causation and deals also with the prevailing circumstantial context of family, commerce and local politics. In a 'whole systems' approach it draws from relevant networks of people and institutions to leverage in whatever configuration of public, private and charitable resources promises to be most appropriate and effective in a particular situation. Most significantly, and again in contrast with the traditional model, it does so without displacing responsibility from recipient to philanthropist. Ownership of the problem, together with at least a shared control over the means for dealing with it, rests with those in need.

In this way, the altruism of the philanthropist, linked to appropriate means of intervention and set within a facilitative charity law structure, can be more effective than the traditional charity model in bridging the gap between the socially marginalized and mainstream society.

The international regulatory framework relating to social inclusion

Recent years have seen an exponential increase in attempts to regulate, on an international basis, various areas of law, policy and practice. A range of legal instruments has been employed for this purpose including conventions, covenants, declarations, protocols and treaties that are legally binding on those States that ratify or accede to them and declarations, principles, guidelines, standard rules and recommendations of varying legal status but without a mechanism for their enforcement. Many of these, such as the conventions relating to the rights and welfare interests of children, for example in relation to intercountry adoption, while undoubtedly relevant to issues of social inclusion, are too narrow, specific and peripheral for present purposes.

The framework

Under the auspices of the United Nations the following legal mechanisms for monitoring and enforcing international human rights have been put in place:

1 the International Covenant on Economic, Social and Cultural Rights (CESCR), which is monitored by the Committee on Economic, Social and Cultural Rights;
2 the International Covenant on Civil and Political Rights (CCPR), which is monitored by the Human Rights Committee;
3 the Optional Protocol to the International Covenant on Civil and Political Rights (CCPR-OP1), which is administered by the Human Rights Committee; and
4 the Second Optional Protocol to the International Covenant on Civil and Political Rights, aimed at the abolition of the death penalty (CCPR-OP2-DP);
5 the International Convention on the Elimination of All Forms of Racial Discrimination (CERD), which is monitored by the Committee on the Elimination of Racial Discrimination;
6 the Convention on the Elimination of All Forms of Discrimination against

Women (CEDAW), which is monitored by the Committee on the Elimination of Discrimination against Women;

7   the Optional Protocol to the Convention on the Elimination of All Forms of Discrimination against Women (CEDAW-OP);
8   the Convention against Torture and Other Cruel, Inhuman or Degrading Treatment or Punishment (CAT), which is monitored by the Committee against Torture;
9   the Convention on the Rights of the Child (CRC), which is monitored by the Committee on the Rights of the Child;
10 the Optional Protocol to the Convention on the Rights of the Child (CRC-OP-AC) on the involvement of children in armed conflict;
11 the Optional Protocol to the Convention on the Rights of the Child (CRC-OP-SC) on the sale of children, child prostitution and child pornography;
12 the International Convention on the Protection of the Rights of All Migrant Workers and Members of Their Families (MWC).

As at June 2004, all 191 member states of the United Nations and one non-member state were a party to one or more of the above. However, only a very few have a broad application to the circumstances of the socially disadvantaged, are legally enforceable and have embedded principles and rights to stand as benchmarks for the future development of charity law in common law nations and elsewhere. Of those, the European Convention for the Protection of Human Rights and Fundamental Freedoms 1950 is undoubtedly the most important.

The International Covenant on Civil and Political Rights 1966

This Covenant was adopted by the General Assembly of the United Nations in 1946 and has subsequently been ratified by many member states. The International Covenant on Civil and Political Rights 1966 came into effect on 23 March 1976 and is monitored by the Human Rights Committee. It articulates principles of considerable importance for sustaining the culture of minority groups. For example Article 27, as qualified by Article 18(3), provides that in states which have ethnic, religious or linguistic minorities, persons belonging to such minorities shall not be denied the right, in community with other members of their group, to enjoy their own culture, to profess and practice their own religion and to use their own language. Article 26 prohibits discrimination on the grounds of race and national origin.

The Declaration of Indigenous Peoples 1993

Article 4 of this Declaration emphasizes the right of indigenous peoples to maintain and strengthen their political, economic, social and cultural characteristics as well as their legal systems while Article 6 states that 'Indigenous peoples have the collective and individual right to be protected against ethnocide and cultural genocide'.

The European Convention for the Protection of Human Rights and Fundamental Freedoms 1950

The European Convention for the Protection of Human Rights and Fundamental Freedoms 1950 (the 'European Convention') provides for the recognition
and protection of the most basic civil rights including: the right to life; freedom
from torture; freedom from arbitrary arrest; the right to a fair trial; the right to
respect for private life; freedom of religion; freedom of expression and; freedom
of association and assembly. It is automatically binding on all signatories to the
Treaty of European Union (i.e. on all 25 members of the EU), is enforced
by the European Court of Human Rights (the Convention's dedicated court)
and by the European Court of Justice.

Social inclusion in the modern western, common law nations that are the
subject of study in Part IV is generally understood as signifying an entitlement to
a higher threshold of civil liberties than is implied by the Convention, but in fact
the latter, at the very least, simply puts in place a floor to catch those occasions
when an omission or breach of the civil liberties of the socially marginalized may
be so significant as to threaten their basic human rights. Moreover, the Convention's relevance is not limited to a safety net function as the ECHR has ruled that
the public authorities of signatory nations, in keeping with the Convention ethos
and principles, must also act proactively to prevent possible breaches of rights and
to promote opportunities for their enjoyment. In fact Convention principles provide a network of benchmarks for all democratic signatory states against which
their individual constitutions, domestic laws and the decisions of public bodies
can be measured. For the socially alienated, the Convention gives permission not
only to challenge State institutions but also to access and use those institutions in
order to increase the effectiveness of that challenge.[7]

There is some evidence that Convention awareness is beginning to generate a
culture of respect for rights which transcends the initial minimalist approach that
focused on avoiding or identifying and then responding to breaches of articles. A
more positive developmental approach is emerging whereby public authorities are
now examining their policies and procedures to Convention-proof them so as to
pre-empt the circumstances giving rise to a potential breach.

The United Nations Security Council Resolution 1373, 2001

On 28 September 2001, the UN Security Council unanimously adopted a wide-
ranging, comprehensive resolution with steps and strategies to combat international terrorism. Two aspects of this resolution carry particular implications for
charities. First, it directed all states to prevent and suppress the financing of
terrorism, to criminalize the 'wilful' provision or collection of funds for such acts
and to freeze the funds, assets and economic resources of those involved. This
directive authorizes at least the inspection of funds flowing into and out of charities in order to detect whether there is any use of funds by or for terrorists.
Second, it required all states to ensure that no asylum seeker is granted refugee

status until satisfied that such person had not planned, facilitated or participated in the commission of terrorist acts. Again this authorizes the use of powers necessary to at least conduct surveillance measures in respect of all immigrants or potential immigrants who may be deemed to be asylum seekers. Resolution 1373 has given rise to a wave of new anti-terrorism legislation across the western world. It remains to be seen how the Resolution's directives, as translated into national anti-terrorism legislation, are more broadly deployed in relation to charities, their funds and activities and in relation to socially disadvantaged immigrants. In particular, the content and effect of all such legislation must also be measured against the protection afforded to fundamental human rights on an international basis by the European Convention and the above United Nations mechanisms and on a national level by relevant human rights and civil liberties statutes (see, also, chapter 6).

Charities and the European Convention

The Convention rights that are most likely to impact on charities are:

- Article 8, the right to respect for private and family life;
- Article 9, the right to freedom of thought, conscience and religion;
- Article 10, the right to freedom of expression;
- Article 11, the right to freedom of association; and
- Article 14, the right to enjoyment of Convention rights and freedoms without discrimination.

Charities as 'public bodies'

The public benefit criterion for charitable status, within a common law context, brings charities within the definition of 'public bodies' and therefore, to the extent that they perform public functions, they are fully subject to the Convention.[8] That such bodies come within the jurisdiction of the European Court was clearly stated by it in *Foster* v. *British Gas:*[9]

> A body, whatever its legal form, which has been made responsible pursuant to a measure adopted by the State, for providing a public service under control of the State and has for that purpose special powers beyond those which resulted from the normal rules applicable in relations between individuals is included among the bodies against which the provisions of a Directive capable of having direct effect may be relied upon.

Moreover, as charities increasingly assume or share responsibilities that were previously borne by government bodies, so they are also increasingly liable to scrutiny to ensure their activities are fully Convention compliant. There are no definitive means of establishing which charities, or which of their activities, come within the 'public authority' umbrella as each case turns on its own facts though, as noted in Tudor, 'the activities of the charity may be so enmeshed with those of a public authority as to be public functions'.[10] However, there are some guidelines. Most obviously any body established by statute or royal prerogative, or vested with statutory powers or to which such powers have been delegated, or that is perform-ing a public function or service or the actions of which are amenable to judicial review is within the definition. The extent to which a charity is dependent upon funding from a government department will also, to that extent, indicate that it is controlled by and is functioning as an arm of that public authority.[11]

The public benefit test

In the common law tradition, application of this test differentiates between bodies (and gifts/activities) entitled to charitable status and those that are not. The test, however, is neither amenable to a standardized definition nor is it applied uni-formly in relation to all charitable purposes: it has a more rigorous application to the fourth *Pemsel* head than to any of the other three; in some countries, such as Ireland, there are statutory provisions preventing its application to organizations (gifts/activities) under the third head (see, further, chapter 9). Moreover, there is a problem in relation to those anomalous classes of case where the test is held to be satisfied even though the beneficiaries are strictly confined by locality or by a private nexus such as 'founder's kin', employer's dependants, etc., which essentially rest on discriminatory decisions.

Any such discriminatory application of a test, capable both of a broad and uncertain range of interpretation while favouring some charitable purposes over others, will be non-Convention compliant unless sufficient justification for its pref-erential application can be adduced. Arguably, the only sure way of achieving compliance is for every Convention signatory common law nation to embed a provision in its statutory law framework for charities, defining the test and requir-ing it to be applied objectively and equally in relation to all charitable purposes.

Emerging key standards

Certain governing standards of social justice are emerging from Convention case law as key building blocks in the gradual harmonization of international human rights jurisprudence. These include, for example, the key standards of 'necessity', 'proportionality' and 'equality of arms' against which relevant national legislative provisions and decision-making processes must now be tested. They have poten-tially far-reaching implications for the socially disadvantaged.

Necessity   The ECHR in *Olson* v. *Sweden (No 1)*[12] explained that to be justifiable, State interference in family life must be 'relevant and sufficient; it must meet a pressing social need; and it must be proportionate to the need'.

Proportionality   An application of the proportionality test to the third of the four *Pemsel* heads, the advancement of religion, might conclude that it is breached by the narrow common law interpretation of what constitutes a 'religion' (the exclusion of non-theistic religions such as Buddhism[13]).

Equality of arms The principle that the State should ensure that those presenting or defending a case are not disadvantaged, relative to the opposing party, by inadequate resources is clearly of considerable importance to the socially disadvantaged.[14]

The emergence of international benchmarks relating to social inclusion

By far the majority of relevant case law principles are those emanating from of the ECHR. However, there have also been a number of important judicial rulings made under the International Covenant on Civil and Political Rights 1966. By grouping relevant case law in accordance with key legal rights, rather than by nation or by international instrument, it becomes evident that the same legal benchmarks are being recognized and underpinned across the common law world and elsewhere.

Freedom of association

A principal hallmark of any democracy is the right of its citizens to form, join or not to join associations. The very existence of non-government organizations is conditional upon this right and it is of crucial importance in the context of social inclusion. Its significance has been recognized by the legislatures of democratic states for centuries and the constitutions of most countries in the world contain articles protecting freedoms of association and assembly.[15]

The International Covenant on Civil and Political Rights (ICCPR) and the Universal Declaration of Human Rights both guarantee freedom of association internationally.[16] The Covenant provides, in Articles 20 and 21, guarantees for the rights of peaceful assembly and freedom of association, permitting them to be restricted only when such restriction is lawful and then only to serve legitimate interests in national security, public safety, public morals or health, or the rights or freedoms of others. The Convention provides in Article 11 that:

1. Everyone has the right to freedom of peaceful assembly and to freedom of association with others, including the right to form and to join trade unions for the protection of his interests . . .

State obligation to avoid breach of right

This fundamental right places a duty on governments to ensure that all laws and practice are compliant with the above Article 11.

The ECHR in *Sidiropoulos and Others* v. *Greece*[17] pointed out that the right to form an association is an inherent part of the right set forth in Article 11, even if that

Article only makes express reference to the right to form trade unions. That citizens should be able to form a legal entity in order to act collectively in a field of mutual interest is 'one of the most important aspects of the right to freedom of association, without which that right would be deprived of any meaning'.[18] The way in which national legislation enshrines this freedom and its practical application by the authorities reveals the state of democracy in the country concerned. While states have a right to satisfy themselves that an association's aim and activities are in conformity with the rules laid down in legislation, they must do so in a manner compatible with their obligations under the Convention and subject to review by the Convention institutions.

Consequently, the exceptions set out in Article 11 are to be construed strictly; only convincing and compelling reasons can justify restrictions on freedom of association.[19] In determining whether a necessity within the meaning of Article 11.2 exists, the states have only a limited margin of appreciation, which goes hand in hand with rigorous European supervision embracing both the law and the decisions applying it, including those given by independent courts. The ECHR does not have to confine itself to ascertaining whether the respondent state exercised its discretion reasonably, carefully and in good faith; it also looks at the interference complained of in the light of the case as a whole to determine whether it was 'proportionate to the legitimate aim pursued' and whether the reasons adduced by the national authorities to justify it are 'relevant and sufficient'. In so doing, the court has to satisfy itself that the national authorities applied standards which were in conformity with the principles embodied in Article 11 and, moreover, that they based their decisions on an acceptable assessment of the relevant facts.

The ECHR found that territorial integrity, national security and public order were not threatened by the activities of an association whose aim was to promote a region's culture, even supposing that it also aimed partly to promote the culture of a minority. The ruling of the court in *Sidiropoulos* was important for social inclusion on an international basis because it emphasized that the existence of minorities and different cultures in a country was an historical fact that a 'democratic society' had to tolerate and even protect and support according to the principles of international law. This principle has clear application both to indigenous minority culture groups (e.g. the Aboriginal people of Australia) and to the more prevalent socially marginalized groups (e.g. the disabled, mentally ill, etc.) within modern democratic countries.

In *The Socialist Party of Turkey and Others v. Turkey*[20] the ECHR ruled that Turkey had once again violated Article 11. The court held that political parties are a form of association essential to the proper functioning of democracy and that in view of the importance of democracy for all countries that were signatories to the Convention, there could be no doubt that political parties came within the scope of Article 11. It noted that an association, including a political party, is not excluded from the protection afforded by the Convention simply because its activities are regarded by the national authorities as undermining the constitutional structures of the State. The ruling emphasized that freedom of speech, assembly and association, as well as pluralism, were the key elements of democracy:

> The Court reiterates that notwithstanding its autonomous role and particular sphere of application, Article 11 must also be considered in the light of Article 10. The protection of opinions and the freedom to express them is one of the objectives of the freedoms of assembly and association as enshrined in Article 11. That applies all the more in relation to political parties in view of their essential role in ensuring pluralism and the proper functioning of democracy.

In a ruling with significant implications for the rights of alienated minorities to access the mainstream socio-political institutions, in order to express their grievances and challenge the status quo, it was firmly stated:

> As the Court has emphasised many times, there can be no democracy without pluralism.[21] It is for that reason that freedom of expression as enshrined in Article 10 is applicable, subject to paragraph 2, not only to 'information' or 'ideas' that are favourably received or regarded as inoffensive or as a matter of indifference, but also to those that offend, shock or disturb. The fact that their activities form part of a collective exercise of freedom of expression in itself entitles political parties to seek the protection of Articles 10 and 11 of the Convention.

More recently the ECHR, in *Partidul Communistilor (Nepeceristi) and Ungureanu* v. *Romania*,[22] held unanimously that Romania had violated Article 11. The case originated in the attempts of Mr Ungureanu, a representative of the Partidul Communistilor (Nepeceristi; PCN), to register the PCN on the special register of political parties. In a judgment, subsequently upheld by the Bucharest Court of Appeal, the Bucharest District Court dismissed his application on the grounds that the PCN was seeking to gain political power in order to establish a 'humane State' founded on communist doctrine, meaning that the applicants considered the constitutional and legal order that had been in place since 1989 as inhumane and not based on genuine democracy.

The ECHR, however, having examined the PCN's constitution and political programme, noted that they stressed the importance of upholding the national sovereignty, territorial integrity and legal and constitutional order of the country, and democratic principles including political pluralism, universal suffrage and freedom to participate in politics. They did not contain any passages that might be considered a call for the use of violence, an uprising or any other form of rejection of democratic principles – which was an essential factor to be taken into consideration – or for the 'dictatorship of the proletariat'. It considered that there could be no justification for hindering a political grouping from registering if it had complied with the fundamental principles of democracy simply because it had criticized the constitutional and legal order of the country and had sought a public debate in the political arena. In conclusion, the court was of the view that a measure as drastic as the refusal to register the PCN as a political party, even before it had commenced its activities, was disproportionate to the aim pursued, unnecessary in a democratic society and therefore constituted a breach of Article 11.

Again, this decision constitutes a powerful benchmark for the rights of minority groups to access the institutional framework of the society in which they are marginalized in order to articulate their grievances and, more importantly, to challenge the status quo and the basis for their marginalization.

State obligation to positively promote enjoyment of right

This Article also carries a requirement that governments ensure that laws and practice positively promote this right;[23] they must 'both permit and make possible'[24] opportunities for citizens to enjoy this fundamental right.

Limitations on exercise of right

The right to freedom of association may be subject to lawful limitations imposed by the State but as the ECHR stated in the *Sidiropoulos* case the exceptions in Article 11(2) are to be construed strictly. In *Refah Partisi* v. *Turkey*[25] the ECHR ruled that a government ban on the Refah Partisi political party was justified under Article 11(2) because the party's proposed political programme would have threatened the rule of democracy in the State and contravened Convention principles. This case illustrates the difficulty in balancing the rights to freedom of association and of expression.[26]

In *RSPCA* v. *Attorney General and Others*[27] the ECHR considered whether the RSPCA was entitled to adopt a membership policy that excluded members who wished to change its policy on hunting. The court held that the organization was entitled to do so because the freedom of association of the RSPCA itself 'embraces the freedom to exclude from the association those whose membership it honestly believes to be damaging the interests of the Society'.

Freedom of expression

The right to freedom of expression is given international recognition in the International Covenant on Civil and Political Rights and in the European Convention.

Article 19 of the Covenant provides that:

1. Everyone shall have the right to hold opinions without interference.
2. Everyone shall have the right to freedom of expression; this right shall include freedom to seek, receive and impart information and ideas of all kinds, regardless of frontiers, either orally, in writing or in print, in the form of art, or through any other media of his choice.

Article 10 of the Convention states that:

1. Everyone has the right to freedom of expression. This right shall include freedom to hold opinions and to receive and impart information and ideas without interference by public authority and regardless of frontiers . . .

Again, this right is one of the hallmarks of a democratic society and is particularly important for the socially disadvantaged who need to present their case and argue for the resources necessary to improve their circumstances. Access to the leverage provided by media exposure is an essential means of courting public sympathy in contemporary society. The traditional common law constraints on political activity by charities are therefore of considerable interest in the context of this right. Certainly, the promotion of human rights is now a charitable purpose and by logical extension, in the absence of evidence that such activity is incompatible with the values of a democratic society, the presumption may be that advocacy on behalf of the socially disadvantaged for a change in law or policy is to be construed as a legitimate charitable purpose.[28]

Upholding the right

The UN Human Rights Committee recently ruled that Angola had violated the right to freedom of expression guaranteed under Article 9 of the Covenant, of a journalist Rafael Marques de Morais, who was arrested and imprisoned in Luanda, on 16 October 1999, following the publication in the Angola newspaper of remarks by him about Angolan President José Eduardo dos Santos. Among other things, Marques said that the President was responsible 'for the destruction of the country' and 'accountable for the promotion of incompetence, embezzlement and corruption'. Marques was detained for 40 days without charges, ten of them incommunicado, and then tried and convicted of the charge of 'abuse of the press' resulting in 'injury' to the President. In its ruling the Committee said:

Given the paramount importance, in a democratic society, of the right to freedom of expression and of a free and uncensored press or other media, the severity of the sanctions imposed on the author cannot be considered as a proportionate measure to protect public order or the honour and the reputation of the President, a public figure who, as such, is subject to criticism and opposition. In addition, the Committee considers it an aggravating factor that the author's proposed truth defence against the libel charge was ruled out by the courts.

The Committee also found violations of several other rights under the ICCPR, including the following:

•   Marques's arrest and detention – 'neither reasonable nor necessary, but at least in part of a punitive character' – were 'arbitrary', in violation of ICCPR Article 9(1).

- He was not informed in a timely manner of the reasons for his arrest, in breach of ICCPR Article 9(2).
- His ten-day period of incommunicado detention without access to a lawyer impaired his right to be brought promptly before a judge, in violation of ICCPR Article 9(3).
- Together with his detention without access to a lawyer, the Supreme Court's failure to adjudicate on a habeas corpus claim made on his behalf violated his right to judicial review of the lawfulness of his detention, guaranteed by ICCPR Article 9(4).

This is a strong, if unenforceable, ruling by the Committee which upholds the important right of an independent press (and, by logical extension, the advocacy rights of any independent person or group) to challenge government policies and demand change, particularly in developing countries where corrupt policies have direct consequences for those already socially disadvantaged.

The ECHR has upheld both the right to lobby for a political party by distributing leaflets prior to an election[29] and the right to receive information relating to birth control[30] as protected by Article 10. In *Steel and Morris* v. *The United Kingdom*,[31] which concluded the longest-running court case in English history (generally referred to as the 'McLibel Case'), the ECHR ruled that two environmental activists (members of London Greenpeace) convicted of defaming the McDonald's Corporation in 1997 were denied freedom of expression (Article 10) by the British government and did not receive a fair trial (Article 6). McDonald's had launched its libel action against the two campaigners 15 years earlier, alleging that they were involved in the production of a leaflet asserting that McDonald's exploited children, harmed the environment, and its food was unhealthy. McDonald's won the original verdict in 1997. In 2000, the defendants went to the European Court, which expressed the view that in a democratic society even small and informal campaign groups, such as London Greenpeace, had to be able to carry on their activities effectively. There existed a strong public interest in enabling such groups and individuals outside the mainstream to contribute to the public debate by disseminating information and ideas on matters of general public interest such as health and the environment. The free circulation of information and ideas about the activities of powerful commercial entities, and the possible 'chilling' effect on others were also important factors to be considered in this context. The ECHR ordered Britain to pay the campaigners a total of €35,000 and offer them a retrial.

This case is an important benchmark for the rights of individuals and small groups to actively campaign for peaceful change and to disseminate their views through the media.

Limitations on exercise of right

Although Article 10 is the most heavily qualified provision in the Convention, the ECHR has made it clear that there is a substantial onus resting on an applicant to justify limits being placed on this right. A test frequently applied by the ECHR, when considering restrictions on Article 10, is whether they could be 'justified in a democratic society'.

Freedom from discrimination

The right not to be discriminated against, traditionally associated with religious differences, is a most important aspect of life in a democratic society and is now generally extended to afford protection from discrimination on the grounds of gender, age, race and from differences arising from other such status designations. This right is given international recognition in the International Covenant on Civil and Political Rights, the Convention on the Elimination of All Forms of Racial Discrimination, the Convention on the Elimination of All Forms of Discrimination Against Women and in the European Convention.

Article 26 of the Covenant provides that:

> All persons are equal before the law and are entitled without any discrimination to the equal protection of the law. In this respect the law shall prohibit any discrimination and guarantee to all persons equal and effective protection against discrimination on any ground such as race, colour, sex, religion, language, political or other opinion, national or social origin, property, birth, or other status.

This provision makes a powerful and unequivocal statement of the legal right of all persons to equality of treatment and to protection from discrimination. It is rather different in that respect from the equivalent provision in the European Convention.

Article 14 of the European Convention provides that:

> The enjoyment of the rights and freedoms set forth in this Convention shall be secured without discrimination on any ground such as sex, race, colour, language, religion, political or other opinion, national or social origin, association with a national minority, property, birth or other status.

This provision has no independent validity as it comes into play only after a substantive Convention right has been breached. It deals only with discriminatory treatment based upon the personal characteristics that distinguish people. As Kennedy L.J. observed in *Southwark LBC* v. *St Brice*:[32]

> In order to establish a claim under Article 14 an individual must show that he has been discriminated against on the basis of 'a personal characteristic

("status") by which persons or groups of persons are distinguishable from each other'.[33]

It must be shown that an applicant is: subject to a difference in treatment from others in a similar situation; in the enjoyment of one of the rights protected by the Convention; which difference cannot be objectively and reasonably justified, having regard to the concepts of legitimate aim, proportionality and margin of appreciation. There is no definitive list of matters constituting discriminatory treatment.

There is a sense in which Article 14 rights function as a dimension of the substantive rights of other Articles, that 'it is as though Article 14 formed an integral part of each of the articles laying down rights and freedoms whatever their nature'.[34] In many cases, once the ECHR had found that there had been a breach of rights under a substantive Article, it did not go on to decide whether Article 14 had also been breached; there was a presumption that this logically followed. For example, the court in *Dudgeon* v. *United Kingdom*,[35] having held that a law in Northern Ireland, which criminalized all homosexual activity, was in breach of Article 8, did not consider it necessary to rule on the ancillary issue of whether the law also discriminated on the grounds of sexual orientation. The Council of Europe has drawn up Protocol 12 to give the independent status to the prohibition on discrimination; this has yet to become law.

Religion

Within the common law tradition the advancement of religion has long been a most important charitable purpose carrying at least an implicit presumption (explicit in the statute law of some countries such as Ireland) that gifts to and the activities of religious organizations are for the public benefit and are therefore de facto charitable. The interpretation of 'religion' within this tradition has suffered from being construed in narrow terms, has often been applied inconsistently and has tended to exclude non-theistic religions. The Convention now requires that any interpretation of 'religion' be applied objectively, have reasonable justification[36] and be non-discriminatory; any differential treatment must comply with strict standards.[37] This legal benchmark for non-discrimination in matters of religion is underpinned by Article 14 and supported by Article 9 (the right to freedom of thought, conscience and religion) and by Article 1 of the First Protocol (the right to peaceful enjoyment of property). It has the effect of requiring governments and other public bodies to give parity of recognition to Christian and non-Christian religions such as Buddhism and Hinduism.

Other matters constituting discrimination

In *Lithgow* v. *United Kingdom*[38] the ECHR held that discrimination in essence occurs when the law differentiates between people 'placed in analogous situations' or more precisely when individuals in similar or analogous situations are treated differently without any adequate justification.[39]

Direct discrimination

An applicant will have established direct discrimination and a breach of Article 14 if he or she can show that: other persons in a similar or analogous situation, as evidenced by the set of facts governing each situation, are being treated differently to the applicant; and there is no justification for the difference in treatment. So, for example, in *Abdulaziz, Cabales and Balkandali* v. *United Kingdom*[40] the three female applicants successfully argued that they had been discriminated against because of their gender. This was a case where the husbands of married non-national women were prevented by UK immigration rules from remaining in the UK with their wives in circumstances where the wives of non-national men would have been granted such permission. The applicants claim that the immigration rules breached their Article 8 rights (right to respect for privacy and family life) was rejected by the ECHR but it held that they had been discriminated against on the basis of sex,[41] which constituted a breach of Article 14 when taken in conjunction with Article 8. As noted by Quint and Spring:[42]

> Thus to the extent a State undertakes to provide some privilege, right or benefit to one group, even though not required to do so under a particular Article of the Convention, it must treat all similar groups equally and provide them with the same privileges, rights and benefits, unless there is justification to support the difference in treatment. . . .

Indirect discrimination

As has been explained by the ECHR, 'the right not to be discriminated against in the enjoyment of the rights guaranteed under the Convention is also violated when States without an objective and reasonable justification fail to treat differently persons whose situations are significantly different'.[43]

The effects of indirect discrimination were examined in *Thlimmenos* v. *Greece*,[44] where the ECHR considered the effect of a blanket ban, imposed by a professional body, on the employment of anyone with a criminal record. The case concerned an applicant who had such a record due to his objection, on religious and conscientious grounds, to military service. The court ruled that the ban had a disproportionate effect on the applicant and could not be justified. For minority groups, this is an important decision as it recognizes that Article 14 also operates to afford protection from legal provisions that, although applied equally to all, have an adverse effect and discriminatory consequences for a few.

Access to justice

This is a composite right that addresses such matters as that: relevant information is available and can be readily understood; appropriate processes and proceedings exist and are accessible; there is an opportunity to avail of such resources as may be necessary for effective representation; the proceedings are conducted independently, fairly, with a right of appeal; and that the outcome is fully and fairly enforced. Access to justice is central to the rule of law and a prerequisite for the recognition and enforcement of other rights. It is a right of fundamental importance for the socially disadvantaged.

The right to a fair trial

Article 14 of the Covenant provides that:

> 1.   Everyone has the right to liberty and security of person. No one shall be subjected to arbitrary arrest or detention. No one shall be deprived of his liberty except on such grounds and in accordance with such procedure as are established by law.

Article 6 of the European Convention states:

> 1.   In the determination of his civil rights and obligations or of any criminal charge against him, everyone is entitled to a fair and public hearing within a reasonable time by an independent and impartial tribunal established by law. . . .

For the socially disadvantaged, the right to a fair hearing of grievances relating to their civil rights is crucially important. The ECHR has warned that there can be no justification for taking a restrictive approach to this right.[45]

Due process

An essential element of a 'fair hearing' is the provision of appropriate legal representation which may include access to legal aid.[46] The concept of 'equality of arms', introduced by the ECHR, 'implies that each party must be afforded a reasonable opportunity to present his case – including his evidence – under conditions that do not place him at a substantial disadvantage vis-à-vis his opponent'.[47] These and such other requirements as 'access', 'impartiality', 'lack of delay' and 'public hearing' ensure that the process (whether judicial or administrative) does not add further to the disadvantage suffered by those attempting to assert their civil rights.

Cost can be an obstacle to accessing justice. In *Steel and Morris* v. *The United Kingdom*,[48] the applicants were refused legal aid and so represented themselves throughout the trial and appeal, with a little help from volunteer lawyers. They claimed that they were severely hampered by lack of resources, not just in the way of legal advice and representation, but also when it came to administration, photocopying, note-taking, and the tracing, preparation and payment of the costs and expenses of expert and factual witnesses. McDonald's, on the other hand, were represented throughout the proceedings by leading and junior counsel, experienced in defamation law and by one or, at times, two solicitors and other assistants.

The trial lasted for 313 court days and subsequently the Court of Appeal rejected the majority of the applicants' submissions as to general grounds of law and unfairness. The damages awarded by the trial judge were reduced, leaving Ms Steel liable for a total of £36,000 and Mr Morris for a total of £40,000. Leave to appeal to the House of Lords was refused. The applicants then brought proceedings before the ECHR alleging a breach of their rights under Article 6 as they had been denied a fair trial because of the lack of legal aid.

The ECHR considered that the question whether the provision of legal aid was necessary for a fair hearing had to be determined on the basis of the particular facts and circumstances of each case and depended *inter alia* upon the importance of what was at stake for the applicant in the proceedings, the complexity of the relevant law and procedure and the applicant's capacity to represent him- or herself effectively. In terms of what had been at stake for the applicants, although defamation proceedings were not, in this context, comparable to, for instance, proceedings raising important family-law issues, the financial consequences had been potentially severe. As regards the complexity of the proceedings, the trial at first instance had lasted 313 court days, preceded by 28 interlocutory applications. The appeal hearing had lasted 23 days. The facts of the case, which the applicants had to prove, had been highly complex, involving 40,000 pages of documentary evidence and 130 oral witnesses. Nor was the case straightforward legally. Extensive legal and procedural issues had to be resolved before the trial judge was in a position to decide the main issue.

Against this background, it was necessary to assess the extent to which the applicants were able to bring an effective defence despite the absence of legal aid. The court was of the view that in a case of such complexity, neither the sporadic help given by the volunteer lawyers nor the extensive judicial assistance and latitude granted to the applicants as litigants in person, was any substitute for competent and sustained representation by an experienced lawyer familiar with the case and with the law of libel. The very length of the proceedings was, to a certain extent, a testament to the applicants' lack of skill and experience.

In conclusion, the ECHR found that the denial of legal aid to the applicants had deprived them of the opportunity to present their case effectively before the court and contributed to an unacceptable inequality of arms with McDonald's. There had, therefore, been a violation of Article 6(1).

This decision clearly provides an international benchmark for the right of those who are championing a social cause to access the State resources necessary for them to represent their cause and have a fair hearing. The principle applies equally to the decision-making processes of all public bodies be they courts or administrative bodies.

The right to respect for private and family life

Article 17 of the Covenant states: '1. No one shall be subjected to arbitrary or unlawful interference with his privacy, family, home or correspondence, nor to unlawful attacks on his honour and reputation.'

Article 8 of the European Convention states: '1. Everyone has the right to respect for his private and family life, his home and his correspondence . . .'.

Essentially this right aims to provide protection for an individual against arbitrary action by public authorities,[49] but it has been applied and upheld in a wide variety of diverse circumstances. It places an obligation on the court to ensure that the rights of an individual are properly secured and are protected against infringements by other individuals,[50] while also requiring that public authorities exercise fairness in their procedures. Article 8 of the Convention together with Article 6 are construed as imposing on a court not only a duty of watchful vigilance, to ensure that the rights enumerated are properly taken into account when determining proceedings, but also as imposing an obligation to be satisfied that any orders then made are given effect in a manner which continues to satisfy those rights.[51] This combination of Articles, arguably, places a positive obligation on the State, once it is made aware of a breach, to intervene and secure the safety of the subject. In effect it has no discretion, once it is put on notice it must follow through with proactive steps.

The prohibition on public authority interference is permissible where to do so is: (a) in accordance with the law; and (b) is necessary in a democratic society[52] (i) in the interests of national security, public safety or the economic well-being of the country, (ii) for the prevention of crime and disorder, (iii) for the protection of health or morals or (iv) for the protection of the rights and freedom of others.

Application in relation to procedural fairness

Article 8 carries an inherent requirement that states ensure their public authorities have and implement procedures that provide citizens with a fair hearing on matters concerning them. For example, Article 8 rights will be breached where a public authority has failed to sufficiently involve the subject in a decision-making process affecting his or her interests[53] or failed to disclose information that may have had a material bearing on the outcome of their case.[54]

Application in relation to sexual orientation

Managing the tension between protecting the traditional legal position of the heterosexual, monogamous, marital family unit while accommodating the rights of same gender couples has been an item on the social inclusion agenda of common law nations as with other modern western societies. The ECHR case law relating to Article 8 has developed an unequivocal approach to this matter: the definition of 'family' is not to be restricted to one based on marriage; it may include unmarried couples, non-marital children and lesbian or homosexual relationships depending as a matter of fact on the existence of actual close family ties.

In *Smith and Grady* v. *United Kingdom*[55] the court rejected the claim by the Ministry of Defence that its action in conducting a formal inquiry into the sexual orientation of members of the armed forces and its subsequent dismissal of a number of those with a homosexual orientation was necessary to maintain the morale of its fighting forces. Similarly in relation to the rights of transsexuals, the ECHR in *Goodwin* v. *United Kingdom*[56] held that the applicant's Article 8 rights had been breached by a refusal to adjust the gender specified on their birth certificate, which constituted a failure to respect their private life.

Application in relation to State surveillance

The protection that Article 8 affords to private life extends also to curbing unwarranted and intrusive State surveillance techniques which can be deployed to monitor the activities of the socially marginalized as well as suspect criminals. For example, in *Malone* v. *United Kingdom*[57] and in *Halford* v. *United Kingdom*[58] the ECHR ruled that the 'bugging' of private calls (even when made to and from an office phone) constituted a breach of this Article. A plea that the relevant statutory provisions were widely or vaguely framed, far from allowing the State to claim in defence a belief that it had a margin of discretion in the exercise of its powers, will itself provide grounds for a finding of non-compliance:[59]

> In view of the attendant obscurity and uncertainty as to the state of the law in this essential respect . . . the law of England and Wales does not indicate with reasonable clarity the scope and manner of exercise of the relevant discretion conferred on the public authorities. To that extent, the minimum degree of legal protection to which citizens are entitled under the rule of law in a democratic society is lacking.

The defence of 'justification' for conduct that would otherwise constitute a breach of human rights is only available where that conduct is governed by clear and specific regulatory provisions.

This is an important right for socially marginalized groups and individuals. The principles applied to the circumstances of those prevented from enjoying rights of privacy and family life because of their sexual orientation apply also to those unable to do so for reasons associated with, for example, disability, mental health, learning disability, etc. This principle may well in time also be brought to bear on the circumstances of those such as asylum seekers, who are consigned by public authorities to living conditions that do not respect their rights to a private and family life.

Freedom of thought, conscience and religion

Article 18 of the Covenant states: '1. Everyone shall have the right to freedom of thought, conscience and religion.'

Article 9 of the European Convention states: '1. Everyone has the right to freedom of thought, conscience and religion . . .'

Article 9 offers only weak protection for this right and has rarely been invoked. The first time it was invoked to limit State action with regard to freedom of religion was in 1993.[60] Moreover, except for two cases, until 1995 the European Commission on Human Rights has always denied applications from religions that could be called 'new', 'minority', or 'nontraditional'.[61] However two important cases have recently raised the profile of Article 9: *Kokkinakis* v. *Greece*[62] and *Manoussakis* v. *Greece*.[63]

In the *Kokkinakis* case it was held that the Greek anti-proselytism law, as applied to Mr Kokkinakis, impermissibly interfered with his freedom of religion. The court distinguished between proper and improper proselytism: if the first is the essential mission of any religious association the second is 'corruption and deformation of it'. The court noted that proselytism (or true evangelism) should be compatible with the respect for the freedom of thought, religion and conscience of others. The use of violence, brainwashing, offers of material and social advantages, as well as putting improper pressure on people in distress or in need are examples of improper proselytism. The court thus recognized the right to proselytize, when it is exercised with respect for freedom of religion of others, and said that it is protected by Article 9 of the European Convention. Moreover, according to Justice Pettiti, 'religion is one of the foundations of a democratic society within the meaning of the Convention and the pluralism that cannot be disassociated from a democratic society depends on religious freedom'.[64] In the *Manoussakis* case the court stated: 'The right to freedom of religion . . . excludes any discretion on the part of the State to determine whether religious beliefs or the means used to express such beliefs are legitimate.'

These cases affirm the significance of freedom of religion for modern democratic states. Given that many contemporary socially disadvantaged groups, cultures and indeed whole communities (e.g. in Northern Ireland) coalesce around a set of religious beliefs, it is clearly a matter of considerable importance that all public bodies are required to impartially facilitate their right to practise in accordance with their religious beliefs.

Indigenous communities

Some modern western nations include within their borders distinct indigenous cultural groups, each established over many centuries and maintained in accordance with traditional customs, that have survived relatively intact into the twenty-first century. This is the case, for example, with indigenous people in Australia, New Zealand, Africa, and North and South America. These indigenous cultural groups are, to a varying degree, coherent entities founded on rules and traditions governing relations within and between families and applying to the functioning of their social system as a whole. They co-exist alongside and in an uneasy relationship with the prevailing western culture, sharing time, territory and the necessities of life but often very little in the way of values, knowledge and social infrastructure.

Having hitherto been silent on the subject, in recent decades international legal instruments have begun to recognize indigenous communities wherever located as sharing many of the characteristics of other socially disadvantaged minority groups but with additional features of historical abuse, cultural alienation and now requiring specific legal protection. International acknowledgement of the rights of indigenous communities first became evident in the Indigenous and Tribal Peoples Convention 1989 (No. 169) and the Declaration on the Rights of Persons Belonging to National or Ethnic, Religious and Linguistic Minorities. While attracting specific international protective measures, indigenous people naturally also benefit from the general rights and case law principles of other international legal instruments, particularly those of the European Convention.

The Declaration of Indigenous Peoples 1993

This international statement of principles can offer a basis for negotiation between indigenous communities and the adjacent mainstream social infra-structure when issues arise. Article 4 emphasizes the right of indigenous peoples to maintain and strengthen their political, economic, social and cultural charac-teristics as well as their legal systems, while Article 6 states that:

> Indigenous peoples have the collective and individual right to be protected against ethnocide and cultural genocide, including the prevention and redress for:
> (a) removal of indigenous children from their families and communities under any pretext.

The Permanent Forum on Indigenous Issues

In April 2000, during the International Decade of the World's Indigenous People, the Commission on Human Rights adopted a resolution to establish the Perman-ent Forum on Indigenous Issues. Three months later the Permanent Forum came into formal existence when ECOSOC, the Economic and Social Council, endorsed the resolution. The Permanent Forum is an advisory body to the Economic and Social Council. Its mandate is to discuss indigenous issues related to culture, economic and social development, education, the environment, health and human rights.

Conclusion

The European Convention is only one of a growing number of international legal instruments that now constitute a framework of external reference for con-temporary charity law. However, because of its broad endorsement by many modern western nations and the enforceability of its provisions by the ECHR, this Convention has become a very powerful means for benchmarking the prin-ciples and standards now required of the public bodies in all signatory states. The law, policy and practice of philanthropy in such states is plainly subject to Convention rights as articulated through the constant stream of ECHR case law, while that of non-signatory states may be subject to equivalent national and/or international provisions and in any event may be measured against the yardstick provided by Convention requirements.

Social inclusion, or the requirement that equal and equitable treatment be extended to all law-abiding persons and minority groups, is central to the Convention and is specifically addressed by many of its provisions. The capacity of charity law with its common law legacy to deal with contemporary issues of social inclusion, whether of a domestic or of an indigenous culture nature, in a Convention compliant manner is set to become an important challenge for philanthropy. This challenge is not confined to proofing existing law against the above Convention rights and ECHR principles, although this is the most basic and pressing duty. Increasingly, judgments of the ECHR show the court exploring the extent to which the public bodies of signatory states should not just react in a protective fashion but should also be proactive in asserting rights, creating opportunities for social inclusion and in predicting and circumventing situations in which minority groups may be adversely affected by legal provisions of general benefit to others. This potential application of Convention principles, together with the above established benchmarks, will be examined further in the country-specific profiles of Part IV.

Part IV

Contemporary law
and practice

Chapter 8

Charity law and social inclusion in England and Wales

Introduction

The United Kingdom comprises England, Scotland, Wales and Northern Ireland. Within the UK, England and Wales form a single jurisdiction and the subject of this chapter. It is singled out because of the unique contribution made by its monarchy, legislature and courts to the development of the common law and because each of the much smaller jurisdictions has a distinct charity law framework and is engaged in a separate charity law reform process, making a composite UK study too complicated and unnecessary for present purposes.

This chapter deals with contemporary law, policy and practice in England and Wales. It begins with a brief national socio-economic profile, examines the size and significance of the charitable sector and considers current social inclusion issues with particular reference to concerns following the London bombings in July 2005. It continues the developmental history of charity law as outlined in Part II and builds upon emerging themes. It then applies the template of functions (see, further, chapter 6) to identify and assess the characteristic features of the charity law environment in this jurisdiction, the key definitional matters, the legal structures for charities, registration and the regulatory framework, financial matters and the legal constraints on the development of philanthropy.

The chapter examines the outcomes of the protracted charity law review process and analyses the implications arising for social inclusion issues. It concludes with a summary of the more distinctive characteristics of charity law in England and Wales.

Charities and social inclusion

In England and Wales, as elsewhere in the UK, the government has made a considerable political investment in conducting high-profile social inclusion policies, to be pursued largely through the Social Exclusion Unit.[1] Its success or failure will be measured particularly by the extent to which it is able to address the concerns of ethnic minorities. The involvement of charities (as well as other non-profit organizations), whether acting in partnership with government as service providers or in opposition as advocates for the socially disadvantaged, may well be crucial to that outcome.

The country

The UK has a current and growing population of approximately 60 million of which approx 53 million live in England and Wales. Although the majority by far is white Caucasian and Christian, this jurisdiction has a well-established multi-cultural and multifaith society. Since the late 1990s, immigration has significantly increased and is now an important factor in population growth.

A leading trading power and financial centre, the UK is one of the largest and most powerful economies of western Europe. Over the past two decades the government has greatly reduced public ownership and contained the growth of social welfare programmes. Agriculture is intensive, highly mechanized, and efficient by European standards. It has large coal and natural gas reserves and until 2005 had been self-sufficient in oil. Services, particularly banking, insurance and business services, account by far for the largest proportion of GDP while industry continues to decline in importance.

The economy is one of the strongest in Europe; inflation stands at 1.4 per cent, interest rates are low and unemployment at 4.8 per cent is also relatively low. The relatively good economic performance has complicated the government's efforts to make a case for Britain to join the European Economic and Monetary Union (EMU). In the meantime, the government has been accelerating the improvement of education, transport and health services at the cost of higher taxes.

The charitable sector

The voluntary (or not-for-profit, or voluntary and community) sector, of which charities form a large part, is a healthy, vibrant and confident entity in this jurisdiction. The Charity Commission report[2] notes that at the end of June 2005, there were 167,022 'main' charities on its Register which in total had an annual income at the second quarter of the financial year of £37.099 billion. It profiles the wealth of charities as follows:

- the majority of registered charities have an income of £10,000 or less; they represent nearly two-thirds of registered charities but have less than 1 per cent of the income recorded;
- under 8 per cent of charities receive 90 per cent of the total annual income recorded;
- the largest 546 charities (0.33 per cent of those on the register) attract over 46 per cent of the total income.

There are also some 100,000 charities that are either exempt or excepted from registration with the Charity Commission. The level of charitable giving in the

UK in 2000 has been estimated at between 0.63 per cent and 0.77 per cent of GDP (compared with 2.1 per cent of GNP in the United States) but:

> Unlike the United States, both giving levels and participation in giving declined in Britain during the later 1990s, despite an increasingly strong economy. Total charitable donations in 1997 were £4.51 billion, down from £5.3 billion in 1993, a fall of 31% in real terms.[3]

The social inclusion agenda

There are significant variations in the distribution of wealth in this jurisdiction with some areas (e.g. Cornwall and Liverpool) being sufficiently economically depressed to qualify for EU regional aid.

A recent research project funded by the Joseph Rowntree Foundation,[4] surveyed the evidence on the impact of policies towards poverty, inequality and social exclusion since the Labour government was elected in 1997.[5] It reports that in 1997 poverty and inequality stood at levels unprecedented in post-war history. More than one in four UK children lived in relative poverty, compared with one in eight in 1979. Income inequality had widened sharply, and many indicators of deprivation were either deteriorating or high in international terms. It then details the range of government programmes designed to tackle these problems. It notes that one of the most prominent and ambitious has been the commitment to cut (relative) child poverty by a quarter by 2004–5, to halve it by 2010–11, and to 'eradicate' it within 20 years – or at least to be 'amongst the best in Europe'. However, research conducted by Barnardo's[6] indicates the extent of government failure in this area. The Barnardo's report[7] finds that one in four children in the UK lives in relative poverty, once eradicated diseases such as scabies and rickets are now to be found in deprived areas of Britain, diagnoses of TB have risen by 25 per cent in the past ten years and that the UK is now fifth from the bottom in the league of European child poverty rates.[8]

Another prominent government target noted by the Rowntree-funded research project was the aim of the neighbourhood renewal strategy that, within 10–20 years, no one should be seriously disadvantaged by where they live. The renewal of poor neighbourhoods has become a primary focus of concern for the government's Social Exclusion Unit and across the jurisdiction many Health Action Zone projects have sought to concentrate and co-ordinate resources to deliver better health outcomes in specifically targeted deprived housing estates.

The report points out that by setting such targets the government is holding itself to public account in a way that few predecessors have done, but also notes the lack of targets for working-age poverty (or for poverty of the population as a whole) and for overall inequality (except insofar as monitored at EU level). In addition, there are areas where policy (let alone impact) appears to be lagging behind analysis and target-setting. In the case of asylum seekers, for example, it observes that government policy has actively increased exclusion along dimensions considered key for other groups (employment, income and housing).

Need for a more inclusive agenda

In England and Wales the social inclusion agenda has recently undergone considerable change in relation to both well-established domestic issues and as regards ethnic minorities. The issues of equal opportunity, non-discrimination and equity of treatment that formed the agenda of those disadvantaged by race, disability, gender, age, etc., have now largely been addressed through law and policy measures (accelerated by obligations under EU law and the European Convention on Human Rights) and are being broadly consolidated in practice. Although by no means finally and uniformly resolved, such baseline issues have recently been displaced by contentious debate regarding the participation of service users in relevant decision-making processes. No longer confined to participation in models of service delivery, some organized socially disadvantaged groups are now involved in policy development and in the framing of legislative provisions. User representation in or control of the many forums and processes that affect their interests are now the subject of negotiation within and between charities and government bodies at various levels throughout this jurisdiction.

However, it is in relation to ethnic minorities, specifically young males in the Muslim communities, that the government's social inclusion agenda is currently facing its greatest challenge. The long-established policy of alleviating ethnic inequalities, promoting ethnic diversity and building a multicultural society in England and Wales is now in danger of unravelling.

The realities of housing and employment opportunities, coupled with the natural tendency for extended families and ethnic groups to coalesce in local communities have, in recent years, led to a considerable 'ghettoization' of new immigrants in impoverished housing estates. The Barnardo's report points out that minority ethnic families have a higher rate of poverty: 29 per cent of white children lived below the poverty line in 2000, while the figure for Pakistani and Bangladeshi children was 73 per cent and 63 per cent for black African children.[9] Some of these communities have been subjected to exploitive labour practices and racial attacks. There have been serious riots and complaints of police harassment. The failures and racial bias of police activity were fully documented in the Macpherson report.[10]

Against this background, fuelled by controversial media attention given to migrant labour and asylum seekers, the government in recent years has introduced measures to restrict immigration, contain and deport unlawful immigrants and to strengthen the citizenship of new immigrants through such means as knowledge tests and oaths of allegiance to queen and country.

The London terrorist atrocities in July 2005 have undoubtedly exacerbated an already strained relationship between the Muslim communities of this jurisdiction and the State. The national security measures subsequently introduced by the government have led to increased use of stop and search police powers and a corresponding growing sense of alienation in those communities.

Government policy

In England and Wales the contribution made by charities to addressing the social inclusion agenda is well recognized by the government. As the then Minister responsible for charities declared:[11]

> Charities are a major force for good in society. They can reach out to some of our most marginalised and deprived communities and provide a strong voice for those who need it . . . The Government is committed to a diverse, expanding and vibrant voluntary sector. We are achieving this by helping charities to realise their full potential to change lives and help transform communities.

History, definitional matters and legal framework

This jurisdiction, the original common law nation, established itself with the Statute of Charitable Uses 1601[12] as progenitor of the charity law framework which, along with a body of related case law precedents explicating crucial definitional matters, it subsequently bequeathed to its colonies.

Historical outline

As explained in Part II, the history of charity law in this jurisdiction can be traced to at least the 1601 Act and has evolved from concepts associated with religion, property rights and the respective responsibilities of citizen and State (see, further chapters 1 and 2). The development of the common law in England and Wales is somewhat different from that of the USA, where the concepts of the 'deserving poor' and self-help rather than charity held a greater appeal[13] and is tied more closely to the law of property (i.e. gifts and trusts) rather than the law of organizations.[14]

The common law

Lord Macnaghten in the *Pemsel* case[15] endorsed established judicial interpretations of charitable purposes as these had evolved from the time of the 1601 Act. The *Pemsel* classification of charitable purposes defined such purposes as being those which were exclusively charitable and which could be grouped under one of four heads:

1   the relief of poverty;
2   the advancement of education;
3   the advancement of religion; and
4   certain other purposes which could not be accommodated within the first three.

Before and after that decision, however, when determining whether or not a purpose could be construed as charitable, the judiciary relied on the 'spirit or intendment' rule for guidance.

The 'spirit or intendment' rule[16]   Broadly speaking, if it could be shown that a new purpose sufficiently approximated an established charitable purpose, so that it could be viewed as an extension of it or as analogous to it, then the court would hold the new purpose to be charitable on the grounds that it lay within the broad intention of the initial legislation (see, further, chapter 3). This rule has until recently underpinned the development of charity law in England and Wales, as it continues to do in other common law nations, giving the judiciary some discretion to adjust the law to fit contemporary social circumstances. However, whereas any such development of the law in other jurisdictions remains dependent upon a significant volume of cases coming before their courts, here this is very largely the responsibility of the Charity Commission, which is empowered to take a more strategic approach.

The legislation

For the best part of four centuries, charities and their activities in England and Wales constituted a legislative backwater; administrative matters were left to be resolved by the relevant agencies and legal issues determined on an ad hoc basis by the High Court. Legislation affecting charities tended to do so only incidentally, statutes being directed mainly towards education, property ownership, trustees, religious organizations, public service provision, taxes, etc., with a marginal relevance for charities. The few significant milestones on the road to constructing a modern legislative framework for charities served mainly to reinforce, regulate and improve the administration of the existing common law approach.

The Charitable Trusts Act 1853   This legislation included provision for establishing the Charity Commissioners for England and Wales.

The Mortmain and Charitable Uses Act 1888   Perhaps the most significant aspect of this statute is that by s 13(2) it explicitly preserved the Preamble (see, further, chapter 3 for the law relating to mortmain).

The Recreational Charities Act 1958   Introduced primarily to close a legal loophole exposed by the court.[17] Section 1(1) of the 1958 Act declared 'it shall be and be deemed always to have been charitable to provide, or assist in the provision of, facilities for recreation or other leisure-time occupation, if the facilities are provided in the interests of social welfare'. It added as a governing principle that only a trust or institution established for the public benefit would be charitable. This legislation otherwise left untouched the common law approach to charities and was reproduced in Australia and other common law jurisdictions.

The Charities Act 1960   Following the recommendations of the Nathan

Committee[18] and the issue of a White Paper,[19] the government introduced the 1960 Act to provide a new legislative platform for regulating charities in England and Wales. It was virtually replicated by legislation in Scotland and Northern Ireland[20] and to a large extent also in the Republic of Ireland,[21] though the law continued on a somewhat different path in Scotland.[22] This statute repealed the last vestiges of the 1601 Act together with the law of mortmain and the Mortmain and Charitable Uses Act 1888 and it charged the Charity Commissioners with the duty of 'promoting the effective use of charitable resources by encouraging the development of better methods of administration, by giving charity trustees information or advice on any matter affecting the charity and by investigating and checking abuses'. It also introduced compulsory registration with the Charity Commission. However, by providing for the continuation of the common law interpretation of 'charity' and 'charitable purpose', the 1960 Act ensured continued reliance on established principles and did nothing to change the substantive law.[23]

The Charities Act 1992   Following the recommendations of the Woodfield report,[24] the 1992 Act sought to improve the monitoring, supervision and support of charities by providing the Charity Commission with enhanced registration and regulatory powers. Again, however, the legislative intent to avoid interference with established common law principles was clearly evident from the view expressed by the government in its White Paper that:[25]

> the government consider that any attempt to define charity (by any of the suggested means) would be fraught with difficulty and might put at risk the flexibility of the present law which is both its greatest strength and its most valuable feature.[26]

The new provisions in Part III of the Charities Act 1992 to regulate fundraising were never brought into force.

The Charities Act 1993   The 1993 Act, consolidating the reforms of the 1992 Act with the provisions of both the 1960 Act and the Charitable Trustees Incorporation Act 1872, essentially improved the registration and regulatory processes by vesting new powers in the Charity Commissioners and provides the current charity law framework. It declared that 'charity' means 'any institution, corporate or not, which is established for charitable purposes' while 'institution' includes any trust or undertaking and 'charitable purposes' means 'purposes which are exclusively charitable according to the law of England and Wales'. This formulation served to continue the established common law approach to defining charities and their activities.

The law as now stated in the Charities Act 1993 is about to be amended as a result of the recently completed law reform process that commenced with the recommendations of the Charity Law Association, the Charity Commission, the National Council for Voluntary Organizations and other bodies[27] (see, further, below).

Definitional matters

In this, the original common law jurisdiction, the main elements in the legal definition of charity emerged from the context of trusts and continue to characterize
modern charity law.

Charitable intent

In England and Wales the judiciary, when determining charitable status, will look
to the purpose to which the gift is to be put rather than to the intention of the
donor[28] as is the case in Ireland (see, further, chapter 9). A charitable intention is
insufficient to attract charitable status for a gift if it is given for non-charitable
purposes or could possibly be so used[29] (see, further, chapter 3).

Public benefit

The public benefit test, differentiating between private and charitable trusts, has
been a fixed common law principle in England and Wales that has received
statutory recognition rule.[30] In common with other jurisdictions, the burden of
proof in relation to the 'benefit' requirement varies across the four *Pemsel* heads,
being presumed satisfied under the first three heads. In determining whether or
not a gift satisfies the public benefit test, the judiciary will apply an objective test.
The awaited new legislation will introduce several more heads of charity
(see, further, below).

Unlike all other jurisdictions, however, the responsibility for determining what
activities constitute a contemporary interpretation of public benefit sufficient to
justify the conferring of charitable status lies with a non-revenue-driven government body, the Charity Commission. Following the publication of the Deakin
report,[31] the Commission launched a rolling review of registered charities with a
view to updating the application of the public benefit criterion.

Exclusively charitable

This long-established principle was reiterated in *Att.-Gen. of the Cayman Islands* v.
Wah-Hansen,[32] when the Privy Council determined that a trust, the income from
which was paid to 'any one or more religious charitable or educational institution
or institutions operating for the public good', was in breach of the exclusivity rule
and therefore void. The term 'public good' was wider than public benefit for
charitable purposes and like 'philanthropic' and 'benevolent' could not therefore
be construed as exclusively charitable (see, further, chapter 1).

Independent

An important aspect of trust law as it developed in this jurisdiction is the importance attached to the independence of trustees and their overriding duty to further

the best interests of their charity ('trust'). However, the requirement of trustee independence is increasingly being compromised by government control and by the pressures of the modern market place (see, further, below).

Non-governmental

The dividing line between the public benefit service provision of government bodies and that of charities has now become difficult to draw with any certainty. The Charity Commission has advised that:[33]

> it is not a bar to charitable status that a new body has been created with a view to discharging a function of central or local government, provided that the new body was established for exclusively charitable purposes (which may coincide with a governmental authority's function) and not for furthering the non charitable purposes of securing and implementing the policies of any governmental authority.

Also that:[34]

> trustees cannot normally use a charity's funds to pay for services that a governmental authority is legally required to provide at the public expense. However, trustees might use a charity's resources to supplement what a governmental authority provides.

As government policy in this jurisdiction continues to promote the partnership ethos there is good reason to believe that this distinction will become increasingly blurred. Complicity between government and charities in addressing social need is an attractive and often effective proposition for both parties but if the latter allows itself to become merely the agent of the former then it may forfeit its right to charitable status.

The Charity Commission has emphasized that the governance of the charity must as a matter of practice be independent from the governmental authority. It advises that any charity planning to deliver public services must continue to comply with the following key legal principles:[35]

- Charities must only undertake activities that are within their objects and powers. This is essential. Charities must not stray from their objects in pursuit of funding.
- Charities must be independent of government and other funders. An organisation must be a separate and independent legal entity to be eligible for charitable status.
- Trustees must act only in the interests of the charity and its beneficiaries.
- Trustees must make decisions in line with their duty of care and duty to act prudently.

In a recent and landmark decision[36] the Commission would seem to have reviewed and adjusted its position somewhat on the above guidance. Having come to the view that charities can deliver public services which public authorities have a statutory duty to provide but have chosen to 'hive off' to voluntary associations, it then permitted the Trafford Community Leisure Trust and the Wigan Leisure and Culture Trust to be registered as charities. Its decision was based on evidence that in both cases the charities were sufficiently independent from the respective local authorities and that the trustees retained their discretion to use charitable funds to provide/subsidize a government service if they judged this to be in the best interests of the charity and complied with its objects. In this jurisdiction the boundaries of traditional government service provision are being rapidly eroded as schools, hospitals, all forms of community care and now possibly prisons acquire charitable status.

Non-profit distributing

In this jurisdiction the restrictions on profit distribution have inhibited the development of entrepreneurial philanthropy.

The recent introduction of community interest companies (CICs) is an interesting development. These are intended to be tailor-made vehicles for social entrepreneurs who are willing to accept a statutory asset lock on the application of assets for purposes that are not for the community benefit. It would seem that while charities are eligible to be formed as CICs, they will lose their charity status if they do so, the reason for this being that the government wishes to clearly distinguish the CIC 'brand' from charitable status.[37]

Charitable purposes

These remain as first identified in the 1601 Act and later classified in *Pemsel*, although subsequent judicial precedent guided by the 'spirit and intendment' rule has broadened the categories (see, further, chapter 3) while the outcome of the charity law reform process promises further enlargement. This list has always been treated as indicative rather than prescriptive. Its extension within the common law has been guided by analogy rather than by principle and has accommodated an exponential increase in the range of charities with purposes that are fitted under the fourth head. The 'public benefit test' has an unequal application across the four heads, gives rise to quixotic interpretations and has resulted in the exclusion of some contemporary manifestations of social need (see, also, chapters 3 and 4 and further p. 29).

The Charity Commission's review of organizations listed on the Register[38] which it began in 1997, together with its issue of advisory leaflets, has broadened the range of activities now entitled to charitable status.[39] Its capacity to do so has been assisted by an approach which seeks to identify the intrinsic public benefit component of an activity rather than continuing the traditional reliance upon the 'spirit and intendment' rule. This has resulted, for example, in the extension of charitable status to organizations established to promote urban and rural regener-ation,[40] to provide relief for the unemployed,[41] and to develop community capacity building.[42] The latter, as pointed out in Tudor, has a particular relevance for the socially marginalized:[43]

> Community capacity building here means developing the capacity and skills of members of a community in such a way as that they are better able to identify and help meet their needs and to participate more in society. The relevant community may be geographical or may be a community of interest, for example, membership of a particular ethnic group.

Legal structures for charities

Contemporary charitable activity in England and Wales is housed in a range of different structures but is still largely oriented around its initial form – the trust. Government-controlled bodies, religious organizations and foundations as well as the more traditional trusts, unincorporated associations and incorporated char-ities are now all likely to be claiming tax exemption on the grounds of their charitable activities. Industrial and Provident Societies, Friendly Societies and corporations (whether established by Royal Charter, statute or by Church meas-ure) may also, provide structures for charitable activity (see, further, chapters 3 and 6). An exotic and unlikely addition to such forms has recently emerged – the hedge fund. These alternative structures are important: many local voluntary organizations use the Industrial and Provident Societies model especially in fields like community transport; the Scout and Guide movement is established by Royal Charter and in turn creates thousands of separate Royal Charter charities for every local group or pack. In the Church of England, every local PCC (of which there are approximately 25,000) is incorporated by act of Parliament and by the powers of the Church Commissioners.[44]

Charities are thus subject to different governance arrangements and their trust-ees subject to a different set of standards depending on the legal structure involved.

Types of structure

There is at present no prescribed form for a charity; though the Charities Bill 2005 makes provision for the introduction of Charitable Incorporated Organiza-tions (see, further, below). In practice they normally take the form of an association (the simplest, with incorporation to give legal personality possible under the Charities Act), trust or charitable company limited by guarantee while some have been established by royal charter or act of Parliament. The American Com-munity Foundation successfully transferred to this jurisdiction in the late 1980s and has since prospered. Recently the government has been experimenting with social enterprises. This is a business with primarily social objectives whose sur-pluses are principally reinvested for that purpose in the business or in the com-munity, rather than being driven by the need to maximize profit for shareholders and owners. Some social enterprises are registered charities. The government is proposing to introduce the Community Interest Company which will provide an alternative to charitable status.

In this jurisdiction the structures for charity, like the law, has tended to strongly favour trusts. The Charity Commission does seek to satisfy itself as to the adequacy of the constitutional structure proposed for a charity on registration.

Regulatory framework

The Charity Commissioners are central to the legal framework for charities in England and Wales, notwithstanding the involvement of other government agencies and the role of the courts. It is the role of the Commission in relation to the Inland Revenue – Her Majesty's Revenue and Customs (HMRC) – that determines the contemporary parameters of charitable purposes.[45] The Charities Act 1993, which modernized and strengthened the Commission's powers, considerably reinforced charity regulation in this jurisdiction.

Charity Commissioners

The Charity Commissioners have statutory duties to register, regulate and support charities (see, also, chapters 3 and 5). This body, for most purposes, has a jurisdiction and exercises powers concurrent with those of the High Court[46] and Commissioners are vested with the same powers as the Attorney General (see, further, chapter 3) as regards taking proceedings in relation to charities.[47]

Registration

Charity Commissioners are responsible for registering and maintaining a public register of charities. The Charities Act 1993, in keeping with established precedents,[48] requires a charity to be set up under the jurisdiction of the law of England and Wales if it is to be eligible for registration. If it operates wholly or partially within the jurisdiction, but is incorporated and registered elsewhere, it will not qualify as a charity for the purposes of the 1993 Act.[49] Charitable purposes may, however, extend beyond the jurisdiction of the courts of England and Wales as, for example, is the case with Oxfam and many other such humanitarian relief agencies.

It is in the exercise of its registration function that the Commission is empowered to broaden the interpretation of charitable purposes. By registering (e.g. faith healing)[50] or deregistering (e.g. gun clubs)[51] in accordance with a contemporary interpretation of the public benefit test, the Commission is able to respond flexibly and reasonably promptly to changing definitions of social need and now does so without being unduly constrained by the 'spirit and intendment' rule.

The Central Register of Charities was established under the provisions of the Charities Act 1960.[52] It makes the purpose and constitution of charities publicly available, together with annual reports of activities and accounts to the prescribed form. All charities in England and Wales not specifically exempted or excepted from registration are required to register with the Commission and registered charities with an income over £10,000 are also required to send a set of their latest accounts and the trustees' annual report. It is important to note that being excused from the requirement to register is not confined to small charities with limited income; the churches and old universities are similarly privileged.

Regulatory role

All registered charities are required to draw up and submit to the Charity Commission an annual report of activities undertaken in pursuit of their objects, together with annual financial accounts, the complexity of which is determined by the size of the charity (measured in terms of income). Examination or audit requirements are likewise set according to turnover. The majority of registered charities (those with a turnover of less than £10,000 a year) are only required to have their annual report and accounts (in simple form) publicly available. Charities with a turnover of over £10,000 a year are required to submit their report and accounts to the Charity Commission. The Commission's regulatory role is restricted by the fact that 70 per cent of the 167,022 'main' charities registered in England and Wales have an income below the £10,000 limit and are therefore not required routinely to submit annual accounts and statutory annual returns to the Charity Commission, although they all are obliged to make accounts available to the Commission or members of the public on request. The accounting regulations for unincorporated charities require an independent examination for those with an income between £10,000 and £250,000, and a professional audit is only required where income exceeds £250,000. The reporting requirements for charities are set out in the Statement of Recommended Accounting Practice (SORP).

The Commission has extensive statutory powers to institute inquiries and appoint receivers, to investigate suspected misconduct, mismanagement and to protect a charity. It may appoint a receiver and manager to act in the place of trustees. Its remedial powers include replacing trustees and requiring restitution of charity money improperly used. It does not, however, have powers to prosecute abuse (a referral to the police is made if a criminal activity is suspected) or to impose punitive sanctions.

The new Charity Database and integrated monitoring system have improved the Commission's regulatory role, as did the coming into effect in 1998 of the reporting requirements in the Charities Acts 1992 and 1993.

Support

The Commission regards its support role as its main function. The Chief Charity Commissioner said in evidence to the Public Accounts committee: 'Our fundamental role as set out in the Charities Acts certainly from 1960 has been to enable charities to operate, to use their resources more effectively. In that sense, it is a promotional and support role first and foremost.'[53] He also referred to the Commission's original function of replacing the Chancery Court in providing legal services to charities.

The High Court and the Attorney General

In England and Wales the traditional common law powers of the High Court and the Attorney General – to protect, supervise and where necessary to amend charitable trusts – have now been largely statutorily transferred to or assumed by the Charity Commission since the Charities Act 1993. While the High Court shares a dual jurisdiction for most purposes with the Commission, it retains its powers of adjudication in relation to certain matters and will hear cases on appeal from the Commission.

Other agencies

A number of other agencies may have a regulatory role in relation to charities.

1 *The Inland Revenue* (now HMRC) An organization, claiming exemption from tax liability on grounds of charitable activity, may be investigated by the Inland Revenue which can direct submission of records etc. for scrutiny.
2 *The Registrar of Companies* Charitable companies have to file an annual report and accounts and make an annual return under the Companies Act 1985 (in most cases, this is the same document that they file with the Charity Commission). The ancient common law office of 'visitor', which allows for the appointment of a person to undertake the supervision of an organization's internal affairs, is most often associated with companies.
3 *Customs and Excise* (now HMRC) The Commissioners of Customs and Excise may exercise their powers under the Value Added Tax Act 1994 to carry out investigations for the purpose of establishing whether a charity is attempting to evade liability for VAT payments.

Regulating the fiscal environment

In England and Wales, responsibility for managing tax matters as they relate to registered charities rests with the Inland Revenue; other agencies are also involved in various aspects of the financial environment.

The Inland Revenue

This body has overall regulatory responsibility for matters relating to tax liability. It has no particular remit in relation to charities beyond ensuring that, like any other claimant, a charity meets the eligibility criteria for tax exemption and otherwise complies with normal legal and administrative requirements. It has a department designated for charitable matters, the HMRC Charities Unit, which has a specialist role particularly in terms of processing applications for repayment of tax on gift aid donations (Finance Act 2000). Where there is any doubt regarding the charitable status of an organization the Inland Revenue will refer and defer to the Charity Commission.

Tax and rates

There is no general exemption from tax. Charities can qualify for exemption from income tax and corporation tax under the Income and Corporation Taxes Act 1988 (Schedules A, C, D and F), from capital gains tax under the Taxation of Chargeable Gains Act 1992, and may also be eligible for exemption from inheritance tax and stamp duty. The Value Added Tax Act 1994 governs charitable exemption from VAT (a European Union tax imposed by the EC Sixth VAT directive which the UK is obliged to implement). The Local Government Finance Act 1992 provides charities with limited exemption from rates liability.

Donation incentives

The Income and Corporation Taxes Act 1988, as amended by the Finance Act 2000, entitles a company or an individual to tax relief on donations made by way of a gift aid scheme to charities. Gift aid by individuals is much more significant in scale and practical impact because the charity reclaims the tax paid by the donor; payroll giving is also significant. Total tax relief to charities on donations has been estimated at £1 billion for 2004–5.[54]

Cy-près

In addition to giving authoritative advice on legal matters and drawing on its experience of governance, administrative and financial issues, the Charity Commission has legal powers to amend the purposes and constitutions of charities through 'schemes' without the charity having to apply to the courts. Neither court nor Commission have the power to terminate a charity which still holds funds but is no longer able to further its purposes; although the Commission can deregister a charity that is no longer active or which has ceased to be charitable (e.g. some rifle clubs are no longer considered to promote the efficiency of the armed forces). However, under section 16(1) of the 1993 Act, both now exercise a concurrent jurisdiction to create *cy-près* schemes enabling the funds of such a charity to be administered, perhaps consolidated with those of other similar defunct charities, and be directed towards a new set of similar but viable objects. Until 1960 *cy-près* schemes were quite restricted, but the Charities Act 1993 now allows amendment or transfer not only when the original use is rendered impossible or impracticable but also when it is no longer effective (see, also, chapter 3).[55]

Fundraising

The provisions of the Charities Act 1992, which came into effect in 1995, are directed towards 'charitable institutions' defined as 'a charity or an institution other than a charity which is established for charitable benevolent or philanthropic purposes'. Parts II and III, the latter not yet in force, provide the main body of legislative provisions governing fundraising by charities. The aim of the new statutory requirements relating to 'professional fundraisers' and 'commercial participators'[56] is to ensure transparency and accountability where fundraising is being undertaken for profit.[57] The Act requires a written agreement between the charity and the professional fundraiser or commercial participator; a statement to potential donors as to the proportion of their donation going to the fundraiser, or the extent of benefit to the charity through involvement with the commercial participator; and that the funds raised must be passed to the charity. The fundraising regulations will be amended by the forthcoming charities legislation (see, further, below).

The Charity Commission has a purely advisory role in relation to fundraising[58] although it does have jurisdiction over funds collected in the name of charity, whether or not collected by a charitable body, and can act to protect funds so raised, e.g. by freezing bank accounts. The rules governing street collections and house-to-house collections on behalf of charity have been consolidated in the Part III provisions, are subject to regulations and are supervised by the local authority. In the case of raising money or selling goods for charity in the streets or public places a permit is usually required from the local authority. Similarly a local authority licence is normally required for house-to-house collections. Alleged criminal activity involving a charity (e.g. in the context of fundraising) will necessitate police enquiries and possible criminal proceedings in the normal way.

The National Lottery

The National Lottery Act 1993, as amended in 1998 (and to be replaced by new legislation in 2006), governs the raising and distribution of National Lottery funds for charities and other good causes.

Trading

The key issue for a charity undertaking commercial or enterprise activities is whether it is doing so as either:

1   primary purpose trading, or
2   trading for fundraising purposes.

Most cases of contracting with the public sector, for example, fall within category 1 and are then exempt from income or corporation tax. Most other trading including charity shops, selling cards and souvenirs, or fundraising events with admission charges falls in category 2 and is potentially liable to corporation tax. However, within category 2 there are various exemptions, the main ones being:

- trading by beneficiaries;
- sales of donated goods (this includes charity shops if only selling donated items);
- fundraising events, subject to certain limits on size and frequency; and
- other non-charitable trading up to prescribed limits (max £50,000 income).

If an activity falls within category 2 but is outside the exemptions above then it is necessary to establish a non-charitable trading subsidiary company. The main bar to a charity undertaking permanent non-primary purpose trading is that the government regards such tax-exempt profits as constituting 'unfair competition' with the private sector. Under the Income and Corporation Taxes Act 1988 (Schedule D), a charity will be eligible for tax exemption on profits from its trading activity[59] provided that these are applied to further its charitable purposes and either the trade is in furtherance of its primary purposes or is conducted by its beneficiaries.

Constraints on modern philanthropic activity

The Labour Party in this jurisdiction, now in its third term of office, has invested much government energy in building a partnership between State and charity. The cornerstone of this policy was laid decades earlier in the Goodman report.[60] It is a policy, however, that is not without risk for the charities concerned and its effectiveness as a means of focusing philanthropic resources on social inclusion issues is inhibited by certain constraints.

Policy constraints: partnership with government

In order to formalize the partnership strategy, the Deakin report specifically recommended a concordat between central government and the voluntary sector.[61] This was accepted by the Labour Party which made a General Election commitment to establish a 'compact' with a clear statement of the principles that would govern relations between central government and the sector and with a task force of ministers to oversee its implementation.

The compacts

Following the accession of Labour to government in May 1997 four separate compacts (for England, Scotland, Wales and Northern Ireland) were then developed.[62] These 'compacts' set out to clarify the respective roles of government and the voluntary sector in the context of the shared values and principles that underpin their partnership.

The compact is a framework document and a process negotiated initially between central government and a cross-section of representatives of the voluntary and community sector (i.e. national and local charities and non-charitable and community bodies). The framework document sets out the principles under which partnerships between public authorities and voluntary and community bodies should be developed. In particular it seeks to entrench the independence of voluntary bodies and ensure that the relationship is genuinely one of partnership. The compacts set the parameters for that partnership. While they relate to the wider voluntary and community sector, not only to charities, and while there is always the danger that they will function as aspirational declarations of intent rather than as an enforceable code of conduct, they do represent a further stage in the development of the centuries-old relationship between government and charities in their mutual commitment to promoting the public benefit. However, it remains the case that the partnership and the compacts are driven more by the interests of government than charities.

Government grants and contracts

Charities are increasingly being compromised by their need to engage in the 'contract culture', develop 'brand-driven' strategies and to compete with commercial organizations for market position. Mostly this is evident in the growth of partnership arrangements with government bodies which has been criticized by some as resulting in a 'muting of dissent'.[63] The increasingly close relationship between some charities and public authorities, particularly through service contracts, has prompted the Charity Commission to issue guidance about maintaining independence:[64]

> As independent regulator of charities, the Commission's position on whether charities engage in public service delivery is neutral; we neither encourage nor discourage it. We are concerned with ensuring that charities retain their independence, remain focussed on their objects and properly meet the needs of their beneficiaries.

It would seem, however, that there are limits to this policy. For example, when community interest companies were introduced the government said that it viewed them as suitable for assisting in the delivery of social services at the local authority level but did not envisage that they should be used to deliver centrally directed public services such as health and education.[65]

The National Lottery

The difficulty in drawing a line between the responsibilities of government and charity is well illustrated by the current controversy surrounding the use of Lottery funds for child care and health care services instead of promoting the arts, culture and national heritage. The 'additionality principle', intended to govern disbursement of funds by ensuring that projects funded would be supplementary to government services, has been undermined and instead a considerable proportion of annual funds are being channelled towards subsidizing the running costs of mainstream government services such as health care. This results in less money being available for charitable purposes.

International aid

In this jurisdiction, the government and prominent charities such as Oxfam are accustomed to working both jointly and independently to provide aid for underdeveloped nations and for those recovering from the effects of war or natural disaster. State aid has tended to be on a government-to-government basis and targeted towards developing social infrastructure. Charities, on the other hand, have tended to feel free to respond to need as and where they see fit, usually with basic food delivery and community development programmes. This arrangement is, however, subject to certain constraints.

First, while there is no doubt that charities in this jurisdiction have a well-earned and wholly legitimate reputation of contributing to the relief of the socially disadvantaged elsewhere,[66] there is uncertainty as to whether in some circumstances this must be accompanied by evidence of that contribution also generating benefit within the jurisdiction. The uncertainty, articulated by Lord Evershed MR in *Camille & Henry Dreyfus Foundation Inc.* v. *Inland Revenue Commissioners*[67] and subsequently reinforced by the Charity Commission,[68] would seem to rest on the issue of whether schemes of general public utility (e.g. roads, bridges, and other developmental projects) contribute directly to the relief of poverty in a specific locality or are of a more open-ended nature intended to generally improve the social infrastructure. The latter activity would appear not to warrant charitable status.

Second, charitable intervention in a foreign country may well have a political impact in that country where it could be seen by some as reflecting badly on prevailing government policies leading to resistance by those parties or in their unwarranted interference with the charity's role and resources. In such circumstances the decision in *McGovern* v. *A-G*[69] indicates that in this jurisdiction the charity would then also be vulnerable to a challenge of engaging in political activity with possible serious consequences for the organization's charitable status.

Finally, and most obviously, as all modern western nations look to their national security interests, there is growing government scepticism about what is seen as the poorly regulated role of international charities in channelling funds to socially disadvantaged countries where they might be misused for subversive purposes. There is a fear that the tightening of international anti-terrorism measures could be undermined by lax supervision of international charities.[70]

Common law constraints

In England and Wales the common law characteristics are obviously more deeply embedded than in other jurisdictions. While the constraints of some have been considerably alleviated by the clear statutory separation of Charity Commission and Inland Revenue functions, in other respects the traditional characteristics remain very evident and continue to restrain the development of philanthropic activity.

Role of the courts

The High Court retains its traditional inherent jurisdiction over charities and its protective remit in respect of charitable trusts, but this has now very largely fallen into abeyance, displaced by statutory powers vested in the Charity Commission, the consent of which is required, under section 33, Charities Act 1993, to any proceedings concerning the administration of a charity. Although the court can and does hear cases where proceedings are initiated by or against a charity, involve complex legal issues or are on appeal from the Commission, and continues to exercise its powers to make *cy-près* schemes or schemes for the administration of charities, it now does so very rarely. This applies equally to the role of the Attorney General who traditionally represented the Crown's *parens patriae* jurisdiction (see, further, chapter 3) and continues in most cases to be made a party to proceedings involving a charity but would now seldom initiate proceedings for the protection of trusts. In England and Wales, in keeping with the experience of other common law jurisdictions, the capacity of the courts to have an ongoing role in developing the guiding principles necessary to ensure an appropriate fit between charity law and contemporary social inclusion issues has faded. Unlike other jurisdictions, however, that role has instead been transferred to another agency equipped with the powers and responsibility to be proactive in giving effect to it.

Legal structures

In this jurisdiction charitable trusts constitute the largest number of charities on the register and this structure constrains their capacity to put in place effective governance models and to respond swiftly and flexibly to the demands of the modern market place.

Governance issues   Whether a charity takes the legal form of an unincorporated association, a trust or a charitable company has considerable implications for its governance thereafter and has been a matter of concern for the Charity Commission.[71] In all cases the directors and staff/members are subject to the common law rules but in the latter case, they are also fully subject to company law and to the principles and statutory duties that govern their roles and relationships. The management model available and the reciprocal rights and duties of directors and staff will differ significantly depending on the legal structure adopted.

The resulting constraints are particularly important in the context of community-based self-help schemes which are frequently initiated in this jurisdiction. In such enterprises the representation of 'users' in the management structure is rapidly becoming a necessity. More radically, many self-help groups now insist on exercising full control over their organizations. However, the strength of such situations, resting in the deliberate fusion of personal and organizational interests, is also their biggest weakness in terms of eligibility for charitable status.

Type of structure As has often been pointed out, the types of legal structures available in this jurisdiction are not ideally suited to give effect to charitable purposes.[72] The difficulties tend to be in the area of legal personality: how best to ensure limited liability for trustees while also equipping the charity to enter into contractual relations with third parties? The present means of coping with this is to opt for incorporation, which brings with it the full burden of administrative and regulatory requirements appropriate to commercial companies. There is a need for a new legal vehicle more tailored to the needs of charities such as 'the Charitable Incorporated Organization' and greater use could be made of existing vehicles such as endowed foundations (see, further, chapter 3).

Restrictions on advocacy/political activity

In England and Wales, as in other common law jurisdictions, the continuing inhibiting effect of this traditional constraint on charitable activity has been illustrated in a number of leading cases.[73] It is certain that an organization may not acquire charitable status and highly probable that it will be unable to retain it if one of its primary purposes is to campaign for changes in the law or government policy. This is a serious deficit in the capacity of charity law to address the circumstances of the socially marginalized. The strategy whereby a charity sets up a separate non-charitable organization to undertake such campaigning activity on its behalf is illogical and (like trading activities) may serve to obscure responsibility and accountability and detract from coherent and effective pursuit of charitable purposes (see, also, chapter 5).

The origin of these restrictions lies in the legal nature of charities, being 'trusts' enforceable by the courts – which have traditionally regarded changing the law and government policy as the responsibility of parliament, not the courts. Although the Charity Commission has issued guidance emphasizing that charities have a wide discretion to campaign and otherwise undertake political activities in pursuance of their charitable purposes[74] the restriction is nonetheless very evident. Thus, while charities like Oxfam, the RSPCA and Shelter are able to engage in political campaigning on issues concerning developing nations, animal welfare and homelessness quite vigorously, organizations such as Amnesty and Greenpeace are denied charitable status in this jurisdiction.

Fiscal issues

In this jurisdiction the government's traditional concern to regulate charities so that tax avoidance is minimized and the management of their finances accords with principles of transparency and accountability has been balanced by an interest in providing for the development of charitable purposes that meet a contemporary interpretation of public benefit. The separation of these functions, particularly after the 1993 Act, has clarified and focused the responsibilities of the agencies concerned, with the result that England and Wales now has the singular distinction of being the only common law jurisdiction in which the legal frame-work for philanthropy is not solely or even mainly driven by government concerns to protect its tax revenue base. However, some of the more traditional character-istics of the law continue to exercise a constraining effect on fiscal aspects of philanthropic activity.

Eligibility for charitable tax exemption   Section 506 of the Income and Corporation Taxes Act 1988 includes, as a definition of charity, a form of words similar to those used by the House of Lords in *Pemsel*.[75] This in effect continues the common law definitional restrictions, safeguards the charitable status of registered charities and ensures their exemption from tax liability in the absence of any contrary evidence.

The doctrine of cy-près   This ancient device for redirecting the resources of charities, with enormous potential in the context of adjusting philanthropy to address modern issues of social inclusion, remains constrained by several common law rules including the three certainties test etc. (see, further, chapter 3).

Fundraising and trading etc.   The regulatory framework for fundraising lacks coherence and is unable to satisfactorily accommodate the proliferation of modern fundraising methods which now include the National Lottery, telethons and professional fundraiser companies. Some enterprises with brief but global impact, blending political and entertainment functions, have enormous capacity for informing, fundraising and for affecting change in the circumstances of the socially disadvantaged, but it is uncertain where they fit in terms of charity law and the fundraising regulations (e.g. 'Live 8' and 'Make Poverty History').

The requirement that a charity sets up a separate and subsidiary organization to undertake trading activity on its behalf is unnecessarily cumbersome and can obscure accountability.

Public benefit matters

In addition to the above-mentioned definitional aspects of the public benefit test there are other matters associated with this test which act to constrain the activities of charities.

Uneven application of the public benefit test   The fact that the test has an uneven application across the four *Pemsel* heads, falling with particular stringency on fourth-head charities, is itself a constraint on the evolution of new forms of philanthropy.

Moreover, the continuance and spread of anomalous exceptions to the test, such as those accommodated under the 'poor relations' rule, creates uncertainty.

Exclusion of matters clearly in the public benefit   As mentioned earlier, the fact that certain purposes such as addressing the causes of poverty, the pursuit of justice, and the promotion of peace and reconciliation are denied recognition in charity law as being for the public benefit and thus warranting charitable status is clearly illogical and counter-productive in the context of social inclusion.

Modern law constraints

In England and Wales the separation of functions dealing with policing tax revenue returns and developing charitable purposes has allowed charity law to be more responsive to emerging patterns of social need than in other jurisdictions.

Forum for developing charitable purposes

The powers and responsibilities of the Charity Commission, as strengthened by the 1993 Act, have equipped this agency to exercise effective leadership in adjusting charitable purposes to meet contemporary social need. Because of its concurrent High Court jurisdiction coupled with intensive ongoing engagement with matters of principle and practice the Commission has been able to move somewhat beyond the confines of the 'spirit and intendment' rule in its efforts to address emerging areas of need. However, the Commission is far from having a free rein in such matters. Its discretion remains confined by the straightjacket of established precedent: new charitable purposes must still be analogous to those already recognized by the law.

Human rights, anti-terrorism and social justice legislation

The Human Rights Act 1998, incorporating the Convention, came into force in the UK on 2 October 2000. From that date all 'public bodies', including courts, local authorities and the Charity Commission, have been required to ensure that their processes and decisions are Convention compliant.[76] All case law resulting from decisions of the European Court of Human Rights (ECHR) has since had a direct relevance for the courts in the United Kingdom.

However, in the political climate set by the UN Security Council Resolution 1373 and the realities of the UK being a combatant nation in Iraq, the government introduced measures to tighten national security that have stretched the limits of compatibility with the European Convention. Indeed, as clearly emphasized by the House of Lords, measures such as detention without trial breached the government's human rights obligations.[77] That House of Lords ruling prompted some political debate as to the desirability of the UK formally derogating from its Convention commitments. Following the London terrorist atrocities in July 2005,

Westminster Parliament passed tough new anti-terrorism legislation including police powers of surveillance, stop and search, summary arrest and deportation, which as noted earlier are in practice implemented in a discriminatory manner, perhaps necessarily.

In this jurisdiction, the effect of current government security measures threatens the real achievements of previous decades in building a multicultural society – achievements marked by a comprehensive programme of social justice legislation, underpinned by a core of anti-discrimination statutes which showed the way for similar legislation in other nations. The potential for effective philanthropic intervention must now be viewed in the context of constraints on civil liberties emanating from the government's preoccupation with matters of national defence.

Charity law review and social inclusion

England and Wales, in keeping with the other two jurisdictions that together constitute the United Kingdom, has in recent years been engaged in a protracted process of charity law reform. This process, which began with publication of a report by the National Council of Voluntary Organizations (NCVO) in 2001,[78] is now drawing to a close. The recommendations initially proposed in the review of the legal framework for the voluntary sector[79] were, after a period of public consultation, accepted by the government.[80] The resulting draft Charities Bill[81] was introduced to the Houses of Parliament in May 2005. The proposals are now finally to be translated into legislative provisions. Of the Bill's three parts, two deal with regulatory provisions for fundraising and with definitional matters.

Proposed changes to definitional matters and legal structures

In keeping with the recommendation made in the Deakin report,[82] the present draft bill proposes to enact for the first time a general statutory definition of charity for the purposes of the law in England and Wales.[83] The intention, essentially, is to preserve the existing meaning of charitable purposes as developed by the courts while permitting the development of new ones to the extent that they are analogous to those already in existence. It is proposed that in future a 'charity' will be an organization with exclusively charitable purposes which fall within the list of twelve descriptions of purposes contained in the Bill and which are for the public benefit.

Charitable purpose

The government proposes that the new legislation will extend the current classification of 'charitable purposes' from four to twelve categories. Under section 2 of the Charities Bill, a 'charitable purpose' is one that is for either:

(a)   the prevention or relief of poverty;
(b)   the advancement of education;
(c)   the advancement of religion;
(d)   the advancement of health or the saving of lives;
(e)   the advancement of citizenship or community development;
(f)   the advancement of the arts, culture, heritage or science;
(g)   the advancement of amateur sport;
(h)   the advancement of human rights, conflict resolution or reconciliation or the promotion of religious or racial harmony or equality and diversity;
(i)   the advancement of environmental protection or improvement;
(j)   the relief of those in need by reason of youth, age, ill-health, disability, financial hardship or other disadvantage;
(k)   the advancement of animal welfare; or
(l)   any other purposes within subsection (4).

The additions are essentially a restatement of the purposes that in recent decades have come to be recognized as charitable. The main exception is the promotion of amateur sport as a charitable purpose in its own right rather than as a means of advancing other existing charitable purposes.[84]

Public benefit

The key proposed change is the removal of the public benefit presumption applicable to the first three *Pemsel* heads of charity, in keeping with the NCVO recommendation in 2001 that the single criterion for charitable status should be the public benefit test as under existing common law. Under section 3 of the Charities Bill, charitable status in all cases and under all of the above heads will in future, therefore, be dependent upon an ability to establish that the purpose of the organization specifically meets the public benefit test. The meaning of public benefit as developed by the courts will remain unchanged but all charities will now have to pass that test.[85]

Legal structures

A new form of corporate body, the Charitable Incorporated Organization (CIO), is to be introduced which can be established with limited or unlimited liability but only for charitable purposes. The Charity Commission will be solely responsible for the incorporation and registration of the CIO and for assisting existing charitable companies limited by guarantee or Industrial and Provident Societies to convert to a CIO.

Proposed changes to the regulatory framework

The lead role of the Charity Commission in developing the capacity of the charity sector in England and Wales is to continue, but will be strengthened by the statutory broadening of its powers in respect of definitional matters and its regulatory function.

Primary regulatory body

The legal status of the Charity Commission will change. In future it will be a statutory corporation with the following new objectives:

- increasing public confidence;
- increasing compliance with legal obligations;
- encouraging the 'social and economic impact' of charities; and
- enhancing accountability.

In furtherance of these objectives the Commission is to have the following general functions:

- determining charitable status;
- facilitating better charity administration;
- identifying, investigating and remedying abuse;
- obtaining, evaluating and disseminating information; and
- giving information, advice and proposals to ministers.

The Commission's dual role as regulator and facilitator of charities is to continue.

Registration

The registration requirement is to be extended to include those larger charities previously exempt or excepted. As a starting point, where such a charity has an annual gross income exceeding £100,000 and is not subject to another regulator, it will be required to register with the Charity Commission. It is intended that this monetary threshold will be lowered in stages until all charities with an annual income of more than £5,000 will be required to register. Where a charity has an annual gross income of less than £5,000 it will be allowed to register on a voluntary basis.

Charity Appeals Tribunal

This new body is to be established to hear appeals against decisions of the Charity Commission, including decisions on charitable status. The tribunal will consider the decision afresh and can admit new evidence.[86] This promises to be an important development as critics of the present system have often made the point that a specialist court could do much to improve the development of the common law and would be in a position to ensure greater consistency in charity law judgments. Appeals can be made to the High Court against the tribunal's decision on a point of law.

Proposed changes to financial matters

Fundraising

Regulating fundraising, and thereby increasing public confidence in the sector, is clearly among the legislative priorities. Most of the provisions in Part 3 of the draft Bill are intended to implement the Home Office's proposals to introduce a unified system to regulate public charitable collections throughout England and Wales.[87] A public charitable collection is defined as a collection of money or other property which takes place in any public place or by means of visits to houses or business premises. The definition is intended to be wide enough to cover all appeals for 'good causes', whether or not charitable, and will apply to collections by or on behalf of campaigning organizations. The promoters of a public charitable collection will be obliged to apply for a Certificate of Fitness which will be issued by the local authority. Local authorities will have limited powers to refuse or withdraw a certificate in appropriate circumstances, and these powers will be subject to a right of appeal. The draft Bill also provides a new reserve power for the Secretary of State to issue regulations to impose good practice requirements on those persons responsible for a charity's fundraising activities. The present policy of the government is to await and review the outcome of the charity sector's efforts to develop an effective policy of self-regulation of fundraising practices before deciding whether to make use of this power.[88]

Implications for social inclusion

As recently stressed by the relevant government minister, the charity law reform process is intended to have direct implications for social inclusion.[89] After much hesitation, this process has taken the route of introducing a statutory specification of definitional matters. This will not entail abandoning the common law basis for determining charitable status as the body of established precedents will continue to guide the future interpretation of such matters, particularly in relation to issues arising under the four *Pemsel* heads, and the vast majority of registered charities will continue to be so. However, with the passage of time it can be anticipated that the new bearing of the public benefit test, together with a build-up of case law principles relating to the broader range of charitable purposes, will gradually alter the relevance of the common law legacy.

Strengths of reform proposals

A number of the changes introduced by the Charities Bill have positive implications for the future capacity of charities to address the social inclusion agenda.

The public benefit test   Removal of the public benefit presumption in respect of the first three *Pemsel* heads will in future require bodies such as public schools, independent hospitals, religious organizations and those established under the rules relating to 'poor relatives' and 'poor employees' to demonstrate that their services are also to some degree accessible to the poor or otherwise socially marginalized if they are to acquire or retain charitable status. This and the fact that the test will be applied objectively must serve to increase the number and range of marginalized people involved in mainstream social activity.

The prevention of poverty   While this includes preventing those who are poor from becoming poorer and preventing persons who are not poor from becoming poor, it remains to be seen how or to what extent it will facilitate organizations dedicated to eradicating the causes of poverty. Nonetheless, this provision must increase the numbers benefiting from localized schemes for dealing strategically with embedded poverty within the jurisdiction and in developing countries.

The advancement of health or the saving of lives   The specific recognition now given to this charitable purpose must again give a particular boost to those organizations involved in mass child inoculation programmes and in combating AIDS and other diseases in developing countries.

The advancement of citizenship or community development   The capacity of charities to contribute towards building social capital and promoting or sustaining the growth of civil society will be enhanced by this provision. Encompassing as it does activities that promote urban and rural regeneration, community capacity building, civic responsibility and good citizenship, it should serve to encourage those organizations working with ethnic minorities and other deprived communities in this jurisdiction.

The advancement of human rights, conflict resolution or reconciliation or the promotion of religious or racial harmony or equality and diversity   On the face of it this provision marks a most important development in charity law as it relates to social inclusion. The recognition given to the role that could be played by mediatory organizations – locally, regionally, nationally and internationally – in negotiating with those who perceive themselves to be alienated, to find a positive way forward and thereby forestall a drift towards conflict, lies at the heart of the challenge to make philanthropy relevant to social inclusion in the twenty-first century. The reference to promoting 'religious or racial harmony or equality and diversity' has a particular resonance in the present global context of a growing estrangement between Islam, or some of its followers, and the western democracies. It is a reference that also encourages mediatory activity on behalf of those who in a more domestic context feel discriminated against for reasons of race, disability, age, sexual orientation, etc. In addition, it would seem to accommodate activities intended to identify and address causes as well as effects of alienation or mutual estrangement. It has a strong preventative dimension. However, clearly this new charitable purpose sits uneasily alongside the common law constraints on political activity by charities and until we see how the tension between the two is resolved it is difficult to estimate the potential impact of this purpose on the social inclusion agenda. In particular, this purpose may not gain acceptance in other common law jurisdictions.

The relief of those in need, by reason of youth, age, ill health, disability, financial hardship or other disadvantage   Again, like the advancement of citizenship etc., this charitable purpose is one with particular application to the domestic social inclusion agenda. It maintains the very traditional focus of charity on those in need for reasons that have attracted compassion, protection and resources throughout the duration and extent of the common law. It accommodates relief in the form of specialist advice, equipment, care or accommodation and specialist housing, care centres, drop-in centres, etc.

Other purposes currently recognized as charitable and any new charitable purposes which are similar to another charitable purpose   Finally, this default provision continues the function provided by the fourth *Pemsel* head, although in future any extension will be statutorily tied to the rule that a new purpose must be analogous to one already existing and, by implication, the 'spirit and intendment' rule is discontinued. This purpose also carries over into the new legislative era the established capacity for partnership between government and charity by allowing for the continuation of charitable status in respect of those organizations that make a public service type contribution. So, the provision of public works and services and the provision of public amenities (such as the repair of bridges, ports, havens, causeways and highways, the provision of water and lighting, a cemetery or crematorium, as well as the provision of public facilities such as libraries, reading rooms and public conveniences) are all thereby endorsed as charitable. Organizations and gifts for the relief of unemployment, for the social relief, resettlement and rehabilitation of persons under a disability or deprivation (including disaster funds) and for the benefit of a particular locality (such as trusts for the general benefit of the inhabitants of a particular place) will similarly continue to be entitled to charitable status.[90]

Weaknesses of reform proposals

It remains to be seen whether the changes resulting from an objective application of the public benefit test across all charitable purposes and the development of new purposes in accordance with the analogous rule will be sufficient to modernize the charity law framework. However, at this stage it is possible to note that from the perspective of its capacity to address this jurisdiction's contemporary agenda of domestic and international social inclusion issues, the Charities Bill has some weaknesses.

It fails, for example, to deal specifically with certain long-standing areas of difficulty.

Partnership with government   A continuation and strengthening of the partnership between government and charity to address public service and civil society matters is at least implicit in some of the proposed charitable purposes. It is not clear how this is to be achieved without compromising the independence of charities.

Legal structures   While the proposed introduction of a new structure – the Charitable Incorporated Organization – is very much to be welcomed, more perhaps could have been done to encourage the creation of such other appropriate structures as the endowed charitable trust. Moreover, the challenge posed to existing structures by the rise in user-dominated governance models has yet to be addressed.

Restrictions on advocacy/political activity   The opportunity would seem to have been missed to bring statutory clarification to this contentious matter, which is central to the relationship between charity law and social inclusion. In particular it is regrettable that provisions were not introduced to clearly empower charities to have as a primary purpose the discretion to lobby for change in law and policy.

Fiscal issues   The above-mentioned constraints relating to fundraising, trading and the use of *cy-près* schemes continue to be problematic. There also remain issues regarding such matters as donation incentive schemes, the role of private finance and the rules governing global enterprises such as 'Live 8' and venture philanthropy initiatives (see, also, chapter 2).

Conclusion

Charity law in a common law context emanates from this jurisdiction. It has guided the development of that law in the common law nations and in all probability, as statutorily reconfigured, will continue to shape the future legal framework for philanthropy in those nations. The changes proposed in the Charities Bill will have significance far beyond their immediate impact on charity law in England and Wales.

The proposed statutory changes are important but the principal jurisdictional characteristics of the law will continue. In particular the institutional separation of the revenue-driven functions from those of determining and developing charitable purposes, represented by the Inland Revenue and the Charity Commission respectively, will remain as the key distinguishing hallmark of the regulatory framework in this jurisdiction. The body of case law precedents and principles relating to the four *Pemsel* heads will also remain in place, as will the trust foundations for modern charities and the institutional administrative framework. The practice developments already underway in relation, for example, to partnership arrangements between charities and government and experimentation with new legal structures, will carry through to the new era and may well prove to be as significant as the legislative developments. The statutory definition and extension of charitable purposes, coupled with the uniform application of the public benefit test, will introduce change over time but the 400-year-old common law legacy is not being abandoned. The new legislation will by no means mark a fresh start to charity law in this jurisdiction.

The social inclusion agenda can only benefit from the proposed changes. But it will not benefit as much as it could have done. The restrictions on advocacy/political activity and on fiscal issues relating to trading, *cy-près* schemes, etc., will continue to inhibit the development of a strategic role for philanthropy. In particular, however, the increasing tension between human rights and anti-terrorism measures may well exercise a more fundamental constraint on philanthropic activity – locally, regionally, nationally and internationally.

Chapter 9

Charity law and social inclusion in Ireland

Introduction

Charity law in Ireland is rooted in the common law and anchored on the Statute of Pious Uses 1634[1] and its English predecessor the Statute of Charitable Uses 1601.[2] It has developed to become more facilitative than interventionist in nature, is dependent upon a legislative framework that is 40 years old and is given effect through a range of government bodies and legal structures which have quite traditional legal functions.

This chapter explores the reality of the fit between charity law and social inclusion in contemporary Ireland. It begins with some background information, briefly outlines the size and significance of the charitable sector and considers the profile of current social inclusion issues. It then examines Irish charity law by applying the template of functions (see, further, chapter 6) and methodically assessing, to the extent that they differ from those of England and Wales, the key definitional matters, the legal structures for charities, registration and the regulatory framework, financial matters and the legal constraints on the development of philanthropy. The chapter takes stock of the current charity law review process and analyses the implications arising for social inclusion issues. It concludes with a summary of the more distinctive characteristics of Irish charity law and highlights some concerns regarding its future capacity to address social inclusion.

Ireland, charities and social inclusion

The country

The Republic of Ireland is a small country of 68,890 square kilometres with a population estimated at 3,917,336 persons in the April 2002 national census.[3] The modern State dates from the Anglo-Irish War of Independence of 1919–21 and the subsequent Anglo-Irish Treaty of 1921, which ended almost eight centuries of political domination by neighbouring Britain. The treaty partitioned the island of Ireland into two jurisdictions: the overwhelmingly Roman Catholic 26-county Irish Free State in the south, which covered 80 per cent of the island's land area and which had a large degree of independence, and the six counties of Northern Ireland, which had a Protestant majority and remained part of the UK.

In 1937 the Irish Constitution, renamed the Irish Free State as Ireland (or Eire) and in 1948 the southern jurisdiction officially became the Republic of Ireland. In the northern jurisdiction, a protracted 30-year period of civil unrest with its roots in the division of the island and which impacted on the politics and economy of Ireland has recently drawn more or less to a close.[4]

Since the early 1990s, after a long period of decline relative to the rest of north-west Europe, Ireland has been enjoying an unprecedented and relatively continuous economic boom which in the year 2000 resulted in the highest rate of GDP growth ever recorded in an OECD member country. During this period it has also undergone considerable socio-demographic changes. The rural/urban balance in population distribution was reversed from its previous 60:40 ratio and was accompanied by a corresponding switch in emphasis from an agriculturally based economy to one that is now much more service based, is host to a large number of multinational manufacturing companies and has a well-educated workforce concentrated in the high-tech sector. The population increased significantly due partially to substantial and sustained non-Irish immigration from the mid-1990s onwards including, from the late 1990s, a rise in the number of asylum seekers. It changed also from being a homogenous monocultural society, coalesced around the Catholic Church and with the highest level of regular church attendance in Europe, to a much more multicultural and multifaith society.

These changes were largely due to the ending of Ireland's isolationist policy with its focus on nurturing a newly found political identity and fostering the growth of an indigenous Irish Catholic culture. In 1973 Ireland joined the European Economic Community (EEC), now the European Union (EU), in 1979 the fixed link between the Irish pound and sterling was broken when Ireland joined the European monetary system (EMS) and in 2002 it distanced itself further from sterling when it abandoned its native currency for the euro. Ireland also became a member of the UN, the OECD and the Council of Europe. The Irish economy has benefited greatly from its enthusiastic commitment to the EC and as its borders have been opened up to an internal EC immigrant workforce so Irish society has become quite suddenly Europeanized.

The charitable sector

The voluntary (or not-for-profit, or voluntary and community) sector, of which charities form a large part, has always played a prominent role in the socio-economic infrastructure of the Republic of Ireland.[5] In particular, the facilities for providing education, health and social care services were very largely established and staffed by the sector with religious organizations providing the bulk of the resources. Since the introduction of national welfare services, the State has either assumed responsibility for delivering such services or is doing so in partnership with the sector.[6]

The voluntary sector, however, continues to play a leading part in the socio-economic life of the nation[7] as was illustrated in a fairly recent study.[8] In 1995 the sector contributed £3.24 billion or 8.2 per cent of GDP and 9.3 per cent of

GNP. Inclusion of the added value contributed by volunteers raises the figures to £3.7 billion, 9.45 per cent and 10.66 per cent respectively. In total, the sector contributed more to the national economy in that year than agriculture and fishing combined and twice that of public administration and defence. However, the lack of any registration system makes it difficult to differentiate between charities and other not-for-profit bodies in terms of their relative contributions to the economy.

Ireland has a particularly rich and diverse range of not-for-profit organizations. While the customary broad division between mutual benefit and public benefit applies, this accommodates a wide spread of non-government organizations including co-operatives, charities, trade unions, residents' associations, foundations, self-help groups, etc. In addition to its NGOs, Ireland also has a significant and growing number of other types of not-for-profit bodies. Since acquiring independence, the national strategy for promoting Irish economic growth and development has depended to a considerable extent on a core of State and semi-State bodies with their distinctive rules governing profit distribution. Then there are the usual social infrastructure bodies established and managed by the government to deliver public benefit services such as transport and health care. Within the sector there are probably upwards of 5,000 charities[9] and the importance of their contribution to the economy in Ireland has been stressed:[10]

> Charities play a vital role in the provision of essential services, and ensuring the participation of Irish citizens in the development of a real civil society. They rely on three main sources of income to enable them to carry out their work effectively and efficiently: State aid and public sector grants and payments; public donations; and earned income (which includes subscriptions, membership dues and the intake from charity shops). The White Paper states that public sector support of the community and voluntary sector amounted to £895.924 m in 1999, which is significant.

Economic growth and the social inclusion agenda

In this jurisdiction, the economic phenomenon known as the 'Celtic tiger' has been well documented. Since 1993 the Irish economy expanded rapidly, with annual rates of growth in excess of 8 per cent averaged over the 1993–7 period. Total employment grew by 25 per cent between 1993 and 1998 and by 1998 the unemployment rate had fallen to less than 8 per cent – below the EU average.[11] Now the immediate domestic concern is to manage the consequences of this last decade of unprecedented economic growth and to ensure that the rising tide of the nation's increased prosperity lifts all boats. There are many indications that this is not happening and, if anything, wealth is now even more unevenly distributed.

Need for a more inclusive agenda

In contemporary Ireland there are pockets of rural deprivation, the 'travelling community' continue to suffer the poorest standards of health, housing and longevity while real poverty continues to oppress a sizeable proportion of the population.[12] There are other indications of latent social inequity. The booming economy has attracted large numbers of immigrants and for the first time in centuries the national census reveals a considerable increase in population,[13] particularly in the labour market sector. This has brought with it much evidence of racial discrimination, problems relating to asylum seekers,[14] homelessness and drug abuse.

In addition, the roles ascribed to those traditional bulwarks of a stable and conservative Irish society – the marital family unit and the Roman Catholic Church – have undergone great changes in the past couple of decades.

Government policy

The Irish government acknowledges the problems associated with poverty and the need for a more inclusive agenda.

In 1986 the Combat Poverty Agency was established by statute under the Combat Poverty Act with the following four main functions: to advise and make recommendations to the Minister for Social Welfare on all aspects of economic and social planning in relation to poverty in the State; to initiate and evaluate measures aimed at overcoming poverty in the State; to examinae the nature, causes and extent of poverty in the State and to promote, commission and interpret research; and to promote of greater public understanding of the nature, causes and extent of poverty in the State and the measures necessary to overcome it. The Agency is now involved in a range of programmes and activities to combat poverty and funds a number of representative national voluntary anti-poverty networks including the Community Workers Co-operative, the European Anti-Poverty Network, the Irish National Organization of the Unemployed, Irish Rural Link and the Irish Traveller Movement.

The Office for Social Inclusion, a government office with overall responsibility for developing, co-ordinating and driving the National Action plan against poverty and social exclusion, became operational in January 2003. In July 2003 the government submitted its National Action plan against Poverty and Social Inclusion for 2003–5 to the EC. The National Anti-Poverty Strategy's *Building an Inclusive Society* set targets for government bodies in respect of social inclusion programmes for up to 2007. In its second National Action Plan against poverty and social exclusion, for the period 2003–5, the government identified the following vulnerable groups: women; children and young people; older people; people with disabilities; travellers; prisoners and ex-prisoners. It recognized that urban poverty and rural disadvantage together with migrants and ethnic minorities were particular focal points for exclusion.[15]

*Government, charities and preparations for a new
regulatory framework*

The government, in response to a number of earlier reports,[16] declared in the *Agreed Programme for Government* (2002) its commitment to reform the law relating to charity: 'a comprehensive reform of the law relating to charities will be enacted to ensure accountability and to protect against abuse of charitable status and fraud'.[17] This is currently being conducted in partnership with the voluntary and community sector. It is anticipated that the charity law review process will lead to the introduction of new legislation in 2006. Charity law reform in Ireland is being undertaken in the context of a government policy to promote social inclusion: 'Government is strongly committed to building an inclusive society in which community and voluntary groups can play a vital role'.[18]

Definitional matters and legal framework

The Charities Acts of 1961 and 1973 provide a statutory framework for charities and charitable activities in Ireland. Other not-for-profit organizations (e.g. Industrial and Provident Societies) are subject to legislation specific to their needs and their activities may also come within the scope of statutes such as the Companies Acts of 1963 and 1990, the Tax Consolidation Act 1997 and the Freedom of Information Act 1997.

Statutory definition

In Ireland, the contemporary legislative framework fails to provide a definition of 'charity', fails to identify where responsibility lies for determining charitable status and fails also to specify whether the test to be applied to determine such status is to be applied objectively or subjectively. To some degree these legislative gaps have been bridged by *Pemsel*, the 'spirit and intendment' rule and related case law.

The common law

In Ireland, the counterpart to the Statute of Charitable Uses 1601[19] was the Statute 10 Car. 1 sess. 3 c. 1 entitled 'An Act for the Maintenance and Execution of Pious Uses 1634',[20] which sought to address the problem of the misappropriation of funds, donated for religious purposes. Sir Edward Sugden LC in *Incorporated Society* v. *Richards*[21] held that the Irish statute of 1634 and the English one of 1601 were to be treated as being of similar effect, though in fact the Irish statute differed in some respects from the English. The *Pemsel*[22] classification of charitable purposes was thus accepted in Ireland and their judicial interpretation, aided by the 'spirit or intendment' rule has developed along much the same lines as in England and Wales.

Statute law

In practice the question of whether the activities of an organization can be defined as charitable will arise when it seeks exemption from liability to pay either taxes or rates on the grounds that it is a charity. Applications for the former are determined by the Revenue Commissioners and the latter by the Valuation Office, both acting quite separately and independently of each other and unassisted by statutory definitions.

Charitable exemption from tax   In the absence of any statutory definition in the Charity Law Acts of 1961 and 1973, the Revenue Commissioners employ the above common law interpretation of charitable purpose to determine exemption. However, charitable purposes at law are wider than those for which the Revenue has traditionally granted tax-exempt status.[23]

Charitable exemption from rates   Again there is no statutory definition to guide decisions. The statutory provisions governing the eligibility of premises for exemption from rates, on the grounds that they are being used for charitable purposes, remain rooted in mid-nineteenth-century legislation.[24] The grounds are not synonymous with those required to substantiate eligibility for charitable exemption from tax. A significant volume of reported judgments clearly distinguishes the law governing charitable exemption from rates in this jurisdiction from that prevailing elsewhere in these islands. In this jurisdiction, it is a common occurrence that an organization will be recognized as a charity but a claim that its premises be exempted from rates because of the charitable activities of the occupier will be denied.

Elements of definition

These are very largely the same as for England and Wales and have evolved similarly (see, also, chapter 8). However there are one or two significant points of difference.

Charitable intent

In Ireland, the judiciary adopts a subjective test in determining whether or not a gift satisfies the public benefit test.[25] The courts will pose the question 'Did the donor believe that the purpose to which he or she was directing a gift was of a charitable nature?' As explained by Keane J in *In re the Worth Library*:[26]

> In every case, the intention of the testator is of paramount importance. If he intended to advance a charitable object recognised as such by the law, his gift will be a charitable gift.

This is quite different from the more restrictive approach of the UK judiciary in similar circumstances where the focus is firmly on deducing the nature of the gift from an objective appraisal of the facts.

Public benefit

The public benefit test, differentiating between private and charitable trusts, has long been a statutory rule in England and Wales[27] but except in relation to religion has never received statutory recognition in Ireland. Indeed, in common with other jurisdictions, the burden of proof in relation to the 'benefit' requirement varies across the four *Pemsel* heads, but in Ireland it is statutorily exempted from having any application to trusts for the advancement of religion.

Exclusively charitable

In Ireland, the judiciary always applied the rule requiring exclusiveness in charitable purposes with some equivocation[28] until statute law placed the matter beyond doubt. The Charities Act 1961, s. 49, now provides that:

> Where any of the purposes of a gift includes or could be deemed to include both charitable and non-charitable objects, its terms shall be so construed and given effect as to exclude the non-charitable objects and the purpose shall, accordingly, be treated as charitable.

However, while the Revenue Commissioners are guided by this provision when determining eligibility for charitable exemption from tax, the rule continues to be applied by the Valuation Office when determining charitable exemption from rates.

Non-governmental

In Ireland many large semi-State bodies have been established by the government as charities. However, when providing public benefit services such bodies are constrained in their capacity to do so by their political masters; they cannot act independently in marshalling resources to satisfy user-identified need. Such charities are clearly vulnerable to pressure to become government agents in the delivery of a government agenda.

Charitable purposes

These conform to the *Pemsel* classification and have evolved similarly, with some significant differences, to those of England and Wales (see, also, chapter 8).

Relief of poverty

The existence of a difference in the relative legal standing statutorily assigned to 'poverty' in the Statute of Pious Uses (Ireland) 1634 and the Statute of Charitable Uses 1601 has long been recognized. The relevant wording used in the Irish statute refers to the relief and maintenance of 'poor, succourless, distressed or impotent persons' whereas the corresponding English provision referred to 'aged, impotent and poor people'. The clearly distinct categorization of potential recipients of charity in the former spared the courts in Ireland from the debate in England which has lingered around the issue of whether they should be construed in a disjunctive manner. As a consequence, there has never been any challenge to the presumption that each named category can be considered independently (the 'poor' for example, are not also required to be 'impotent'). As in England and Wales, 'the requirement of public benefit has all but disappeared in the context of trusts for the relief of poverty'.[29]

The advancement of education

In Ireland, religion and education have always been closely linked. The history of charity law, as it relates to trusts for the advancement of education, is tied closely to the history of religious organizations. Unlike the position in England and Wales, a large part of the educational infrastructure in this jurisdiction has been and continues to be provided by religious bodies. Elsewhere in these islands, the importance of this branch of charity law has faded as the role of voluntary organizations in education has been displaced by State provision. In Ireland, as many of the buildings and teachers comprising the educational system are provided by religious bodies or to a lesser extent by other independent organizations, trusts for the advancement of education continue to have a real significance.

The public benefit test: the 'public' requirement   Determining the minimum number of possible beneficiaries necessary to meet an acceptable definition of 'public' has proved difficult. In *Re Worth Library*,[30] Keane J was certain that three named persons was insufficient but could only suggest that to satisfy a definition of 'public' the number should not be 'negligible'.

In Ireland, the rule governing membership of a class remains as stated prior to the ruling of the House of Lords in *In re Baden's Deed Trusts*[31] when it was generally accepted that the objects of a trust must be certain: the language employed must be certain; and the trustees must at any time be able to ascertain definitively the persons who would have a vested interest in the capital and income of the trust property. On the other hand where the trustees were not bound by a trust but merely had a power or discretion to confer or withhold a benefit then the requirement of certainty was recognized as being far less stringent.[32] In this juris-diction the judicial view is that the House of Lords decision *In re Baden's Deed Trust* is not to be preferred to the previously established case law. Both Budd J[33] and

Murphy J[34] have declared that they will continue to place greater reliance on the established authorities than on the *ratio decedendi* of *In re Baden's Deed Trusts*.

In Ireland, there has been no equivalent to an extension of the 'founder's kin' class in line with the ruling in *Re Koettgen's Will Trusts*.[35] Instead the rule remains confined to its original interpretation based on 'blood ties' or personal nexus.

The Irish judiciary have also taken a different approach to their English counterparts in relation to the significance of 'dissemination' in the context of trusts for the advancement of education. Keane J in the *Worth* case held that a gift for the advancement of scholarship or academic research, and thus for the advancement of learning, which might reasonably be regarded as for the public benefit, would not be deprived of charitable status merely because such scholarship or research was not combined with teaching or education.[36]

The public benefit test: the 'benefit' requirement   In Ireland, the judiciary are unlikely to substitute an objective assessment for the donor's subjective view but, as was apparent in *Re Worth*, they will insist that the public benefit test is satisfied. Keane J, in that case,[37] had cause to examine the requirement for a public benefit component in gifts for the advancement of education. He conceded that the gift of a library which is open to the public would be charitable,[38] as would be a gift which was conducive to the attainment of a charitable object such as one for the purchase of books for Trinity College, Oxford,[39] where it was held to be for the advancement of education. However, in this instance he expressed his view that the gift of a library, comprising a large and valuable collection of eighteenth-century books, would be unlikely to come within the legal definition of charitable in an education context. The gift would fail the 'public' branch of the test because access to the library was restricted 'for the use, benefit and behoof of the physician, chaplain and surgeon for the time being of the said hospital . . .'. It would also fail the 'benefit' branch because as he pointed out:

> even if it could be said that the bequest was for educational purposes (and, given the insignificant proportion of the library devoted to medicine and surgery, that would involve some straining of the concept of 'education' even beyond the liberal limits of the modern decisions), it would be impossible to hold that this was an educational charity for the benefit of the public.

But, as can be seen on page 232, he then went on to construct a novel interpretation of 'benefit' which, under a different heading, he found to be satisfied by the tranquil setting of the library.

The advancement of religion

In Ireland, Article 44 of the Constitution makes special reference to the Christian nature of the State[40] while the advancement of religion is further underpinned by s. 45 of the Charities Act 1961, which states that 'in determining whether or not a gift for the purpose of the advancement of religion is a valid charitable gift it shall be conclusively presumed that the purpose includes and will occasion public benefit'.

The public benefit test   Section 45 of the Charities Act 1961 gives statutory effect to the ruling in *O'Hanlon* v. *Logue*[41] where Palles CB established that a gift for the saying of masses[42] whether in public or private satisfied the public benefit test and, being affirmed by the subjective judicial approach,[43] was determinative of a donor's charitable intent. Gifts of this nature have long been a distinctive characteristic of Irish charitable activity, traditionally distinguishing it in particular from the non-charitable status of such activity in the United Kingdom.[44] This has been evident also in gifts to closed contemplative religious orders, as opposed to those actively engaged in good works in the community.[45] The decision taken by the Irish courts in *Re Howley*[46] stands in direct contrast to that taken in *Gilmour* v. *Coats*.[47] In Ireland, as a consequence of s. 45 of the 1961 Act, the public benefit test has no application to trusts for the advancement of religion.

However, religion no longer holds its traditional very special position in this increasingly secular society; it has diminished considerably since the introduction of the 1961 Act and more so since the Constitution with its Roman Catholic ethos was introduced. Ireland in the twenty-first century is not the homogenous Catholic society it once was. Moreover, religion on this island has become a demonstrably divisive influence, polarizing communities and hindering the consolidation of a pluralist civil society. Further, the activities of some religious organizations, particularly those entrusted with providing residential care for children, highlights the risks inherent in not subjecting such activities to the 'public benefit' test.

Beneficial to the community and not falling under any of the preceding heads

As already stated, this *Pemsel* head has accommodated by far the largest volume of new charities particularly in the field of health and social care.

The public benefit test   It is in relation to gifts under this *Pemsel* head, as in England and Wales, that the test is applied most rigorously. In Ireland the most distinctive feature of the public benefit test is its subjective nature. It was in relation to gifts under this *Pemsel* head that the subjective approach was first articulated. In *Re Cranston*[48] Fitzgibbon LJ argued that gifts for certain vegetarian societies were charitable and came within the category of gifts for other charitable purposes. This view was endorsed by Lord O'Brien LCJ in *Attorney-General* v. *Becher*,[49] by Barton J in *Shillington* v. *Portadown UDC*[50] and finally by Keane J in *Re Worth Library* when he set the seal of the Irish judiciary on this issue.

Another singular characteristic relates to the quotient of 'benefit'. The deliberations of Keane J in *Re Worth Library*[51] shed an interesting light on judicial interpretation of when the public benefit element of a gift is sufficient for it to acquire charitable status within this category. Two different approaches were considered. First, Keane J rejected the proposition that such a gift was charitable *per se*.[52] On the facts, it failed to satisfy the 'public' requirement because the donor was most explicit that access be restricted to the physician, surgeon and chaplain. It also failed to meet the 'benefit' requirement because the books that comprised the library were on subjects that could only be of marginal interest to the designated beneficiaries. Therefore he determined that in this instance the gift of a library did not *per se* constitute a charitable trust within the fourth category. Second, he considered the possibility that the gift might so qualify on the grounds that as it was directed exclusively for the use of hospital staff it could be construed as intended as a gift for the hospital which would normally be charitable.[53] Again, on the facts, he held that in this instance the terms of the gift were so conditional as to debar the gift from vesting in the hospital generally. Having thus ruled out the possibility of the gift acquiring charitable status on either of the two grounds presented, Keane J then advanced a further possibility – that the library itself 'in its beautiful setting would have provided a haven of quiet intellectual relaxation for the beneficiaries'. The necessary 'benefit' quotient was supplied by the intrinsic quality of the library environment, despite the restricted access to it. Keane J held that the requirements of the public benefit test were accordingly satisfied and ruled in favour of the gift's charitable status within this category on the ground that it furthered the capacity of the charity represented by the hospital.

Judicial application of the subjective approach together with the latitude illustrated by the importation by Keane J of 'tranquillity' as an indicator of 'benefit', allows for a much more liberal if not quixotic interpretation of the test than is permissible in England and Wales. In other respects the law and practice under this head has unfolded somewhat similarly in both jurisdictions, including the maintenance of restrictions on political activity by charities.

Legal structures for charities

In Ireland, charitable activity is housed in much the same range of structures as in England and Wales, with the same marked reliance on trusts (see, further, chapter 8). It is likely, however, that the proportion of government-controlled bodies and religious organizations claiming tax exemption on the grounds of charitable activity is higher in this jurisdiction.

Types of structure

In Ireland the range of not-for-profits includes large government bodies and other non-government organizations such as co-operatives, credit unions, trade unions, etc., while the types of legal vehicle available to further the work of charities are very much the same as in England and Wales. Most charities in Ireland at least commence life as an association, though many subsequently became incorporated, while trusts and the law of trusts have been as dominant as in that jurisdiction.[54] In Ireland, as elsewhere, many charities, as they grow in size and complexity, become incorporated and must then comply with statutory registration requirements and have their names entered in the Registry.[55] Foundations may be established under powers available in the Companies Acts, by a special act of the Oireachtas, or by powers available to the Commissioners of Charitable Donations and Bequests under the Charity Acts.

Regulatory framework

The legal framework for charities in Ireland provides more of a facilitative than a regulatory environment. Monitoring and supervision responsibilities continue to rest mainly with the Commissioners for Charitable Donations and Bequests, a benign body that has survived relatively intact since the nineteenth century. In that respect the regulatory framework differs considerably from its counterpart in England and Wales.

Registering charities

In Ireland there is no statutory provision for the registration and inspection of charities. No one government body keeps a register of all 'live' charities and no statutory mechanisms exist for ensuring probity, requiring accountability, setting and monitoring standards nor for ascertaining the effectiveness of charitable activity. In the absence of any single and specific process for confirming the standing of an organization as a charity, the term 'charitable status' is a misnomer in Irish charity law. However, certain bodies have powers or duties to maintain registers in which charities will be listed or they have other related responsibilities.

The Commissioners for Charitable Donations and Bequests

This, the only body with specific responsibility for charities, has no statutory obligation to maintain a register, nor any other duty in relation to noting their creation, termination or to direct publication of their accounts. Unless the Commissioners require the publication of details relating to a charitable bequest in a particular case, a general exemption from publication is available.

The Revenue Commission

This body has no responsibilities in relation to the registration or inspection of charities. It does, however, maintain a list of those bodies that have successfully applied for tax exemption on charitable grounds. There is no requirement that the Revenue publish this list but it is now publicly accessible under the Freedom of Information Act.

Other bodies

A number of other bodies keep lists and/or identifying information on charities.

The Probate Office   This body monitors and collates information on all charitable gifts or bequests contained in wills. This is passed to the Commissioners for Charitable Donations and Bequests.

The Companies Registry Office   Incorporated bodies, including charities, are required to register with the Registrar of Companies, as in England and Wales, and are subject to the same requirements. This provides one of the few legal mechanisms that allow for a measure of transparency in relation to the organizational structure, financial standing and activities of a charity.

The Valuation Office   This body maintains the Valuation Lists containing details of: the current rateable valuation of commercial properties (hereditaments and tenements); and of the rateable valuation of commercial, domestic and land properties from 1852. This includes information on whether or not premises are entitled to exemption from rates on the grounds of charitable use by the occupier.

The Industrial and Provident Society Registrar   An Industrial and Provident Society has to satisfy the IPS Registrar that its purpose can be defined as 'industry, business or trade' before its name is entered in the IPS Register. The regulatory powers of the IPS Registrar also apply to Friendly Societies. Charities with the status of either an Industrial and Provident Society or a Friendly Society must register their particulars in the relevant Register in much the same way required of an incorporated charity.

Regulating charities

Ireland's tradition of reliance upon NGOS has been accompanied by a reluctance to regulate their activities. Partly this is due to the entrenched doctrine of subsidiarity, itself a by-product of the delicate relationship between Church and State, characterized by the vigour with which the former traditionally policed the latter's intrusion into matters it judged to be outside the remit of government. Whatever the reason, no statutory regulatory system now exists for facilitating transparency, monitoring effectiveness and ensuring public accountability in relation to the activities of charities, though some bodies are statutorily vested with related responsibilities. However, in its recent White Paper *Regulating Better*,[56] the government acknowledged the need for better regulation and laid down some key guiding principles and an action programme for developing effective regulatory systems.

The Revenue Commission

The Revenue Commissioners determine whether or not the purposes and activities of an organization are such as to warrant its recognition as a charity for tax exemption purposes under the Taxes Consolidation Act 1997. A charity reference number is issued to bodies which are granted charitable tax exemption and the

Commission maintains and publishes on its website[57] a list of these bodies. This list is not a register of charities. First it establishes whether the activities of the applicant body come within one of the four heads of charity identified in *Pemsel*. Where this is confirmed it then examines the body's 'governing instrument' to establish whether the income and property of the applicant body is exclusively and irrevocably committed to charitable purposes.

The Revenue Commissioners also play a limited regulatory role by checking that income has, in fact, been applied exclusively for charitable purposes and that claims for repayment of tax are properly substantiated. It can also withdraw recognition where it appears that purposes are no longer exclusively charitable, for example where there has been an inappropriate alteration to a founding document or where the body's actual activities do not correspond to those in the founding document upon which charitable status was based. Any accounts furnished to it from registered charities are wholly confidential and are not open to public scrutiny.

The Commission of Charitable Donations and Bequests

This statutory body has certain powers with regards to the administration of charity law, but there are no corresponding duties imposed on charities in terms of accountability or transparency, and indeed some of the Commissioners' statutory powers have never been exercised. The role and powers of the Commissioners are governed by Part II of the 1961 Act as amended by the 1973 Act and do not provide for any procedures in relation to complaints or compliance regarding the activities of charities. While the powers of the Commissioners have been extended they do not differ in any fundamental respect from those conferred under the nineteenth-century legislation. Its powers in terms of monitoring and investigation of charities are much more closely circumscribed than those of its English counterpart. In particular, this body has no specific brief or powers to extend the contemporary interpretation of charitable purposes construed to be in the 'public benefit' and it has no power to require the Revenue Commission to do so.

The High Court and the Attorney General

In Ireland, both these bodies retain their traditional common law functions in relation to charities. Reserved for the courts are matters referred by the Attorney General[58] and/or by the Commissioners where the issues are complex, involve a fine point of law, require interpretation or where a *cy-près* scheme concerning property valued at £250,000 or more is needed. When dealing with definitional matters the High Court will resolve issues by referring to the *Pemsel* classification, associated precedents and in compliance with the 'spirit and intendment' rule. In this jurisdiction, the High Court continues its traditional role in respect of charities and remains the only body vested with sufficient powers to broaden the interpretation of public benefit and thereby able to adjust the definition of charitable purposes to meet the contemporary pattern of social need.

Other bodies

Several government departments and an array of government bodies have varying and largely unco-ordinated responsibilities in respect of charities.

The Department of Community, Rural and Gaeltacht Affairs   Initially, responsibility for charity law matters rested with the Department of Justice and continued with the Department of Justice, Equality and Law Reform when it was established in 1998. In 2001, responsibility transferred to the Department of Social, Community and Family Affairs and in 2003 it passed to the Department of Community, Rural and Gaeltacht Affairs. The latter now has responsibility for regulating charities and for implementing the Charities Acts 1961 and 1973. It is currently reviewing the law governing matters relating to charities following the recommendations made by the Costello report[59] and subsequently by the Advisory Group.[60]

The Department of Justice, Equality and Law Reform   This department retains competence with regards to the issue of fundraising permits. In particular it has responsibilities for the operation of the Gaming and Lotteries Act 1956 (which provides for the issue of Garda permits and court licences, respectively, in relation to lotteries) and the Street and House to House Collections Act 1962 (which provides for the issue of police permits to take up collections in specified areas).

The Probate Office   Under s. 58 of the 1961 Act, the Probate Office is required to furnish the Board, annually, with particulars of every charitable devise or bequest contained in any will. This duty requires the Probate Office to first identify a charitable bequest and differentiate between it and all other forms of bequest.

The Valuation Office   This body determines eligibility for rates exemption on charitable grounds as governed by certain nineteenth-century legislation but otherwise has no general regulatory function. The Valuation Tribunal, established by the Valuation Act 1988, rules on matters affecting the rateability of individual charities and its register of judgments provides valuable guidance to circumstances where charities are not fully compliant with eligibility criteria.

The Companies Registry Office   Where a charity is registered as a limited company then annual returns, including a statement of accounts, must be made to the Registrar. Failure to comply with the requirement to make annual returns will lead to a company being struck off the register[61] and where the Registrar is able to confirm improper, irregular or illegal behaviour (usually following police investigations) then sanctions as provided by the Companies Acts may be applied. There are no accounting or filing requirements for charities that are not incorporated.

The Garda Síochána   Evidence of criminal activity will give rise to an investigation by the Garda Síochána, the national police force, in the normal way. This is really the only form of regulatory intervention that an unincorporated charity is likely to encounter. The Gardaí play a statutory role in the issuing of permits for street and house-to-house collections.

Regulating the fiscal environment

In Ireland the regulatory system for managing the financial environment as it relates to charities is the orthodox revenue-driven model, resting primarily on the role of the tax collection agency which also determines charitable status. Although the High Court and the Commissioners for Charitable Donations and Bequests share important if traditional responsibilities in respect of creating *cy-près* schemes, it is the inspectoral and supervisory powers of the Revenue Commission and the Garda Síochána that impact most directly on charities.

The Revenue Commission

This body, the government agency statutorily vested with responsibility for maximizing the accrual of tax revenue, determines the tax exemption eligibility of organizations claiming charitable status. It does so in relation to income tax, corporation tax, capital gains tax, deposit interest retention tax, stamp duty, capital acquisitions tax, probate tax and sundry lesser liabilities. The question as to whether or not the purposes and activities of an organization are charitable in nature only arises in the context of its tax liability.

Fundraising and trading

In Ireland, fundraising is governed by legislation that addresses fundraising for charitable and for other purposes and is more concerned to outline authorizing procedures than to identify and proscribe abuses. It deals with such traditional methods of fundraising as raffles, church collections, door-to-door and street collections for traditional purposes such as service provision for the destitute, elderly and infirm and for disaster relief within Ireland and overseas. The lack of integration between legislation regulating fundraising and that governing charitable activity in general is a characteristic feature of Irish charity law.

The usual fundraising activities of charities are largely governed by two statutes, the Street and House to House Collections Act 1962 and the Casual Trading Act 1995. Both assign responsibilities to the Garda Síochána regarding the issue of permits for collections. Fundraising through the National Lottery is governed by the National Lotteries Act 1986. In addition, many charities develop commercial activities as a method of raising funds and these are subject to their own specific rules and regulations. Although telethons have become extremely popular, at present such activity is outside statutory control.

Registering and regulating fundraising activities

In this jurisdiction, the absence of adequate provisions to ensure transparency and accountability, particularly as regards telethons and the activities of professional fundraisers, is a deficiency in the current regulatory framework. Regulating fundraising activities is currently left to the Gardaí who, after granting the necessary permits, will rarely intervene unless presented with evidence of a crime such as fraud.

In 1996 the Irish Institute of Fundraisers was established as a self-regulating body to monitor and protect standards and promote good practice in fundraising.

Commercial activities

Irish tax law provides for a 'trading exemption' in respect of profits that charities derive from trading. The Revenue Commissioners define trading as 'generally involving the sale of goods or services to customers with a view to generating a profit'. To qualify for a trading exemption the relevant body must have charitable status and the income derived from trading must be applied solely to the purposes of the charity. In addition, the trade must be a primary purpose of the charity or the work in connection with the trade must be carried on mainly by beneficiaries of the charity.

Tax and rates

Tax exemption is governed largely by the Tax Consolidation Act 1997 and the Finance Act 2002, is determined or authorized by the Revenue Commissioners and in the event of dispute an appeal can be made to the courts. Rates exemption is governed by, and s. 2 of The Valuation (Ireland) Acts 1852 and 1854 and the Valuation Act 2001 is determined by the Commissioner of Valuations, and in the event of dispute an appeal can be made to the Valuation Tribunal and ultimately to the courts.

Tax

To avail of tax exemptions a charity must be established in Ireland.[62]

Exemption from income tax and corporation tax is granted under the Taxes Consolidation Act 1997 in respect of certain income of an organization established for charitable purposes and in respect of income applied exclusively for those purposes. Although there is no general exemption for charities from VAT the Value Added Tax Act 1972 gives the Revenue Commissioners authority to exempt some activities.[63] Again, while there is no blanket exemption, charities may be exempt from such taxes as capital acquisitions tax, discretionary trust tax, stamp duty and capital duty. In addition, the Finance Act 1995 instituted tax relief in respect of individual donations to charities focused on developing nations while the Finance Act 1998 instituted the scheme for tax relief on corporate donations to certain voluntary organizations.

Rates

In Ireland, not all entities recognized as charitable for general tax and legal purposes will qualify for rates exemption in respect of their premises.[64] To be eligible for charitable exemption from rates a property must be used for charitable purposes or for public purposes as defined in section 2 of The Valuation (Ireland) Act 1854 and the Valuation Act 2001.[65]

Donation incentives

The Finance Act 2001 introduced a uniform scheme of tax relief for donations to approved bodies, which includes a body of persons or trust established for charitable purposes where the income is applied for charitable purposes only. The charity must have held tax-exempt status from the Revenue Commissioners under the Taxes Consolidation Act 1997 for not less than three years prior to the date of its application. No ceiling is imposed on the amount which may qualify for a deduction and no differentiation is made between charities.

Basically, Irish law recognizes the special place held by charities in society by applying more favourable rules to charities than to other entities and the special role of charities is also recognized by the Irish tax code at present. However, no provision is made for targeting incentives towards charities with a social inclusion agenda and new charities, which are more likely to have such an agenda, are penalized by the three-year rule.

Cy-près

Perhaps one of the most important powers available to the Commissioners for Charitable Donations and Bequests is the ability under section 8 of the 1973 Act to apply a charitable fund *cy-près*, without the necessity of a High Court application. Under s. 47 a *cy-près* order may be made where the original purposes have ceased to provide a 'suitable and effective method' of utilizing the property, having regard to the spirit and nature of the gift.[66] Usually a general charitable intention on the part of the donor must be shown to exist before property can be applied *cy-près*.

Three brief observations may be made in relation to the present use of *cy-près* as a means of adjusting a charity's objects. First, notwithstanding the judgment in *Worth*, the rationale behind section 47 of the 1961 Act to ensure that *cy-près* jurisdiction could be exercised whenever it was necessary or desirable has been to some extent frustrated by the courts' rather restrictive approach in interpreting a 'general charitable intention'.[67] Second, by applying a subjective test to determine the applicability of the *cy-près* doctrine, the judgment of Keane J in *Worth* demonstrates an important divergence between the judiciary in this jurisdiction and their counterparts elsewhere. Third, although the ceiling for Board jurisdiction was raised from £25,000 to £250,000 in 1995,[68] removing the ceiling completely would undoubtedly facilitate greater use of *cy-près*.

Constraints on modern philanthropic activity

Ireland's particularly strong tradition of joint Church and State involvement in public service provision has matured into the present broad and formal partnership arrangement between State, business and the community and voluntary sector which now forms the basis for planning the future socio-economic development of the nation. This is the policy context within which the future role of philanthropy will be determined. In the meantime, Ireland continues to provide a characteristically facilitative legal environment for philanthropic activity. The current quite dated legislation relies upon traditional institutions exercising their customary functions in relation to charitable purposes as classified in *Pemsel* and extended by case law precedent. This naturally results in some tensions due both to the continuation of deficiencies inherent in the traditional common law approach and to the inadequacy of dated legislative provisions as a means of addressing the new pressures generated from within the contemporary philanthropic environment.

Partnership with government: the constraints

In Ireland, over recent decades, successive governments have carefully formulated and implemented a policy of formal partnership with the community and voluntary sector.[69] This is to much the same effect as similar more recent policies in England and Wales except that the roots of this relationship are deeper in Ireland, particularly as regards the involvement of religious organizations in providing and staffing the State's health and education facilities. The grounds for concern regarding the possible constraints on the independence of charities resulting from their being drawn into policies of partnership with government, which have been the focus of considerable debate in England and Wales,[70] are more substantial in this jurisdiction. The terms of reference for such a partnership are more likely to be weighted in favour of protecting the interests of Church and State and less likely to accommodate and promote the interests of the broad range of more radical secular charities representing marginalized minority groups.

Government grants and contracts

The difficulties for charities in maintaining their independence and avoiding being compromised, as they compete for and undertake government service provision contracts or become ever more dependent upon government grants, are much the same as for their counterparts in England and Wales. The relative weakness of charities in the modern business environment leaves them particularly exposed in the current contract culture climate where partnership arrangements with government bodies are difficult to resist but may fatally compromise the independence of charities, threaten their sustainability and inhibit assertive advocacy on behalf of the socially disadvantaged. Again, however, the dominant position of the Catholic Church, relative to other charities, reinforced by a statutory presumption of public benefit, adds further complications in this jurisdiction.

International aid

Ireland has long played a very active role in the provision of international aid to underdeveloped countries. Of the few charities with an almost omniscient presence in third world sites of human tragedy and distress, at least one will be wholly Irish (e.g. Trocraire); others will be manned by Irish volunteers and some will be initiated and led by the Irish. This role has traditionally been strongly associated with the Catholic Church and was often set within the missionary work of that Church. The delivery of international aid from Ireland, which in recent decades has acquired a much more secular emphasis, has not been accompanied by adjustments to the regulatory framework necessary to facilitate such charitable activity.

Common law constraints

In addition to the constraints imposed by its traditional definition (the 'spirit and intendment' rule and the four *Pemsel* heads) as mentioned above, philanthropy in Ireland is hindered by other typical common law characteristics.

Role of the courts

The High Court and the office of the Attorney General, both traditionally crucial for adjusting the fit between charity law and social need, are now of random and peripheral significance while the use of *cy-près* schemes remains underdeveloped. As in England and Wales and other jurisdictions, the constraints of expense, time and media exposure result in the court having very few opportunities to exercise its traditional role in relation to charities. Most issues affecting charities never reach the courts. Unlike England and Wales, however, there is no other body with the power or responsibility to compensate for the contemporary deficit in judicial involvement.

Legal structures

As in England and Wales, the continued reliance on a very traditional range of legal structures is a constraint on the modernizing of charitable activity (see, also, chapter 8).

Restrictions on advocacy/political activity

In Ireland charities are restrained from engaging in advocacy/political activity to much the same extent as in England and Wales. The extent of the constraint is evident from the interpretation given to 'political activity' by O'Sullivan J in *Colgan* v. *Independent Radio and Television Commission, Ireland and the Attorney General.*[71] It was held that the phrase 'political end' would include activity which:[72]

> is directed towards furthering the interests of a particular political party or towards procuring changes in the laws of this country, or countering suggested changes in those laws, or towards procuring changes in the laws of a foreign country or countering suggested changes in those laws, or procuring a reversal of government policy or of particular decisions of governmental authorities in this country, or countering suggested reversals thereof, or procuring a reversal of governmental policy, or of particular decisions of governmental authorities in a foreign country, or countering suggested reversals thereof.

Arguably, for a nation on an island that has suffered so much from violent community divisions (not unrelated to politics, laws and policy), an embargo on such a wide span of activity by charities amounts to a particularly severe constraint on philanthropy.

Fiscal issues

In Ireland there is a particularly traditional approach towards charities.

Revenue driven   The Revenue Commission continues to dominate the tax-oriented but supportive legal environment for charities. Essentially the Revenue Commission is therefore left to exercise its restricted common law role in relation to philanthropy as a subsidiary to its main function of maximizing the return of tax revenue due to the State.

The doctrine of cy-près   The use of *cy-près* schemes in Ireland is similar in principle and law to that in England and Wales but in practice it is more problematic. Unlike the latter jurisdiction, there is no dual jurisdiction shared between the High Court and the Commission: the *cy-près* brief of the Commissioners for Charitable Donations and Bequests, as noted above, is limited. This mechanism offers a potential means for applying the assets of a defunct charity, such as the many city-zoned and very valuable property sites of retracting religious organizations, to address contemporary social inclusion issues. However, as illustrated by the last two major charity law cases,[73] both of which concerned *cy-près* issues, the considerable assets of venerable but redundant institutions can simply end up being diverted to supplement existing government expenditure on public services.

Fundraising and trading, etc.   The constraints regarding the capacity of charities to raise revenue through these means are similar to those affecting their counterparts in England and Wales, but though the latter has abolished the traditional distinction between 'street' and 'house-to-house' fundraising, this continues in Ireland. These difficulties are exacerbated by largely out-of-date legislative provisions and poor co-ordination between government agencies (see chapter 8).

Public benefit matters

In this jurisdiction the long-standing charity law deficiencies regarding the uneven application of the public benefit test and the exclusion of matters clearly in the public benefit are as for England and Wales (see, further, chapter 8).

The legal presumption favouring religion   Philanthropy in Ireland continues its traditional and singularly (among modern western nations) close relationship with religion and its reliance on religious organizations as a primary delivery vehicle for charitable activity. In this jurisdiction, where religion promotes homogeneity rather than inclusiveness, the statutory presumption perpetuating the common law preferential treatment of religious organizations is open to challenge.

The legal presumption favouring the donor's intent   Unlike the position in the UK and elsewhere, this traditional common law presumption, long since repealed in other jurisdictions, favouring a subjective interpretation of the donor's intent as determining the validity of his or charitable gift,[74] continues in place in Ireland. Judicial application of the subjective test allows gifts to acquire charitable status and be directed towards such marginal if not questionable areas of need as 'the Dublin Home for Starving and Forsaken Cats'.[75] Again, this presumption does not assist an efficient and effective use of philanthropic resources.

Modern law constraints

The functions of modern charity law in Ireland are constrained by certain pressures, not untypical of other jurisdictions, from within the contemporary philanthropic environment.

The facilitative approach to charities, for example, has led to the present rather lax and fragmentary regulatory regime which fails to provide the rigorous systems of accountability, transparency and governance necessary for the efficient management of all modern organizations. The lack of any synchronization of the rules and procedures applied by the many government bodies involved with charities, particularly between the Commissioner of Valuations and the Revenue Commissioners, is noticeable.

Forum for developing charitable purposes

Unlike England and Wales there is no independent forum capable of developing charitable purposes in response to emerging patterns of social need. This is a particularly significant deficit. Neither the Commissioners for Charitable Donations and Bequests nor any other body has the power or responsibility to proactively cultivate in the not-for-profit sector a capacity to address a more contemporary interpretation of public benefit, nor to require the Revenue Commission to broaden its conservative approach and confer charitable status in circumstances where it has not done so in the past, remove such status where it is no longer appropriate or to prevent unnecessary duplication of charitable activity. This results in the survival of many archaic charities for causes such as the maintenance of burial plots and the 'saying of masses', multiple charities for cancer relief, etc., and none at all for contemporary causes such as peace and reconciliation.

Human rights, anti-terrorism and social justice legislation

The law governing philanthropic activity in Ireland is now also required to take into account related legal developments in Europe, including the Council of Europe's 'Fundamental Principles on the Status of non-governmental organizations in Europe' issued by the Secretariat Directorate General of Legal Affairs, Strasbourg, in April 2002. Issues of human rights and social justice are given specific statutory recognition.

The European Convention   The European Convention for the Protection of Human Rights and Fundamental Freedoms 1950 became part of Irish law when given effect by the European Convention on Human Rights Act 2003 on 31 December 2003. While it would be premature, so soon after that event, to consider possible compatibility issues in relation to Irish charity law and Convention requirements, it is perhaps fair to comment that the legal environment for charitable activity in this jurisdiction is currently vulnerable to challenge under Convention non-discrimination principles. A charity law with a history steeped in promoting religion (not just Christian but specifically Roman Catholic), reinforced by statute and Constitution, may have difficulty in squaring its public benefit principle with the Convention's non-discrimination principle in Articles 9, 11 and especially in Article 14.

Anti-terrorism   Despite a constitutional assertion of neutrality, Ireland has been unable to avoid being drawn into global anti-terrorism concerns; this has been apparent from the public protests against the use of its airports by the US military for troop transport and 'rendition' purposes. In addition to legislation addressing the 30-year-old period of civil unrest affecting the northern part of the island, the government has also recently introduced a law permitting data retention into its Criminal Justice (Terrorist Offences) Act 2005. As was explained by the Minister for Justice, Malcolm McDowell, the retention of such information 'is an essential aid . . . in the fight against crime and in combating terrorism and, . . . the protection and security of the State.'

Social justice   In Ireland human rights also find protection in the Constitution[76] and in a typical range of social justice legislation. The latter includes the Prohibition of Incitement to Hatred Act 1989, the Equal Employment Act 1998 and the

Equal Status Act 2000. In addition two new agencies, the Office of the Director of Equality Investigations and the Equality Authority, have been established with the legislative powers necessary to develop an anticipatory and proactive approach such as the auditing and developing of 'racism-proofing' approaches to institutional and corporate policies and practices in the same way that gender- and poverty-proofing are already becoming standard practice. The National Consultative Committee on Racism and Interculturalism was established in 1998 with no statutory powers but with the aim of promoting a more pluralist and intercultural Ireland.[77]

Charity law review and social inclusion

In Ireland the past 40 years have been a period of considerable social change. This has included exposure to the effects of civil strife in the adjoining jurisdiction, accommodation of multicultural influences and a transition from a rather insular agricultural society with a population steadily depleted by annual emigration to one that is now growing and generally more prosperous, is a high-tech exporter and is firmly part of Europe. This was also a period that saw no new charity legislation enacted. It was widely recognized that contemporary patterns of social need were not readily addressed by a charity law framework designed for the largely rural, Catholic and homogenous society that was Ireland in the mid-twentieth century.

The Department of Community, Rural and Gaeltacht Affairs were accordingly assigned lead responsibility for conducting a review of charity law. This process recently concluded and the department duly published a Consultation Paper[78] which, although conspicuously suffering from the lack of a joined-up government approach, is an important first step towards reform.

Proposed changes to definitional matters

The government is suggesting that a new and clear definition of what constitutes a charity is critical to the establishment of a modern statutory framework.

Charitable purpose

The government proposes that new legislation might redefine 'charitable purposes' so that it would accommodate:

- the advancement of health, which includes the prevention and relief of sickness, disease or human suffering;
- the advancement of education;
- the advancement of community welfare, which include:
  1 the prevention and relief of poverty, distress or disadvantage,
  2 the care, support and protection of the aged and people with a disability,
  3 the care, support and protection of children and young people and

4   the promotion of community development;
- the advancement of religion;
- the advancement of the natural environment;
- other purposes beneficial to the community, which include:
  1   the prevention and relief of suffering of animals,
  2   the promotion and fostering of culture, and
  3   the care, preservation and protection of the Irish heritage.

In this context, 'advancement' would include protection, maintenance, support, research, improvement or enhancement. It is intended that the presence or presumption, as the case may be, of 'public benefit' will continue to be an essential element of a valid charity.

Legal structures

The Consultation Paper notes that charity trustees are currently subject to differing standards according to the legal vehicle chosen to give effect to the charity. It proposes updating and codifying existing legislative provisions to ascribe a uniform role, duty of care, range of responsibilities and duties to all trustees/officers/directors of charities regardless of the legal structure or type of governing instrument used. The Paper suggests that a new form of incorporation for charities might be appropriate and that the Department of Enterprise, Trade and Employment may be engaged in designing such a new legal structure. This might take the form of a 'charitable designated activity company' (CDAC), created specifically and exclusively for charities; existing charities could opt to convert to this structure. No attempt has been made to define a charity as a non-government organization so presumably the existing situation, allowing many bodies established and managed by the government to qualify for charitable tax exemption on the grounds that they satisfy the public benefit test, will continue.

Proposed changes to the regulatory framework

Some of the deficiencies noted above will be addressed in the proposed new legislation.

Primary regulatory body

The Consultation Paper proposes an independent statutory body as the centrepiece of a modern framework that will regulate charities. It leaves open the issue as to whether this will be a new body or whether the statutory functions will be grafted onto an existing body. In either case it is suggested that the new functions might include:

- determining charitable status (with a right of appeal to the High Court);
- maintaining a register of charities;

- ensuring the public accountability of charities;
- regulating and monitoring charities, including their fundraising activities, and ensuring their compliance with relevant statutory provisions;
- providing guidance to trustees and directors of charities;
- investigating possible abuses;
- advising the Minister and informing the public on developments;
- determining *cy-près* applications;
- issuing codes of conduct, best practice guidelines, model constitution documents, etc.;
- receiving notifications of charitable bequests and following up on these as appropriate; and
- issuing performance reports.

This independent regulatory body is to be called Caradas (meaning proactive friendship or alliance) and the Consultation Paper stresses the need to clarify and simplify the lines of communication between such a body and all others currently involved in the institutional framework for charities.

Registration

The Consultation Paper proposes that the regulatory body would be responsible for compiling, publishing and maintaining a register of 'Registered Charities' and that all charities would be required to register and to file annual returns with it. The necessary arrangements would be made with the Companies Registration Office to avoid dual filing requirements. A centralized, computerized database, accessible to the public, will hold registration details and all related information, thereby ensuring that 'as an integral part of a cohesive regulatory framework, registration would amount to a badge of transparency for the individual charity concerned'.[79] However, it is not clear whether the continued registration of a charity will be conditional upon satisfying a regular review process nor whether it will be required to disclose, in its annual returns, the amount of government funding if any it has received.

Where the regulatory body has evidence of fraud, maladministration or other misconduct it will be statutorily empowered to strike the charity off the register, prosecute or refer to the Director of Public Prosecutions. It may also impose lesser sanctions, short of deregistration, where appropriate.

Proposed changes to financial matters

The Consultation Paper avoids dealing with finance-related matters on the grounds that the primary responsibility falls to other departments.

Tax

The role of the Revenue Commissioners in determining tax exemption for charitable bodies is not addressed on the ground that this is a matter for the Department of Finance. Similarly, fundraising permits, gaming and lotteries are not dealt with on the grounds that the responsibility for such matters falls to the Department of Justice, Equality and Law Reform.

Fundraising

In relation to fundraising by charities, the Paper recognizes the need for new legislation and gives an assurance that the regulatory body will require disclosure by charities in their annual returns of permits applied for and funds raised and it will have investigatory powers to detect possible abuses. It acknowledges the need to consolidate the present sets of regulations governing trading, fundraising (professional and otherwise) and promises of money (telethons etc.), and to co-ordinate the related responsibilities of the Garda and local authorities, within the same new body of regulations. The Paper also favours the introduction of a voluntary Code of Conduct as a self-regulatory mechanism for the sector.

Implications for social inclusion

Charity law reform in Ireland is primarily concerned with making some funda-mental adjustments to the relevant institutional framework. The introduction of a registration system, proposed improvements to the regulatory regime and refine-ments to legal structures and financial matters as they relate to charities will create a more efficient and effective legal environment for philanthropy and reduce opportunities for abuse. Much of course depends on the actual distribution of responsibilities between the independent regulatory body and the Revenue Commissioners – will the former have a role and powers resembling those vested in the English Charity Commission? While these improvements will assist char-ities to address contemporary social inclusion issues, it is the proposed changes to charitable purposes that carry the most significant implications for that agenda.

Proposal strengths

The proposed changes to the definition of 'charitable purposes' that promise to be most conducive to strengthening the capacity of charities to address social inclu-sion are those that deal with 'prevention'. In particular, the references to the prevention of 'poverty' and 'disadvantage' under the new category of 'advance-ment of community welfare' offer considerable scope for the setting up of new charities to deal with the causes of social disadvantage in its myriad forms. The fact that certain vulnerable groups are specifically mentioned under that new category is reassuring for the associated charities but gives rise to a risk of exclu-sion for those not mentioned. Again, the specific endorsement given to 'com-munity development' should prove useful to those organizations striving to tackle embedded rural poverty and pockets of chronic unemployment; though much will depend on how this works in practice, particularly as regards the possible involvement of business enterprises. The interpretation of 'promotion and fostering of culture' can, presumably, be stretched beyond the usual subsidies to the arts and allow charities to be established for the purpose of assisting the many immigrant minority groups from eastern Europe and elsewhere which have settled in Ireland to retain their culture and separate sense of identity.

Proposal weaknesses

It must be assumed that the simple restating of the two *Pemsel* heads relating to education and religion is intended to ensure that the associated public benefit presumptions will carry over into the new regime. The government would seem to have decided that this opportunity to assert the integrity of the public benefit test and validate it as an independent standard, objectively and uniformly applicable to the activities of all bodies seeking charitable status, religious or otherwise, is to be rejected. This is regrettable. The twin concepts of 'charitable purpose' and 'public benefit' are central to charity law and the combination of new statutory definitions for both would have served to firmly differentiate between charities and other not-for-profit organizations while bringing more rigour and resulting credibility to future practice. In the case of the advancement of religion, it is clear that the existing favoured position of religious organizations will be maintained and the public is not to have the added reassurance that mandatory compliance with the public benefit test would bring in relation to their activities.

Again, it may be assumed that the reference to 'human suffering' is intended as a catch-all gesture to human rights concerns. However, it is by no means clear that this clause will rectify the deficit in existing law by encompassing purposes such as peace and reconciliation. In this context, it is also noticeable that the government has not introduced provisions to clarify the law relating to the political activities of charities and made clear statements regarding the permissibility of charities advocating and mediating on behalf of the socially disadvantaged. Nor is it clear whether non-resident charities working or fundraising in Ireland would qualify for charitable status in this jurisdiction.

Conclusion

Ireland is an archetypal common law jurisdiction. It has a legal framework for philanthropy accompanied by a range of quite separate institutions that continue to bear all the traditional characteristic features of that legacy. The current legislation is dated, relies on principles and provisions first articulated in the English Charities Act 1960 and is facilitative rather than regulatory in nature. It is encumbered with constraints, inherited from its common law origins and resulting from deficits in contemporary law, that inhibit effective philanthropic intervention. In addition, charity law has retained its initial strong association with religion and in this jurisdiction the fusion between the Catholic Church and philanthropy has led to the provision of significant public service infrastructure under the third *Pemsel* head. It has other singularly Irish features, such as applying the subjective rule when determining charitable intent and a quixotic interpretation of 'benefit' under the fourth *Pemsel* head. These and other weaknesses in the legal framework for philanthropy have been considered in this chapter.

Ireland at the beginning of the twenty-first century has to cope with an interesting array of social inclusion issues. Some of these result from or are associated with the 30 years of violent social unrest that has afflicted the adjoining jurisdiction. Others are more typical of those presenting on the agenda of many modern western nations: the challenges posed by the large-scale migration of distinct ethnic groups including asylum seekers; pockets of rural poverty as agribusinesses displace small farmers; urban deprivation as cities grow but manufacturing is outsourced to developing countries; and the customary domestic range of vulnerable groups including people with disabilities, children, the elderly, etc. There are also issues relating to Ireland's indigenous nomadic cultural group, the 'travelling community'. These issues differ in their causes and effects and require different interventionist strategies.

In Ireland, the current fit between the charity law framework and the social inclusion agenda is not conducive to promoting the forms of philanthropic intervention likely to be most effective in relation to presenting issues. Judging from the Consultation Paper, the ongoing charity law reform process will not significantly alter this basic lack of fit. While the proposed changes will increase the technical efficiency of the charity law framework, reduce opportunities for abuse and permit a more flexible response to some areas of need, they are insufficient to remove existing constraints and appropriately focus the legal functions of charity law. This may be due in part to the government's hesitancy to introduce radical change to the regulatory framework for activities in the voluntary and community sector, particularly changes that might be viewed as challenging the accepted orthodoxy of its relations with its social partners. However, possibly Caradas will be established as an independent statutory body, not dissimilar to the English Charity Commission, and be empowered to offer the leadership and targeting necessary to overcome the weaknesses in the legal framework and facilitate effective philanthropic intervention in relation to contemporary social inclusion issues.

Chapter 10

Charity law and social inclusion in Australia

Introduction

European settlement of Australia began in 1788 with a British penal colony. The British Crown claimed the sovereignty and ownership of the land on the basis of *terra nullius* – that Australia was an empty land belonging to no one. Not unlike other common law nations it subsequently acquired the laws and institutional infrastructure of England and this, to a large extent, continues to provide a contemporary context for charity law and social inclusion.

This chapter deals with the current law, policy and practice of charity law in Australia. It begins with a brief national socio-economic profile and considers current social inclusion issues. The non-profit sector (including charities) is located within this context, with an indication of its size and significance. The chapter examines the limited outcomes of the protracted charity law review process and analyses the implications arising for social inclusion issues. Particular attention is given to the plight of indigenous citizens and the charity law framework. The chapter concludes with a summary of the more distinctive characteristics of charity law in Australia.

Australia, charities and social inclusion

The country

The establishment of a penal colony in New South Wales was followed by five more colonies during the first half of the nineteenth century. The colonies became states with their own constitutional establishment, Acts, parliaments, administration and a considerable degree of sovereignty. In 1901 the six colonies federated to form the Commonwealth of Australia. The Constitution formally divided powers between the two levels of government. The constitutional powers given to the federal government were mainly concerned with external or national affairs such as defence, immigration, currency and marriage laws.

Australia's estimated resident population at December 2005 was just under 20.5 million, an increase of 12.5 per cent over the past decade. Following the financial downturn of the late 1980s and early 1990s, Australia experienced more than a decade of sturdy 4 per cent economic growth in a low inflation environment which bled the OECD countries. The unemployment rate has fallen steadily from 8.1 per cent in November 1995 to a 30-year low of 5.0 per cent in November 2005. Home ownership has risen as in 2000–1 there were approximately 18.9 million people living in private dwellings in Australia, an increase of 7 per cent on the number of people in 1994–5.[1] Despite these trends leading social researcher Professor Peter Saunders estimates that the national poverty rate (in income terms) was around 23 per cent in 1998–9, and if poverty is estimated using expenditure, then 20 per cent.[2]

The charitable sector

Although churches and other religious associations were evident from the early years of the penal settlement, it was not until the nineteenth century that the origins and growth of secular nonprofit organizations can be discerned.[3] It was also the period in which philanthropic foundations began to emerge in the prosperous gold mining state of Victoria.

The early 1970s witnessed an explosion of small, community-based associations involved with delivering child care, citizen advisory services and general social welfare services. This occurred in the context of an expanding welfare state driven by increased federal funding. In the last decade Australia's welfare state has been changing and receding more or less along the broad lines of the UK, US and Canada. This has impacted on many nonprofit social welfare organizations with withdrawal of the direct provision of government services, contracting for services by government and in some areas competitive tendering.

While it is estimated that there are some 700,000 nonprofit organizations in Australia,[4] there are only about 48,000 strictly 'charitable' institutions or funds.[5] An unknown, but probably fairly small number are in the legal form of a charitable trust with the vast bulk being corporations with charitable objects. The nonprofit sector employs 6.8 per cent of Australians in employment (similar to the US, but larger than the UK) and contributed 3.3 per cent to GDP. Its sources of income are about 58 per cent from sale of goods and services, 30 per cent from government contracts and fees and 9 per cent from household transfers.[6] Compared to the US and the UK, the Australian sector is more reliant on fees and charges and has less philanthropic income.[7]

Philanthropy has significantly increased in Australia over the past decade rising to 0.68 per cent of Australian GDP; in the USA, during the same period, it constituted 1.6 per cent of GDP.[8] In 2004 giving by Australians amounted to approximately $A11 billion (excluding the Asian tsunami) with $A7.7 billion from individuals and $A3.38 billion from business. During that year, 41 per cent of Australians volunteered a total of 836 million hours of labour for non-profit organizations of all sizes. This voluntary contribution, equivalent to an additional $A8.9 billion worth of income to the nonprofit sector, including voluntary labour, boosted the sector's contribution to GDP to 4.9 per cent.[9]

Non-profit organizations play a vital role in Australian society. They provide education for over 30 per cent of schoolchildren, over half the private hospital beds, the majority of arts and cultural institutions and community services such as housing, aged care, counselling and emergency aid as well as facilitating sport, leisure and religious interests. Traditional sector areas such as health, aged care and child care are coming under increasing competition from the for-profit sector which is largely facilitated by government procurement policies and lack of access to capital by nonprofit organizations.

The social inclusion agenda

Although poverty has traditionally been measured in terms of income in Australia, social inclusion measures are now recognized and are becoming part of public policy discourse. In 2004, the Australian Bureau of Statistics began to measure social disadvantage in its official statistics identifying patterns of disadvantage over a range of social dimensions.[10] Recognition is now also given to the effect of multiple deprivation, e.g. lone parents with dependent children, those unemployed or living alone often have multiple disadvantages which are significantly worse when they reside in remote areas. However, as Arthurson notes 'the utility of social exclusion as an academic concept to explain poverty and disadvantage and its political use to justify new forms of policy intervention' are not always recognized.[11] This is particularly so with the federal government. Since the current federal government's election to office in 1996, it has adopted a free market approach with a conservative social agenda built on notions of mutual obligation. For example, for those on unemployment benefits, mutual obligation has seen the introduction of requirements that they volunteer for community work, 'work for the dole', or environmental work for a period of time. Throughout this period, the federal government has targeted income transfers and relied increasingly on competitive tendering between government and non-government agencies to deliver its social programmes such as unemployment and community services and health care.

The federal government also established the Reference Group on Welfare Reform (RGWR) in 1999 to develop a new welfare reform blueprint to address welfare dependency.[12] The RGWR approach was that 'the nation's social support system must be judged by its capacity to help people participate economically and socially, as well as by the adequacy of its income support arrangements'.[13] Following the report, the government stated its welfare reform objectives as:[14]

> People who depend for long periods on income support rather than paid work face increased risk of financial hardship and social exclusion. The longer they spend out of work the harder it is to get another job and the more likely they are to lose confidence. This can have negative effects on their personal relationships and lead to a sense of detachment from society . . . The Government believes that Australia is best served by a safety net that encourages participation, through a renewed emphasis on expecting Australians to use all their existing capacities.

The reforms which followed the RGWR tightened the mutual obligation requirements on those receiving unemployment benefit, but this was mitigated by the federal government not having control of the upper house. When the government finally obtained control of the upper house, the 2005 budget announced further reforms to pensions for sole mothers and those with a disability. The key feature of these reforms is a reduction in the 'capacity to work' requirement that will make many recipients no longer eligible, forcing them instead onto the lower benefits. As Professor Saunders comments, 'In the wrong hands, social exclusion can become a vehicle for vilifying those who do not conform and an excuse for seeing their problems as caused by their own "aberrant behaviour" '.[15] States have been controlled over the same period by Labour governments and while not embracing mutual obligation rhetoric they have rationalized their health and welfare services through the imposition of conditional federal funding and adoption of new public management processes.

Asylum seekers

The federal government's approach to asylum seekers has created an alienated section of the population which, being denied basic human rights, is largely held in detention centres for years. If asylum seekers are released on 'bridging visas' into the community, they are often denied the ability to earn an income and ordinary health services and social welfare payments. Many are entirely supported by charity for up to five years while their status is being determined.

The Indigenous people

The Indigenous people of Australia comprise a total of approximately 500 distinct communities from quite diverse cultural groups. The 1996 Census estimated the Indigenous population to be 386,049 or approximately 2.1 per cent of the total Australian population. Compared with other Australians, Aboriginal and Torres Strait Islander people are disadvantaged according to a range of socioeconomic indicators, including education, employment, income and housing, and are therefore at greater risk of ill health.[16] Their plight has been emphasized by researchers 'Indigenous Australians remain the most disadvantaged section of the Australian population'[17] – and by the judiciary – in *The Mum Shirl* case Gyles J expressed the view that:

> An indigenous person with virtually no assets and with all the social disadvantages shown by the evidence needs help in order to break free of the poverty trap . . . Economic, social and cultural barriers exist to successful participation in commercial or administrative life at any level by such persons.[18]

This ruling endorsed existing judicial notice of the fact that Indigenous people *per se* are within the definition of 'necessitous circumstances' and it has construed activity, intended to benefit those in need by providing more strategic leverage, as being worthy of charitable status. The Australian Tax Office (ATO) subsequently chose not to appeal against this ruling commenting only that it will 'seek the earliest available opportunity to test these issues before the court'.[19] The evidence of social disadvantage is extensive and irrefutable.

Recipients of public services   Aboriginal and Torres Strait Islander people are over-represented in several areas of community services. Available data show that Indigenous people were more highly represented in the Supported Accommodation Assistance Programme than non-Indigenous people, and Indigenous children were more likely to be placed under care and protection orders, or in out-of-home care, than their non-Indigenous counterparts. Aged care services were accessed by Indigenous people at younger ages and in proportionally lower numbers than the non-Indigenous population. Indigenous people access disability services at similar rates to the rest of the population.

Housing   In 1999, Aboriginal and Torres Strait Islander people were more likely than the non-Indigenous population to live in conditions considered unacceptable by general Australian standards. In particular, overcrowding, high housing costs relative to income, poorly maintained buildings and facilities, and inadequate infrastructure were major issues associated with the housing of Indigenous people. Aboriginal and Torres Strait Islander people were also less likely to own their own homes than non-Indigenous Australians.

Health   The available evidence suggests that Indigenous people continue to suffer a greater burden of ill health than the rest of the population. Indigenous people suffer from higher levels of many mental and behavioural disorders and their susceptibility to infectious diseases is 12 times higher than the Australian average. In 1998–9, Indigenous people were more likely than other people to be hospitalized for most diseases and conditions; hospital admissions for males being 71 per cent higher and for females 57 per cent higher than for their counterparts in the non-Indigenous population. Diabetes is a disease of particular importance for Indigenous people, affecting 30 per cent of the population.

Health services   There are clear differences between the Indigenous and non-Indigenous populations in the way that health services are accessed. Overall, Indigenous people experienced lower levels of access to health services than the general population.

Mortality   The life expectancy of Indigenous people is 20–21 years less than that of the general population; over the period 1997–9, the life expectancy at birth for an Indigenous male was 56 years, and for an Indigenous female 63 years. Data from national surveys in 1994 and 1995 show that Indigenous people were more likely than non-Indigenous people to smoke, consume alcohol at hazardous levels, be exposed to violence, and to be categorized as obese. Babies of Indigenous mothers were nearly twice as likely as babies of non-Indigenous mothers to be of low birthweight and Indigenous childhood mortality is three to five times higher than that for the population of Australian children; babies of Indigenous mothers are twice as likely to die at birth and during the early post-natal phase.

Need for a more inclusive agenda

The pace of social change in Australia since the nineties has been dramatic with the dismantling of the welfare state, move to new public management styles and the greater reliance on market mechanisms. Nonprofit organizations, particularly those delivering health, education and community services have had to adapt to this new environment in order not only to achieve their mission, but in many cases to simply survive and be relevant to the new environment. For charities that new environment presents particular challenges.

Australia like Canada is a nation experiencing the social tensions associated with both a high level of immigration and unresolved issues in relation to its chronically disadvantaged indigenous population, in addition to a relatively high national poverty rate and the usual domestic social inclusion issues relating to disability, age, gender, etc. The racial riots in Sydney and the fatalistic ennui afflicting many Aboriginal communities in the Northern Territories are indicative of a broad failure on the part of mainstream society to find ways of reaching those who are marginalized. There is a danger that, in the face of the threats from international terrorism, Australia might become less unified and inclusive in nature. This is a time when appropriate adjustments to the regulatory environment for philanthropy could usefully facilitate more focused mediatory intervention.

Government policy

In Australia – as in such other common law countries as England and Wales, Ireland, Canada and New Zealand – governments in recent decades have moved from a position of struggling to maintain a role as central provider of health and social care services to one of openly embracing the opportunity to share such responsibility with the nonprofit or charitable sector. In Ireland and Canada, for example, this policy is enshrined in a formal partnership arrangement. In the US and Australia the lack of any explicit contractual arrangement does not prevent the government from acting on an implicit understanding that such a partnership is in effect. Recognition that the government shared responsibility with the sector was noted in the recent address by the Prime Minister:[20]

> Charitable, religious and community service not-for-profit organisations play a vital role in our community and are pivotal members of the social coalition. The Government has recognised their importance in a range of policy areas, including the business and community partnership, illicit drugs policy, welfare reform and the Job Network.

It was in that context that the government launched the Inquiry into the

Definition of Charities and Related Organizations in September 2000 which reported in 2001 (see, further, below, p. 276).[21]

History, definitional matters and legal framework

The Australian law governing contemporary charities and their activities derived from the English Charitable Uses Act 1601 (43 Eliz. 1 c. 4) and has remained true to its common law origins. As elsewhere in the common law world, the law governing charities and their activities originated as a constituent part of the law of trusts: a trust being the means for giving effect to the charity established by a donor; and requiring the trustee to apply the donor's gift exclusively for charitable purposes. The principles of trust law survived to sit alongside the legislative provisions of company law and tax law to form the legal framework for philanthropy in Australia.

Historical outline

The concept of 'charitable purposes' was central to the law governing gift deductions until the introduction of the Income Tax Assessment Act 1927 (Cth) which divorced 'charity' from gift deductibility and introduced the term 'benevolent institution'.

In 1925 the Australian High Court decided that the meaning of 'charity' in a federal taxing statute was the popular narrow meaning of the word, rather than the wider legal meaning. The decision was overturned on appeal to the Privy Council which relied on *Pemsel*.[22] The federal government at the time responded with the new legislative concept of 'public benevolent institution' (PBI), a subset of charity. Subsequently, in *The Perpetual Trustee Co. Ltd.* v *Federal Commissioner of Taxation*,[23] the High Court defined the term 'public benefit institution' as an 'institution organised for the relief of poverty, sickness, destitution or helplessness'. The component of 'helplessness' has since attracted a good deal of judicial attention, most usually affirmative in nature. From that time Australia has had a double-pronged approach to tax liability: a charity is eligible for tax exemption; while a public benefit institution (PBI) is eligible for donation deduction. Some state jurisdictions have also adopted the public benevolent institution definition for the purpose of their payroll and land tax statutes.

The PBI category has become a distinguishing feature of Australian nonprofit law in that charities generally do not qualify for tax donation deductible status. Gift deductibility is reserved for a restricted subset of nonprofit organizations and only about one-third of charities are PBIs. This makes Australia quite different to the arrangements in the UK, US, Ireland and Canada. Professor Chesterman has recently argued that it provides a model for the UK in restricting charitable purposes.[24]

More recently, the development of charities legislation has been closely modelled on the English Charities Act 1960[25] and the use of *cy-près* has similarly closely followed practice in England.

The common law

Australia received English common law at the time of colonization – both the common law of charitable trusts as well as the Statute of Charitable Uses of 1601 (Statute of Elizabeth).[26] It has not adopted the English specialist regulatory agency model of a Charity Commission, but has generally adopted later statutory initiatives such as the charitable provisions of trust statutes, the extension for recreational charities and the company limited by guarantee.[27] The common law now provides the basis of the definition of charity in Australian jurisdictions and there is no codified statutory definition of charity.

The Australian state and federal jurisdictions have adopted and closely follow the English definition of charity based on the Elizabethan 1601 Preamble. The classification of charitable purposes by Lord Macnaghten in *Pemsel's* case[28] into four heads, being the relief of poverty, the advancement of education, the advancement of religion and other purposes beneficial to the community, is relied upon by Australian courts and regulators. English case authority is consistently used as the basis for Australian law in both federal and state courts. A recent definitive taxation ruling on the meaning of 'charity' for the purposes of the Income Tax Assessment Act 1997 of over 70 pages cites 145 English cases and only 113 Australian with 28 decisions from other jurisdictions.[29] There are some minor statutory extensions which are discussed below.

The legislation

Australia, being a federation of territories and states, does not have a unified and uniformly applicable legislative capacity: each state and territory is reasonably free to legislate for itself; with the exception that some Commonwealth legislation is applicable across all state jurisdictions. Consequently, there are now over 20 federal statutes which use the term 'charity' and over 130 in state and territory jurisdictions. Most adopt the common law definition, but there is some statutory modification. The most prominent statute is the Income Tax Assessment Act 1997, which uses the common law definition of charity as the basis for the exemption regime of certain non-profit organizations from income tax. However, all federal statutes (not just taxing acts) are now modified by the Tax Laws Amendment (2005 Measures No. 3) Act 2005, which extends the common law definition of charity to include certain child care and self-help groups, and closed or contemplative religious orders. Each state and territory has a trust statute which provides minor modifications to the law of equity such as dealing with mixed purpose gifts, *cy-près* applications and some states extend the common law definition to include facilities for recreation or in the interests of social welfare.[30]

The federal jurisdiction provides the Corporations Act 2001 for the registration and regulation of companies limited by guarantee and each state has an association incorporation statute which, although not uniform, are all fairly similar.[31] Each state and territory (except the Northern Territory) has legislation regulating public fundraising with provisions that differ considerably.[32] State courts refer to the definition of charity in respect of the supervision of charity trusts, dispositions in wills, fundraising regulation and in connection with various statutes governing local tax exemptions. However, as the cost of litigation and the sensitivity of nonprofit organizations to adverse publicity have grown, few cases have been pursued to the superior courts over recent years. In fact, the last major case in the ultimate court of appeal (High Court of Australia) occurred 30 years ago.[33] The common law without a vibrant case flow tends to ossification, particularly if there is no quasi-judicial body in the legal environment such as a Charity Commission.

Definitional matters

In the absence of any federal statutory definition of 'charity', the interpretation of what constitutes charitable activity draws heavily on traditional English common law dating back several centuries. As the ATO has explained:[34] 'For a purpose to fall within the technical meaning of "charitable" it must be: beneficial to the community; and within the spirit and intendment of the Statute of Elizabeth.'

Charitable purposes are commonly grouped under the four heads of the relief of poverty, the advancement of education, the advancement of religion and other purposes beneficial to the community. Although the common law continues to serve as a significant basis of the definition of charity, the costs of accessing the superior courts has slowed the development of precedent. The High Court has not only not decided a significant charity law case in over 30 years, as stated, but it has not decided any charity-related case since 1998.[35]

Public benefit

Public benefit remains essential as a common law element of charity in Australia. The purpose must be beneficial in itself, not limited to material benefits, and include social, mental and spiritual benefits as long as they are of some practical utility. The public is taken to mean the general community or a sufficient section of it as *per* the *Compton/Oppenheim* test.[36] The anomalous cases of poor relations, poor employees, closed religious orders and self-help groups, as recognized in England and Wales and elsewhere, are equally part of the Australian common law. Statutory action has now taken place at the federal level to alter the position of closed religious orders and self-help groups.

Exclusively charitable

Australian common law holds to the general principle that a trust expressed for both charitable and non-charitable purposes is invalid, but a charitable institution can have non-charitable purposes that are merely incidental or ancillary to its charitable purposes.[37] In the most recent High Court case on the issue (over 50 years ago), a religious association had objects which when examined independently were both charitable and non-charitable. The non-charitable objects were maintaining philanthropic agencies, and preserving civil and religious liberty. However, when viewed in the context of the constitution as a whole, the court found that the offending objects were ancillary to the appellant's main object to advance religion.

Considerable public debate about this issue was generated during the seven years taken to settle the Australian Tax Office's ruling on the definition of charity. The first draft ruling used the phrase that 'an institution is accepted as charitable if its dominant purpose is charitable', and that 'any non-charitable purposes of the institution must be no more than incidental or ancillary to this dominant purpose'.[38] The second draft ruling omitted the reference to 'dominant' purpose and used the phrase 'wholly, solely and exclusively' charitable.[39] The final ruling settled on 'its sole purpose must be charitable', but 'in carrying out its charitable purpose it can have purposes which are incidental or ancillary to the charitable purpose'.[40]

As to what will happen in the event that a matter comes before a court on this issue is difficult to predict. Australian incorporated bodies that claim to be charitable tend to have loosely drafted constitutions in relation to their objects, often mixed in with powers. This is probably due to their not being vetted at incorporation by a regulatory body such as a Charity Commission or taxing authority.

Non-governmental

Australian common law follows the standard view that government departments cannot be charitable when they are performing statutory duties, and charities must be independent of government or other dictation. However, the range of quasi-government bodies that inhabit a no man's land between public and government sector is growing at an increasing rate. Several cases have come before the Australian courts in relation to bodies such as ambulance, fire brigade and mine rescue authorities involving the definition of public benevolent institution.[41] The quest for such status is often driven by the fiscal advantages attached to such classifications and the federal authorities often perceive this as state governments trying to avoid federal taxes.

A charity case, at the present time before the High Court, produced a surprising result in the lower courts.[42] An independent association of general medical practitioners almost wholly funded by a federal government department was found not to be charitable. The court decided that although the formal objects of the division were charitable and seemingly legally independent, the activities of the organization denied it charitable status. The court noted:[43]

> The purposes and objects of the Division can be regarded as falling within the fourth head of *Pemsel's* case, and whilst the government does not control the Division in terms of determining the composition of its governing body or controlling its day-to-day operations, it is plain enough, as I have said, that it has assumed responsibility, on the national level, for developing the role of general practitioners in providing health care services through the divisions.

It has also been noted that, through the use of OBF [output-based funding] agreements, the government has relevantly controlled the critical standards and outcomes that must be achieved by the divisions.

If the High Court upholds this view of the government/charity boundary, then a significant number of nonprofit bodies will have to readdress their status as charitable organizations.

Charitable purposes

The lack of recent superior court decisions in Australia combined with the absence of any quasi-judicial body such as a Charity Commission has resulted in few departures from the English common law. The 1925 Chesterman decision mentioned above which led to the creation of the term 'public benevolent institution' is the major departure. Courts have ventured to find that the purposes of preservation of native fauna and flora,[44] the elimination of war,[45] the Church of Scientology,[46] adopting electronic commerce,[47] and promotion of a culture of innovation and entrepreneurship[48] are charitable. There has been judicial recognition of assisting Indigenous persons as charitable,[49] their housing,[50] together with a trust to change the law with respect to Indigenous land rights.[51]

The ATO has been a cautious regulator in comparison to the Charity Commission and not pushed the boundaries past the case law. An example of this is for nonprofit child care. While non-profit child care is recognized in other jurisdictions, there was not a significant case on point that could be used by the ATO as a basis of accepting the purpose as charitable and legislation was required as mentioned above.

Statutory definition

It remains the case that there is no statutory definition of 'charity' in Australian law although there are now multiple extensions of the common law charity definition. Legislation in a number of states, but not at federal level, extends charitable status to the provision of recreational facilities.[52] These provisions mirror legislation enacted in England (namely the Recreational Charities Act 1958).

Legal structures for charities

In Australia, charitable activity is largely carried on by entities other than charitable trusts. The charitable trust form is most commonly used in relation to the holding of money or property for charitable purposes by, for example, a grant-making foundation or religious property-holding trust. The trustee is usually corporate, being a company limited by guarantee. These trusts are only required to notify the ATO of their status and address. No further information is collected.

Unlike the UK, there are no corporate law provisions which link the charitable objects of a corporate body to the supervision of a charity regulator or charity law. The matter has been indirectly addressed in the Australian courts through the issue of whether a gift to a charitable corporation is a gift in trust or a gift to the corporation generally for its objects. Although the decisions espouse differing judicial views, it appears that a disposition to a 'charitable' corporation will presumptively take effect as a trust for the purposes of the corporation rather than a gift to the corporation.[53] There are no provisions in corporate law statutes regulating corporate forms such as the company limited by guarantee to prevent the changing of charitable objects to non-charitable objects, altering a non-distribution constraint clause or making new arrangements for the distribution of surplus assets on dissolution. Although such changes usually result in the loss of concessional taxation status.

Types of structure

Corporate entities, such as incorporated associations and companies limited by guarantee, vastly outnumber charitable trusts and charitable activity is mostly undertaken by corporate bodies with charitable objects or purposes. Companies limited by guarantee number approximately 10,000 and are almost identical to their UK inspiration. During the 1980s, all states and territories either reformed or introduced a simple form of incorporation designed specifically for small community associations and sporting bodies known as an 'incorporated association'.[54] These are administered through the Fair Trading Offices of states and territories. There are now over 138,000 incorporated associations in existence, many with charitable purposes.[55]

There are special statutory provisions for co-operatives, Indigenous associations and private acts of parliament for large associations such as religious organizations. Professor Lyons estimates that there are about 700,000 nonprofit organizations in Australia, the bulk of which are small unincorporated associations.[56] Most unincorporated associations with any significant liability exposure have incorporated under incorporated association statutes to take advantage of limited liability and relative ease of obtaining insurance cover in a corporate name.

Regulatory framework

In Australia no government body bears a particular responsibility for administering the law as it relates specifically to charities, nor are there any legal provisions imposing either registration or regulatory requirements upon charities *per se*; though some associated activities, such as fundraising, are regulated on a state-specific basis. Responsibility for charities (via the Attorney General – *parens patriae* – and the courts), for state-based incorporated association regimes (via the Offices of Fair Trading) and for all nonprofit organizations lies with the state and territory governments. Each state and territory has it own laws with respect to fundraising, incorporation of associations and exemption from state taxes such as stamp, land and payroll taxes. Little effort has been made to rationalize the different rules that apply to nonprofit organizations. The federal government, however, controls broad taxation powers thus exercising considerable policy influence through nonprofit fiscal exemptions, which is also bolstered by being a significant funding source of sport, recreation and community services through nonprofit organizations.

As noted previously, the ATO has played a limited regulatory role in relation to the taxation affairs of nonprofit organizations including charities. It has not been as active or dynamic as the taxing authority in either the USA or Canada.

Registering charities

There is no central public registry of all nonprofit organizations and no requirement for filing of financial reports to any central register. In 2000, after the introduction of a value added tax, the ATO was required by legislation to endorse charitable funds, institutions and deductible gift recipients (DGRs) which created a publicly available database of names and tax status.[57] There is no further information available such as data on annual returns.

Regulating charities

In this jurisdiction as in such other common law nations as Canada, the primary regulatory authority is vested in the federal government revenue agency with the courts, Attorney General and other agencies exercising a lighter regulatory role at state/territory level.

Australian Taxation Office

As indicated above, nonprofit income tax exemptions and donor gift deductions are administered by the ATO. It has over the last decade and a half generally pursued decentralization of some of its functions into regional centres and adopted self-assessment strategies. Until 1 July 2000, income tax exemption and donation deductible status for organizations were primarily matters of self-assessment dealt with by individual regional offices. This appears to have led to some inconsistent decision-making. The Industry Commission, a federal government agency, came to such a conclusion[58] and recommended that the definitions of gift deductible organizations should be simplified[59] and that the ATO should introduce a process of regular review of nonprofit organizations' tax status.[60] Neither these recommendations, nor the vast majority of the report's recommendations were ever specifically acted upon at the time. However, the introduction of valued added tax required a more thorough determination of charity and DGR status to ensure the integrity of the taxation system.[61]

The independent inquiry into the definition of charity (commissioned as part of the political deal to pass the value added tax through the upper house) again raised concerns about the lack of consistency in decision-making by the ATO for endorsement of charitable and deductible gift recipients.[62] The ATO submitted to the Committee responsible for the report that it had:

set up a specialist unit known as the Non-Profit Centre, with staff located in a number of regional offices, to provide expert technical guidance on issues relating to charities and other not-for-profit entities. Other specific measures include:[63]

- development of a legal database which includes summaries of key decisions which may be used as precedent by other decision makers;
- an enhanced quality assurance process which rates the quality and appropriateness of decisions by ATO officers; and
- a process for staff to refer significant issues encountered in their decision making to specialist teams in the Non-Profit Centre for advice.

It further submitted to the inquiry, in surprisingly frank language for a revenue agency, that it would rather not be given this task. It stated in its letter accompanying the formal submission:[64]

> However, you will see from our submission that there are significant difficulties with the present system. It is our view that no matter the source of definitions used (common law or statutory or a combination), there will be a continuing need for the making of fine distinctions, and this presents many issues that are both difficult and politically sensitive. Many of the problems we see are virtually without solution.
>
> It is also our view that administration would be better served by a single, independent common point of decision making on definitions leading to conclusions about whether organisations are charitable or non-profit, such as occurs with the Charities Commission in the UK for example.

Despite the report agreeing and recommending that an independent body be established to register charities, review the definitions, monitor accountability, and act as an information source for and about the non-profit sector, the recommendation has not been taken up by government.[65]

The ATO has made substantial progress in reviewing the register of charitable institutions and funds and produced a range of educational materials and rulings on charity definitional matters.[66] As noted above it has been a fairly conservative regulator compared to the Charity Commission's review of the register of charities and its policy statements on contested boundaries such as human rights, political advocacy and the boundary with government.

The courts

The High Court of Australia adjudicates constitutional disputes and is the superior appeal court as appeals to the English Privy Council have been abolished. The scope of the federal government's powers has increased enormously, because of the High Court's constitutional interpretation and referral by the states of their taxing powers.

In the absence of an equivalent to the English Charity Commission, the task of fitting the law to contemporary social need falls exclusively to the courts. However, it has long been a characteristic of charity law in this jurisdiction and elsewhere that the volume of litigation is drying up, primarily because of the heavy costs, the time constraints and the unwelcome publicity that charities are unwilling to tolerate. As the number of cases appearing before the courts decline so too does their capacity to exercise any consistent influence on the evolution of charity law. This issue largely figured in the Charity Definition Inquiry of 2001 recommendation to codify a definition of charity in contemporary terms and for the establishment of an independent administrative body.

The Attorney General

The Attorney General in each state and territory exercises the traditional *parens patriae* role in relation to charitable trusts but there is little evidence of any substantial control or scrutiny being applied to charities. Reported cases involving the Attorney General show, almost without exception, that the proceedings were instigated privately. Inquiries in Victoria,[67] for example, noted very few actions brought by the Attorney General against charities. This is partly due to the lack of interest in respect of charitable matters and to the fact that the bulk of charitable activity is undertaken through corporate entities that are not regarded as coming within the *parens patriae* jurisdiction.

The Australian Securities and Investment Commission (ASIC)

Charities *per se* are not required to register the facts of their existence, location, assets, governance arrangements or dissolution with any public body. However, many charities choose to assume the legal form of a company limited by guarantee and then, in common with all other companies, are required to register with ASIC. This body administers the provisions of the Corporations Act 2001 as it applies to all companies including incorporated charities but it has no specific brief in relation to charities as such.

Other agencies

Each state and territory (except the Northern Territory) has legislation which regulates the conduct of appeals for support to the public by nonprofit organizations.[68] The administration of such legislation is located with the department known as Fair Trading, which looks after general consumer issues and industry licensing. There is quite a variation in the proactive administrative regulation in such departments and they usually respond to complaints from the public.

Regulating the fiscal environment

The Income Tax Assessment Act 1997 in conjunction with the Tax Laws Amendment (2005 Measures No. 3) Act 2005 provides the primary federal source of legislative authority for regulating the fiscal environment. In addition, the individual states and territories each have their own statutes which provide additional regulatory powers.

Australian Taxation Office

The lack of a central regulatory body with the capacity to collate all relevant financial data in ways that promote accountability and transparency is increasingly seen as a deficiency in the Australian regulatory environment of the nonprofit sector.[69]

Tax and rates

The ATO determines liability for income tax, capital gains tax, fringe benefits tax, customs duties, and Goods and Services Tax (GST). State and territory governments are responsible for taxes such as land, payroll and stamp duties. Local authorities levy rates and charges. At each level of government, nonprofits including charities are, to varying degrees, exempt from taxation.

In fact, charitable organizations have remained exempt from income tax in Australia since the first comprehensive state income tax legislation in 1884[70] through to the current Income Tax Assessment Act 1977. Charitable institutions and funds are endorsed by the Australian Taxation Office but they are not required to file any income tax returns.

Donation incentives

Australia – unlike other jurisdictions such as Canada, the UK and the USA – employs a distinctively different set of classifications for charitable contribution deductions. As noted above the charity definition is not used for donation deductions and only a subset of charities is included. Over half the organizations with deductible gift recipient status are public benevolent institutions (PBIs) with the other categories being made up of quasi-government bodies such as educational institutions, scientific establishments and specifically named bodies which may or may not be charitable.

In this jurisdiction, income tax is levied at the federal level and there are provisions for taxpayers to claim a deduction for certain gifts made to specified types of nonprofit organizations (deductible gift recipients). Generally the deductible amount is uncapped, apart from the restriction that the deduction can only be set off against assessable income, so it cannot create a tax loss. Provisions have been recently introduced for taxpayers to average their gift deduction over five years.[71]

The federal government has since 1999 initiated a series of gift deduction reforms. These reforms widen the range of acceptable forms of gifts to property other than cash which is valued by the ATO at over $5,000, conservation covenants, streamlined administrative procedures for payroll giving and the allowance of US-styled private foundations. These new foundations known as Prescribed Private Funds allow families and private individuals to establish charitable trusts which they effectively control, but are also allowed a taxation deduction. Previously a gift deduction was only permitted when the trusts had a publicly controlled board and actually received donations from the general public.

Supplying a service does not fall within any of the gift types. There is no deduction for a gift of a service, as no money or property is transferred to the deductible gift recipient. For example, volunteers' expenses in carrying out voluntary work are not considered tax-deductible.[72] Testamentary gifts are not deductible, except in respect of cultural bequests. A deduction can be claimed for a quid pro quo transaction in respect of a political contribution and certain minor benefits such as fundraising dinners.

Cy-près

Where a charitable trust has been established and a subsequent failure occurs, the trustee is usually obliged by force of law to initiate assistance from the state to alter its purpose and overcome the failure. The state facilitates the unlocking of a trust's perpetual existence and its unalterable objectives. In Australian jurisdictions, the State represented by the Attorney General is empowered to supervise the schemes and there is little administrative machinery such as a Charity Commission.[73] The early UK legislation (1960) found its way into Australian state jurisdictions, but not the later provisions which allow for administrative interventions.[74] Australian courts have inherent powers to deal with subsequent frustrations. However, they have no power to vary a charitable purpose that is defined and legally capable of being executed. The court cannot vary the donor's original charitable purposes to what it considers to be more beneficial to the public, or even what the court may surmise that the founder would have contemplated if they could have foreseen the changes in circumstances.[75]

In New South Wales, the courts are given widened powers to devise *cy-près* schemes where the original purposes have 'ceased to provide a suitable and effective method of using the trust property, having regard to the spirit of the trust'.[76] Queensland, South Australia, Tasmania and Victoria follow New South Wales with slight variations in the statutory wording.[77]

It appears that there is little activity by the courts, as initiated through the Attorneys General, in relation to the reform of frustrated charitable trusts. While all Australian jurisdictions place a positive duty on charitable trustees to bring *cy-près* actions before the court with the joining of the Attorney General, there are few reported cases and most take a long time to be resolved. Attorneys General rarely initiate *cy-près* actions.

Some recent *cy-près* applications do not arouse a great deal of faith in the efficient redeployment of dormant charitable funds.[78] For example, a recent case involved an endowment fund of $64,000 for charitable purposes. Between 1937 and 1950, no meetings of trustees were held and the judge noted:

> Thereafter at various times the incumbent Lord Mayor of Brisbane, officers of the Justice Department, and the present applicant raised questions as to the future management of the trust, the desirability of passing legislation with respect to it, and otherwise debated among themselves the future management of the trust. However, nothing concrete has ever been done.[79]

There is little opportunity for the Attorney General to supervise corporate entities with charitable objects. The matter has been indirectly addressed in the Australian courts through the issue of whether a gift to a charitable corporation is a gift in trust or a gift to the corporation generally for its objects. Although the decisions espoused differing judicial views, it appears that a disposition to a charitable corporation will presumptively take effect as a trust for the purposes of the corporation rather than a gift to the corporation.[80]

Fundraising

The law governing fundraising is in quite an unsatisfactory state, with Professor Dal Pont remarking that the 'lack of uniformity, coupled with the antiquity of the legislation in some jurisdictions, has prompted calls for widespread and wholesale reform of fundraising laws'.[81] The Industry Commission in 1995 made similar comments.[82] National charities must register in each state and comply with differing requirements which add to their compliance burden with little gain in accountability or protection of the public from fraudulent behaviour. Until recently, two jurisdictions contained regulations drawn from a 1908 English fundraising regulation which prevented solicitation of funds using a box on a long pole to reach passing stage coaches. The provisions fail to deal with Internet, email or text messaging appeals and only some deal with 'face to face chugging'.

Trading

The restraints on trading by charitable organizations are similar to those imposed in other common law nations. There is no income tax on unrelated business income and business or commercial activities that are merely incidental to a charitable institution's or fund's purposes do not prevent it from being a charity. This is an increasingly controversial issue as competing sectors of the Australian economy seek competitive neutrality.

Constraints on modern philanthropic activity

In Australia, the law governing philanthropic activity functions in a complex environment. As in Canada, it must respond to its colonial legacy as represented by the needs of its indigenous people and to the cultural tensions arising from difficulties in accommodating the waves of recent non-European immigrants. There are also particular difficulties presented by the challenge of the asylum seekers phenomenon. In addition, Australia shares with all modern western nations the obligation to respond to the needs of those suffering, for example, from poverty, disability, age and gender discrimination, etc. Arguably, the capacity of the relevant law to best address such contemporary pressing social issues is compromised by the distribution of authority between federal and state/territory and by reliance upon a body of common law rules and principles that largely precede the establishment of Australia as an independent jurisdiction.

Partnership with government: the constraints

All Australian governments are moving towards increasing the accountability measures that accompany government funding. In the health and community services sector the relationship is moving towards a procurement model with imposed quality frameworks and competitive tendering. Agreements for state funding often contain harsh conditions such as transfer of liability, appropriation of all intellectual property, refunding of any surpluses and invasive auditing within imposed quality frameworks. In some extreme cases, acceptance of funding often goes with foregoing the right to publicly comment on relevant policy matters or vetting of any press release by the funding agency. This approach by government bodies carries risks for charities.

Whilst the discourse of partnership is constantly used by government, the legal relationship it is developing with the charitable sector is in many instances better characterized as one of master and servant.[83] The Central Bayside case presently before the High Court illustrates the extent of control that some government funders are exercising over nominally independent nonprofit organizations.[84]

The Indigenous people

The continuing and, by all accounts, steadily worsening circumstances of this the most socially disadvantaged group in Australia is a standing indictment of the failure of philanthropy (and other equally fruitless forms of intervention). It is readily acknowledged that arresting the rate of decline involves strengthening the capacity of small communities to be self-sustaining. This would seem to be recognized by the ATO which has stated that:[85]

> A charitable purpose must be for the benefit of the community. Charity is altruistic and intends social value or utility. The benefit need not be for the whole community; it may be for an appreciable section of the public.

However, the application of this principle in the context of Indigenous community development projects has not proved to be so straightforward.[86]

A number of cases have been brought before the courts by local councils and state government revenue authorities disputing property rates exemptions or payroll tax exemptions for indigenous organizations which are in the main devoted to assisting the poorest of the poor.[87] The case of the Toomelah Co-operative Limited is a stark example.[88] The Human Rights Commission produced a report which gained significant publicity for its criticism of the failure of government authorities to supply basic services to the community such as water, sewerage and rubbish disposal.[89] The local Indigenous housing co-operative leased houses to the local population who were members, with no houses having sewerage and one three-bedroom house having between 7 and 15 occupants at a time. Of the 900 Indigenous inhabitants over 95 per cent were unemployed, and only 2 of the co-operative's members were employed. The local council refused rates exemption for the organization's houses and put in argument before the court that as two of the co-operative's members were employed and were occupying co-operative houses this was evidence that the land was not used for 'charitable or benevolent' purposes. Clearly in the circumstances such a view is a less than meritorious argument with little legal basis. Other payroll cases have tried to exclude clerical staff's wages from payroll tax as they were not 'frontline' workers.

Businesses

Community development schemes very often have a business component as disadvantaged communities usually place a priority on projects that may serve to bring in capital and help lift its members out of poverty. Such schemes may not be overtly run for profit but may involve a private financial contribution and/or generate a surplus. They are often set up solely for the purpose of training the unemployed in skills appropriate to the needs of local industries. However, the involvement of private funds and/or the basis for distributing any profits can be fatal to the charitable status of the organization concerned.

Common law constraints

As Australia has stepped back from the proposed bold step to introduce a codified definition of 'charity', the characteristics of the common law legacy operate to constrain its charitable activity in much the same way as in England and Wales (see, also, chapters 3 and 8).

The 'spirit and intendment' rule

As the ATO has emphasized:[90] 'Purposes are not charitable if they lack the required community benefit or are not within the spirit and intendment of the Statute of Elizabeth.' In this jurisdiction, the 'spirit and intendment' clause is a crucial common law determinant in the development of the public benefit test for charitable activity. Those organizations that have purposes which do not fit within the *Pemsel* classification or are not analogous to those listed there must show that they can instead be construed as coming broadly within the legislative intent of the Preamble to the 1601 Act. Four hundred years later it can require some ingenuity and willingness to interpret the public benefit of a modern activity (such as Internet access) to correspond with a Preamble activity (such as repair of highways) and so qualify for charitable status.[91] This is much less likely to happen in Australia where the responsibility for making such interpretations largely falls to the ATO, which adopts a conservative approach to novel purposes with potential to further erode the tax base.

Legal structures

Australia is served by a range of corporate structures designed for use by non-profit organizations. The charitable trust is little used in comparison to the UK. However, there are issues of protecting the stated objects of a corporation from inappropriate alteration and abandonment, particularly those with charitable purposes. This is an avenue for abuse which could lead to a reduction in trust and reputation of the sector.

Restrictions on advocacy/political activity

The ongoing public debate about the role of nonprofit organization advocacy has been raging in Australia over the last decade. Government funders are accused of stifling free speech with harsh contractual terms about public comment and of awarding of contracts to those who do not have an aggressive advocacy platform. Right-wing think tanks complain that strident advocacy groups are unrepresentative and have too much influence with government administration.[92]

The public debate about the introduction of the Charity Bill and its provisions with respect to charities advocating and participating in the public policy process brought left and right to the battlefield and left the possibility of genuine legal reform in tatters. The ATO's finalized taxation ruling on the definition of charity goes some way to clarifying how they will interpret and apply the law in this regard, but it is yet to be seen if the courts will hold to the same view.

Fiscal issues

The greatest constraint on charitable activity is the restriction of gift deductibility to a small subset of charitable bodies (mainly PBIs) which focus on direct alms to the poor. It does not allow preventative and development work to be encouraged by fiscal incentives and this is out of step with other jurisdictions such as the US, UK and Canada. The added layer of tax classification only adds to the regulatory burden.

Public benefit matters

In addition to the above-mentioned definitional aspects of the public benefit test there are others that are particularly counter-productive in the context of Australia's social inclusion agenda.

Uneven application of the public benefit test

As with other common law countries, there is an uneven application of the public benefit test across the four *Pemsel* heads. The non-statutory presumption that the test will be satisfied in relation to gifts to religious organizations is perhaps interpreted by the judiciary and the ATO in a spirit of deference and generosity that is closer to the approach adopted by the equivalent authorities in Ireland than is generally the case among other common law nations.

The Indigenous people and training

While the advancement of education is a charitable purpose not all training schemes will necessarily fit under this umbrella. They may fail to satisfy the 'public benefit' test. The more tightly drawn the criteria for accessing the training, the more likely the scheme will be insufficiently 'public' to qualify for charitable status. The courts, however, have found that Indigenous persons *per se* qualify as disadvantaged:[93] 'many, indeed most, Indigenous persons in Australia could properly be described as "disadvantaged" generally and, in particular, in relation to education and the ability to take a place in the business and professional world of Australia'.

Moreover, training even when narrowly restricted to a rather elitist profession such as 'barrister' would meet the 'public' requirement; at least in relation to the needs of Indigenous people:[94]

> Whilst, at one level, assisting persons to become practicing barristers may be seen by some as a luxury, I see it as the grant of assistance to persons to take a place in the world which the ability of the person would warrant but which might be denied without the assistance provided in order to overcome economic and social disadvantage.

The group targeted for training must be large enough to be construed as sufficiently 'public' in nature. So, while 'Indigenous people' may satisfy the test, any further limitations that restrict access to those of a certain age, clan or locality will probably prevent the training scheme from being charitable.

The Indigenous people and the 'poor relations' rule

The blood-link characteristic of indigenous communities gives rise to the ancillary issue as to whether this constitutes a personal nexus that compromises the 'public' component of the public benefit test. In Australia, as in Canada and New Zealand, this common law rule threatens the capacity of indigenous communities to establish organizations with charitable status or that of charities to work with such communities.

Cultural affirmation

Where a group belonging to a minority culture constitutes an organization to preserve and promote its cultural heritage it will probably not qualify for charitable status because the ATO is likely to regard such activities as essentially social and therefore of insufficient 'benefit' to the community.[95] So, for example, a community centre established in Melbourne to provide for the cultural and social needs of Latvians was held to be non-charitable on the grounds that the needs it addressed were mainly social in nature.[96] Such initiatives may also fall foul of the ATO rule that purposes must not be vague or ambiguous.

Modern law constraints

In this jurisdiction, as in most other common law countries, the main constraints on the development of more relevant and effective methods of philanthropic intervention stem from the fact that the regulatory framework conforms to the archetypal revenue-driven model.

Lack of coherence in charity law administration

The distribution of authority between federal and state/territory levels is unclear except insofar as determination and supervision of tax-exempt eligibility falls to the former, and this function is compromised by the lack of a central register together with mandatory and uniform financial reporting requirements that would enable the ATO to maintain an informed overview of the sector. At state/territory level the disparity between jurisdictions in relation to registration and supervision requirements, the role of the Attorney General, fundraising laws, etc., is confusing and leads to some forum shopping by nonprofits. Confusion also pervades the legal distinction between the status of charity, public benevolent institution and deductible gift recipient (DGR), with few laypersons understanding the difference and grasping the resulting significance for tax exemption privileges. This situation is not helped by legal provisions that fail to harmonize the requirements for those charities structured as companies or trusts. There is a clear need in this jurisdiction for laws that unify and co-ordinate the administrative regime for charities.

Lack of an appropriate forum for developing charitable purposes

The common law is wholly dependent upon a continuous case flow to permit judicial review of principles in the light of practice. The ATO, however, does not have a brief to be proactive in giving recognition to those charities which engage in new forms of public benefit activity and the courts seldom have the opportunity. The fact that no mechanism exists to permit an ongoing review and adjustment of the law to ensure an appropriate fit with new or embedded forms of social disadvantage amounts to a structural flaw in the charity law framework.

Judicial review of principles and precedents occurs so seldom and randomly as to provide little capacity for effectively addressing changes in social need. This is not to deny that the judiciary make important rulings with potential to reset the application of the law. As evidenced by the finding made by Gyles J, in *Trustees of the Indigenous Barristers Trust*:[97] 'In my opinion, the undisputed evidence leads to a finding that, at the time the Trust was settled, and for the foreseeable future, many, indeed most, indigenous persons in Australia could properly be described as "disadvantaged".' However, that judicial notice has been taken, in this and other cases, of the fact that Indigenous people are *per se* socially disadvantaged has not influenced the approach adopted by the ATO. In the absence of an explicit High Court judgment directing a different interpretation of the law, the ATO is free to continue its conservative defence of exemptions from income tax liability on grounds of an organization's charitable purposes.

Human rights, anti-terrorism and social justice legislation

In Australia, as elsewhere in the more developed common law nations, the law governing philanthropy functions against a background of rights-oriented legislation.

Human rights   Although Australia does not have a formal Bill of Rights nor as extensive human rights-based legislation as operates in the European context, it does have a Human Rights and Equal Opportunity Commission (HREOC) established under the Human Rights and Equal Opportunity Commission Act 1986 (Cth) and each state has some sort of human rights commission. Human rights and discrimination legislation in Australia usually exempts religious organizations and often all nonprofit organizations from most of its provisions.

Anti-terrorism   Australia, along with many other countries, has recently introduced new laws to implement anti-terrorism measures. These have an impact on general civil liberties and in particular they seek to control suspect nonprofit organizations. The federal parliament has considered over 47 separate bills on the issue since 2001 and the states have all passed similar legislation. Provisions include preventative detention for up to 14 days, new sedition laws, increased stop, question and search powers, interception of electronic communications, anti-money laundering and financing provisions, banning of organizations and criminalization of membership of certain associations.[98] The potential to abuse freedom of association and expression, which is the foundation of nonprofit organizations, is available to governments and administrations with fewer safeguards and checks than ever before in Australia's history. Whether the opportunity to abuse these freedoms is taken is yet to be seen, but given the secrecy surrounding such action perhaps it will never be seen.

Social justice   Australia has in place much the same set of laws addressing much the same domestic social justice concerns (equity, equality and non-discriminatory practices, etc.) as other modern nations. They are mainly enacted at federal level[99] but some states and territories[100] have an established reputation for initiating independent legislation. A considerable body of case law testifies to the vigour with which social justice issues are pursued, mainly by the Human Rights and Equal Opportunity Commission.

International aid

Charities find it difficult to conduct any substantial activities internationally unless they are specially registered through the taxation system. Charitable organizations must generally be located and conduct their activities 'in Australia' to be income tax-exempt.[101] Nearly all DGRs for the purposes of the taxation legislation must also be 'in Australia'.[102] This generally requires that the DGR is established and operates in Australia and has purposes and beneficiaries in Australia. The limited exceptions are for:

- funds that are overseas aid relief funds;
- public funds on the register of environmental organizations; or
- specifically listed DGRs that when listed in the Income Tax Assessment Act were approved for overseas purposes or beneficiaries.

In practice this dramatically restricts deduction of gifts to non-Australian organizations. Giving to international purposes is largely facilitated through the special category for overseas aid relief funds. There are about 120 approved relief funds. To receive status as a relief fund it must be:

- a public fund, established by an organization declared by the Minister of Foreign Affairs to be an approved organization;
- solely for the relief of people in a country declared by the Minister for Foreign Affairs to be a developing country;
- endorsed as such by the ATO;
- in Australia; and
- declared by the Treasurer as a relief fund.

There are a limited number of countries listed as developing countries and the administrative process for approval is difficult and often expensive. It is possible for expatriates of some countries who have become residents of Australia to make deductible gifts to overseas aid funds by transferring monies to endorsed relief funds in other countries.[103] Laws in some developing countries prohibit or 'block' expatriates of that country from transferring money to Australia, and such monies can be donated to the Australian overseas aid relief fund account in that country.

The Australian deductible gift regime does not permit domestic organizations to serve as a conduit for a foreign charitable organization without discretion and control over the funds transmitted.

Charity law review and social inclusion

Australia came close to adopting a full statutory definition of charity, but the federal government chose to abandon a draft bill after public consultation and public debate. The federal government, in fulfilling a political commitment to an upper house minor party in order to allow the passage of the new value added tax law, commissioned an independent inquiry into definitional issues relating to charitable, religious and community service nonprofit organizations.[104] The inquiry included amongst its recommendations the introduction of a statutory definition of 'charity' accompanied by an independent administrative body.

Proposed changes to definitional matters and legal structures

After considering the inquiry report, the Federal Treasurer released a draft bill and directed the Board of Taxation to consult on the workability of the definition of charity proposed.[105]

Charitable purpose

The draft bill took the traditional four heads of charity and divided them into seven distinct charitable purposes, following the spirit of the inquiry's recommendations. They were:

1   the advancement of health;
2   the advancement of education;
3   the advancement of social or community welfare (including care of young people);
4   the advancement of religion;
5   the advancement of culture;
6   the advancement of the natural environment;
7   any other purpose that is beneficial to the community.

'Advancement' was defined to include 'protection, maintenance, support, research and improvement'. While not adding completely new purposes such as 'amateur sport', it did give legislative clarity to purposes which were regarded by some as on the boundary of charity (such as the care of young people).

Other provisions in the draft bill caused significant public discussion. The bill declared the following to be disqualifying purposes:

• illegal activities;
• advocating a political party or cause;
• supporting a candidate for political office; and
• attempting to change the law or government policy.

Many believed that the draft bill was an attack on their ability to advocate for a political cause or attempt to change the law or government policy. A political debate ensued with little reference to the actual state of the law. The draft bill also sought to prevent any organization that engaged (at the present time or in the past) in a serious criminal offence (no conviction required) from charitable status. There was no means of rehabilitation. It is unclear what the purpose of such a provision was to be, but many assumed it was aimed at activist peace and environment groups who might storm military bases or physically act against industrial polluters or farmers.

Public benefit

The draft bill also sought to alter the public benefit element of the common law definition. Under the first three heads of charity in the common law is a general presumption that, *prima facie*, the element of public benefit is satisfied. Under the draft bill all organizations would have required to positively satisfy the test of having a purpose for the public benefit which:

• is aimed at achieving a universal or common good;
• has practical utility; and
• is directed to the benefit of the general community or to a sufficient section of the general community.

Private schools and religious organizations perceived this as a difficult provision. The Treasurer decided not to codify the definition and merely extended the definition to cover certain child care, self-help groups and closed or contemplative religious orders. It applies to all federal statutes. The states have not followed this Commonwealth lead to date and Australian now has multiple definitional extensions of the common law charity definition.

Legal structures

The draft bill left untouched the existing structures for charities.

Changes to the regulatory framework

The draft bill left the regulatory framework alone. The government failed to introduce a new administrative body, like the Charity Commission in England and Wales, as suggested in the report to it. Another legislative initiative at the same time widened the scope of endorsement of charitable funds and institutions for other taxes, but this public register merely notes the name and tax status of the organization.

The outcome of the process

The Australian charity law review process culminated with an announcement by the Federal Treasurer on 11 May 2004 in the following terms:[106]

> [t]he common law meaning of a charity will continue to apply, but the definition will be extended to include certain child care and self-help groups, and closed or contemplative religious orders. The Government has decided not to proceed with the draft Charities Bill.

Implications for social inclusion

The collapse of the charity review process is a serious setback for the prospects of achieving a better fit between the legal framework for philanthropy and the contemporary needs of the socially disadvantaged in Australia. The statutory extension of the charity law definition to include child care, self-help groups and closed religious orders is not just a minimalist, conservative exercise in political face-saving but more importantly it misses the main issues on the social inclusion agenda. The circumstances of the Indigenous people, the plight of asylum seekers and multicultural or racist tensions are currently among Australia's most pressing social problems, and the outcome of this review process has done nothing to facilitate much needed ameliorative philanthropic intervention. It is also an outcome which threatens to damage government attempts to cultivate an authentic working partnership with the sector.

Among the more significant consequences are the following.

1   *Failure of statutory definition and other inquiry recommendations*   The proposed new statutory definition of charitable purposes promised to significantly broaden the range of charitable activity and would have been generally welcomed in the philanthropic world. The withdrawal of this initiative leaves federal and state jurisdictions unaligned in their definitions so it is possible to be charitable in one state and not in another or charitable for the purposes of federal law, but not state.

2   *ATO is left as the regulator*   The proposal to introduce a new administrative agency, with a role and responsibilities similar to the English Charity Commission, would have been an important strategic step in shaping a new regulatory framework for philanthropy and again would have been generally welcomed. The lack of charity cases passing through superior courts, combined with the absence of a progressive charity regulator or quasi-judicial administrative body does not bode well for charity purpose development in Australia. The ATO is now left as the only likely body that could take a role in this development, but to date it has erred on the conservative side in its interpretation of charitable purposes.

3   *Growing issues of accountability with the public*   The collapse of this process, after several years of negotiation with the sector and after hard-won mutual

undertakings had been secured, is unquestionably a serious setback for future partnership prospects. Government credibility in this context has been damaged and the bona fides of its intentions will be questioned by the sector when the partnership dialogue resurfaces.

4   *Legal structures and charity link*   The traditional legal structures are not best suited as vehicles for modern philanthropic ventures. The confusing mix of trust principles and the statutory provisions of company and tax law continue to generate uncertainty. This has been a missed opportunity to simplify and increase the functionality of the vehicles that deliver philanthropy in Australia.

Conclusion

Charity law must be adjusted to allow philanthropic intervention to promote the social inclusion of marginalized groups such as the Indigenous people and thereby forestall their alienation. Ensuring a better fit between the law, philanthropic resources and the needs of the socially disadvantaged remains a matter of pressing importance for the Indigenous people, for other marginalized groups and for achieving greater social cohesion in Australia.

Chapter 11

Charity law and social inclusion in New Zealand

Introduction

New Zealand completed its charity law review process when parliament passed the Charities Act on 13 April 2005, Part I of which came into effect on 1 July 2005. However, as the operative provisions are confined to definitional matters and establishing the Charities Commission and as no date has been set for introducing the bulk of the Act, the legal framework is considered as at the time of writing.

This chapter begins with a brief overview of the country, its primary socio-economic indicators and of the relationship between charities and social inclusion. This is followed by an outline of the history of charity law in New Zealand as developed through its legislative milestones. The template of functions (see, further, chapter 6) is then applied to identify and assess the characteristic features of the charity law environment in this jurisdiction, the key definitional matters, the legal structures for charities, registration and the regulatory framework, financial matters and the legal constraints on the development of philanthropy. The chapter continues by examining the outcomes of the protracted charity law review process, considers the actual and potential role for the Charities Commission and analyses the significance of the Charities Act 2005 for social inclusion issues. It concludes by reflecting on the distinctive characteristics of charity law in New Zealand.

Charities and social inclusion

New Zealand has a proud tradition of self-reliance: of looking to family and community-based organisations rather than to government for support in times of need.[1] This has allowed or required charities, in common with other not-for-profit bodies, to find their own space and develop as independent entities relatively free from regulatory restraint. Not unlike Ireland, from an early stage the prevailing policy was to encourage charities, usually church-based community groups, to fill the gap and establish the health and social care facilities for the poor, ill or otherwise disadvantaged that the government could not afford to provide. The development of the charitable sector in New Zealand was actively facilitated by legislation that promoted the use of charitable trusts and by the absence of regulatory controls. This history has shaped the modern partnership ethos between government and community as demonstrated in the process and outcome of its recently concluded charity law reform.

The country

This small trading nation based on two main islands and a number that are much smaller (comprising approx 268,680 square kilometres), has a largely urban population of some 4,035,461 consisting mainly of those of European descent and the native Maori, and some mixed ethnic groups with multifaith but mainly Christian religious beliefs.[2] Traditionally an agrarian economy highly dependent upon its exports of agricultural produce to Britain it has, over the past two or three decades, undergone considerable socio-economic changes.

The economy

Since the mid-1980s, the deregulation of the economy, removal of tariff protections, privatization of State assets, labour market reform and the rise of the free market ethos have combined to secure New Zealand the strong competitive role in the global marketplace it needs if trade profits are to continue to fund social progress. In order to further this process of economic reform, government policies have stressed the need to achieve and maintain low inflation, remove economic distortions, lower taxes and exercise fiscal prudence with the primary purpose of enhancing the growth of gross domestic product. By the end of the 1990s, a low inflation rate was achieved and per capita income was increasing annually. By 2004 unemployment stood at 4.2 per cent, exports accounted for 20 per cent of GDP while the GDP growth rate had reached 4.8 per cent.

Health and social care

Arguably, however, success in the pursuit of economic growth was at the price of cutbacks in public sector spending. The welfare state underwent a radical overhaul in the late 1980s and throughout the 1990s. In 1991 most benefits, such as the Sickness, Domestic Purposes Benefit and Unemployment Benefit, were cut by between 5 per cent and 27 per cent.[3] Certain health subsidies, formerly universal, were restricted to low-income families through the introduction of the Community Services Card. The move towards an ever more tightly targeted welfare state proceeded.[4]

The extent of government withdrawal is evident in the current low rate of income tax (39 per cent compared with the OECD average top rate of 47.8 per cent) and of government spending (36.4 per cent of GDP compared with UK 37.8 per cent, Norway 43 per cent, Denmark 52.4 per cent, Germany 44.8 per cent and Canada 42 per cent). In addition this jurisdiction has a Goods and Services Tax, at 12.5 per cent, with no general exemptions except for financial transactions. The resulting negative impact on the socially disadvantaged in New

Zealand society has been charted by various commentators,[5] in reports published by national and international non-government organizations[6] and in regular reports by government agencies.[7]

The charitable sector

Because of the lack of any system for registering their existence, it is difficult to estimate the number of charities in New Zealand let alone gauge their impact.[8] In 1989, the Working Party on Charities and Sporting Bodies estimated that the contribution of the charitable sector could be valued at somewhere between 5 per cent and 10 per cent of GDP.[9] It has been conjectured that the number of charities in New Zealand might be in the tens of thousands.[10]

The social inclusion agenda

The social inclusion issues currently challenging New Zealand have been candidly acknowledged by the government:[11]

> Average material living standards have fallen relative to most other OECD countries; income inequality increased particularly in the late 1980s; the incidence of household poverty is too high; there are wide gaps in ethnic averages across a range of social indicator, there are poor outcomes in health and education among lower socio-economic groups; there are quite sharp divisions in values and attitudes on key socio-economic issues; and there are institutional weaknesses that trouble Crown-Maori aspirations and our levels of social capability more generally. Added to this is a regional picture of increasing deprivation in Northland and parts of Auckland, and stagnation in East Cape. Finally, there is the threat of more skilled young New Zealanders leaving for what they see as more prosperous foreign countries that are putting out the welcome mat for them.

The need to counter these deficits and build greater social cohesion is implicit in the government's key goals which include:

- strengthening national identity and upholding the principles of the Treaty of Waitangi;
- growing an inclusive innovative economy for the benefit of all;
- maintaining trust in government and providing strong social services;
- improving New Zealanders' skills; and
- reducing inequalities in health, education, employment and housing.

The Maori

The Maori, the indigenous people of New Zealand, currently total some 523,000 persons constituting approximately 15 per cent of the population of New Zealand, are expected to represent nearly 20 per cent of the population by the year 2031. The median age for Maori is around 22 years and 55 per cent of the population is under 25 years compared with only 34.6 per cent of non-Maori. More than half of all Maori live in the northern part of North Island, mostly around Auckland (46 per cent). In general, they have lower incomes and larger households than non-Maori and are more likely to be living in one-parent households. Relative to the non-Maori, they are disadvantaged by age, geographical distribution, by low standards of education and skills and by levels of unemployment.[12]

The Indigenous people of New Zealand have a well-developed communal culture. The critical organizational construct is the tribe, an extended kinship organization comprising sub-tribes and extended family groups. The tribal identity was and is the *iwi*. The tribal institutions of *whanua* (extended family or kin group), *hapu* (sub-tribe), *hui* (meeting of the *iwi*) and *marae* (ceremonial centre) remain key features of contemporary Maori culture. Maori belong to diverse communities: some identify with a particular *iwi*, *hapu* and *whanau* irrespective of where they reside; others identify with their tribal connections but do not know their ancestry or *whakapapa*; while others prefer to identify simply as Maori. However, the strength of their communities, built on networks of blood relationships, is also a considerable weakness in terms of charity law. The common law framework has operated to obstruct philanthropic activity on behalf of the socially disadvantaged Maori as acknowledged by the government in its discussion document *The Taxation of Maori Organisations*.[13]

Need for a more inclusive agenda

In the first comprehensive assessment of the status of human rights in New Zealand, the Human Rights Commission noted that the most pressing social inclusion issues were those relating to:[14]

- the poverty and abuse experienced by a significant number of New Zealand children and young people;
- the pervasive barriers that prevent disabled people from fully participating in society;
- the vulnerability to abuse of those in detention and institutional care;
- the impact of poverty on realization of the most basic human rights;
- the entrenched economic and social inequalities that continue to divide Maori and Pacific people from other New Zealanders; and
- the challenge of the place of the Treaty of Waitangi now and in the future.

The action plan proposed by the Commission to address these issues rests very much on a strategic approach to what it views as structural social problems. So, for example, it suggests direct and systematic participation of disabled people in policy development and decision-making. It insists that there should be a focus on the elimination of poverty and that ways are developed to improve democratic participation, including that of children and young people, and widening access to justice. These problems and the proposed methods for tackling them present a real challenge for the future role of philanthropy in New Zealand. The outcomes of the charity law reform process must be set against the nature and scale of this challenge.

Government policy

In New Zealand the government's policy of creating a genuine partnership with community, voluntary and *iwi*/Maori organizations was formally proclaimed in November 2001. The Prime Minister and the Minister for the Community and Voluntary Sector then signed a statement of intent on behalf of the government to signal the government's recognition of the fact that community, voluntary and *iwi*/Maori organizations interact across a range of ministries and departments. By so doing the government committed itself to giving priority to working with the not-for-profit sector to develop co-ordinated, inter-sectoral policies and programmes. The government's vision for the future is one where the State performs its role as a facilitator of a strong civil society based on respectful relationships between government and community, voluntary and *iwi*/Maori organizations.

The Charities Act 2005 is seen as a cornerstone of its partnership policy. As a government minister declared:[15] 'This legislation is a symbol of this government's commitment to growing the relationship between government and the charitable sector.'

History, current legislation and definitional matters

The law relating to charities in New Zealand reflects the history of a non-regulatory but facilitative government approach to organizations established to provide public benefit services.

The early colonial experience promoted self-reliance and the government encouraged the vulnerable to look to their families rather than to the State for assistance.[16] This was illustrated, for example, in the Destitute Persons Ordinance 1846 which imposed obligations on the relatives of the needy and enforced deductions from employers' wages for this purpose. This approach seemed to experience a revival in the last decades of the twentieth century as the government withdrew its support for an inclusive, non-contributory, welfare state and instead introduced means testing for many health and welfare benefits. At both stages it was an approach that proved conducive to promoting the role of community-based health and social care charities.

Outline of legislative history

The understanding of what constitutes a charity has been developed by the common law and is based on the Preamble to the Statute of Charitable Uses[17] enacted by the English Parliament in 1601, as extended by the 'spirit or intendment' rule[18] and on the classification of charitable purposes set out by Lord Macnaghten in the *Pemsel* case[19] (see, further, chapter 3). In New Zealand, as in other common law jurisdictions, the history of charity law can essentially be traced to the 1601 Act. By the time this jurisdiction acquired a measure of independence in 1840, the development of its legal framework for charities[20] was rooted in common law principles and now, under the auspices of the Charities Act 2005, it is clear that its future will continue to be so.

The Religious, Charitable and Educational Trusts legislation

Beginning with the Religious, Charitable and Educational Trusts Act 1856, a series of statutes set out the government's recognition, support and encouragement of charitable trusts established for public benefit purposes. The 1856 Act was extended in 1863 from conveyances to trustees in respect of freehold and leasehold property to also include mortgages and loans. In 1884 legislation provided for the incorporation of the bodies established by such trustees.

The Charitable Funds Appropriation Act 1871

Although introduced to cope with fundraising problems, this statute made a significant contribution to the development of charity law by specifying a list of 11 categories of charitable purposes comprising an uneven mix of health, social care and educational services for the poor or otherwise disadvantaged, with provision of public service utilities, religious activities and insurance schemes. It also introduced provisions to allow funds raised by an organization for a particular charitable purpose, that had subsequently become 'impossible or inexpedient' or 'uncertain or illegal' for the organization to deal with as it had intended, to be applied instead to other charitable purposes. This provision marked the beginning of a process that saw the functions of *cy-près* schemes being accommodated by a statutory procedure.

The Hospitals and Charitable Institutions Act 1885

As the name suggests, this legislation was concerned with health and social care infrastructure. It sought to organize facilities on a localized basis. Included among the schedules to the Act, however, was a list purposes and objects deemed to be charitable.

The Charitable Trusts Extension Act 1886

This statute further developed the measures addressed in the Acts of 1871 and 1885. In particular it continued the process of providing a statutory procedure to enable charities to redirect assets to other charitable ends when original purposes had become impossible, impractical, uncertain or illegal.

The Hospitals and Charitable Institutions Act 1909

This legislation sought to bring the localized facilities established under the 1885 Act into a country-wide health care scheme.

The Religious, Charitable and Educational Trusts Act 1908

This Act, as subsequently amended in 1928, consolidated the law relating to charitable trusts. The latter, as Dal Pont notes, introduced two important measures:[21]

> First, by section 3, 'charitable purpose' was defined as every other purpose which in accordance with the law of England is a charitable purpose. Secondly, a judge of the Supreme Court or the Attorney-General could, under section 5, alter the purposes of an approved scheme under the procedure laid down in the principal Act and even restore the original purposes.

Thereafter, legislation gradually introduced the basic elements of a national health, welfare and benefits system.

Current legislation

As the staged introduction of the long-awaited Charities Act 2005 gradually takes effect, it is becoming clear that in New Zealand the law relating to charities is not, at least in the foreseeable future, going to be radically transformed.

The Charitable Trusts Act 1957

This statute, which remains unaltered by the 2005 Act, provided further consolidation of previous legislative provisions and the rudiments of a supervisory system.

Section 2 explains that 'charitable purpose' means every purpose which in accordance with the law of New Zealand is charitable; and, for the purposes of Parts I and II, includes every purpose that is religious or educational, whether or not it is charitable according to the law of New Zealand. Parts I and II regulate the vesting of property and the incorporation of trust boards.

Section 61A explains that it is charitable to provide, or to assist in the provision of, facilities for 'recreation or other leisure-time occupation, if those facilities are provided in the interests of social welfare'. The requirement that the facilities be made available 'in the interests of social welfare' is not satisfied unless: –

(a) the facilities are provided with the purpose of improving the condition of life for the persons for whom the facilities are primarily intended; and
(b) either:

   (i)   those persons have need of those facilities by reason of their youth, age,

infirmity, disablement, poverty, race, occupation or social or economic
circumstances; or

(ii) the facilities are to be available to the members of the public at large, or
to the male or female members, of the public at large.

This section specifically retains the principle that a trust or institution must be for
the public benefit to be charitable.[22]

In Part IV of the Act, which deals with charitable funds raised by voluntary
contributions, an expanded interpretation of the common law definition of 'charitable purposes' applies. In this context the term is defined in section 38 to mean
every purpose which in accordance with the law of New Zealand is charitable and
includes a number of listed purposes such as 'the promotion of athletic sports and
wholesome recreations and amusements', and 'encouragement of skill, industry
and thrift' whether or not they are beneficial to the community or to a section of
the community.

The Charities Act 2005 [23]

Part I of the Charities Act 2005, which came into effect on 1 July 2005, has
placed the definition of 'charitable purposes' onto a statutory footing. However,
in the absence of any alteration to the substance of the definition or to the
categories of purposes to be recognized as charitable in that statute, the existing
interpretation of 'charity' and 'charitable purpose' will continue. This statute
neither repeals nor significantly amends any previous legislation; it inserts only
slight amendments to the Estate and Gift Duties Act 1968 and the Incorporated
Societies Act 1908.

Interpretation   Under s. 4(1), 'charitable entity' means a society, an institution,
or the trustees of a trust that is or are registered as a charitable entity under this
Act while 'entity' means any society, institution, or trustees of a trust.

Under section 5(1), repeating the definition in section OB 1 of the Income Tax
Act 1994 (as amended by the 2004 Act), 'charitable purpose' is defined as including: 'every charitable purpose, whether it relates to the relief of poverty, the
advancement of education or religion, or any other matter beneficial to the
community'.

Charities Commission   In a break with tradition, the 2005 Act has established a
government body to manage a new registration, support and supervisory system
for charities. The duty to determine charitable status will now fall to this body
rather than, as formerly, to the Inland Revenue Department.

Definitional matters [24]

In this jurisdiction the characteristic common law hallmarks of charity law as
established in England and Wales (see, further, chapter 3) have played their

customary role and, subject to some specific adjustments, will continue to do so in the new era inaugurated by the 2005 Act.

Charitable intent

The presence or absence of a charitable intent will be as determinative in cases of doubt in this jurisdiction as it is in England and Wales.

Public benefit

As in other common law jurisdictions, there is a presumption that the public benefit test is satisfied by gifts made under the first three heads but will require to be proved in relation to the fourth. The test is applied objectively; the fact that a testator believed that a gift was for the public benefit will not prevent the courts from concluding otherwise and denying it charitable status.

The Maori and the public benefit test   From the Maori perspective there are problems with the public benefit test. The main difficulty arises from the fact that the bloodline relationship that characterizes their communities introduces a personal nexus factor that compromises their *locus standi* as charity beneficiaries by breaching the 'public' requirement of the test.[25] There is also the fact that their communities are organized around the small clearly defined units of *iwi* and *hapu* which again may breach the same requirement because of their inherently 'closed' nature.[26]

The government proposal in the *Taxation of Maori Organisations Discussion Document*,[27] is to change the 'public benefit' test so that an entity would not cease to be eligible for charitable status simply because its purpose is to benefit a group of people connected by blood ties. *Whanau* trusts may qualify for a 'charitable' tax exemption if their pool of beneficiaries is large enough and inclusive enough to constitute an appreciably significant section of the public, or if the purposes for which they are established confer a wide public benefit. However, if the entity benefits a few family members only (so that it is actually a private family trust), it will not be regarded as benefiting an appreciably significant section of the public.

The fourth head and the public benefit test   In keeping with the spirit of the above proposal, it would seem that there is a broad willingness to relax the test in relation to 'other purposes beneficial to the community'. This was demonstrated in *Commissioner of Inland Revenue* v. *Medical Council of New Zealand*,[28] which confirmed that the Medical Council's purpose – 'the protection and promotion of the health of New Zealanders' – was charitable.[29]

Exclusively charitable

As in England and Wales and other common law jurisdictions, a purpose must be exclusively charitable if it is to come within the legal definition of 'charity' in New Zealand.[30]

Independent

The independence of charities, a characteristic derived from trust law, is as important in this jurisdiction as in all others that share the common law legacy.

Non-governmental

Again, maintaining independence entails avoiding surrendering autonomy of decision-making by becoming purely an agent of government. This can be as real a danger for charities in New Zealand as in England and Wales and elsewhere in the common law world. The government has issued guidelines intended to encourage the use of better contracting practices by all departments and Crown entities involved in negotiating arrangements with non-government organizations.[31]

Nonprofit distributing

In this jurisdiction, as in other common law nations, it is essential that a charity does not permit any individual to gain a private pecuniary profit or advantage. Where a pecuniary advantage is gained by the charity but this is incidental to its main purpose and does not constitute private profit then its status may be safe.[32]

Charitable purposes

These remain as first identified in the 1601 Act and later classified in *Pemsel*. However, under section 2 of the Charitable Trusts Act 1957, in addition to those purposes recognized under New Zealand law as charitable, all other purposes that are religious or educational are also deemed to be charitable. The development of charitable purposes, unlike the position in England and Wales, is strictly by analogy in keeping with the 'spirit and intendment' rule.

Legal structures for charities

The main vehicles or legal structure for charities are the unincorporated association, charitable trust, the incorporated society, the trust board and the limited company. The well-established legal characteristics of a charitable trust are that it is for purposes rather than persons, it will not fail for uncertainty if a clear general charitable intent is evident, it is exclusively charitable and it may be perpetual[33] (see, further, chapter 3). At 30 November 2000 there were 21,444 registered incorporated societies and 11,582 registered trust boards in New Zealand. The number of organizations listed each year is growing steadily currently at about 30 per cent per annum.

Types of structure

Charities normally take the form either of an association, a company or a trust board.

Unincorporated association   In New Zealand, unincorporated associations are not recognized by common law, statutes or rules of court as separate legal entities.

Company   At an early stage, this jurisdiction adopted the incorporated society which became the dominant non-profit legal structure instead of the trust. A society that has a minimum of 15 members who are associated for any lawful purpose but not for pecuniary gain, may apply to become incorporated under the Incorporated Societies Act 1908. To incorporate the group must be registered at an office of the Registrar of Incorporated Societies. Both charities and not-for-profit organizations may incorporate under the Incorporated Societies Act 1908, but only societies which exist exclusively or principally for charitable purposes may apply for incorporation as a board under the Charitable Trusts Act 1957. Following introduction of the Companies Act 1993, companies limited by guarantee were abolished and were required to reregister as companies limited by shares.[34] The traditional distinction between private and public companies was also removed and as a consequence all companies are treated equally.

Trust board   The trustees of a charitable trust or the members of an unincorporated society that exists exclusively or principally for charitable purposes may incorporate as a board under the Charitable Trusts Act 1957.

Regulatory framework

Until the partial introduction of the Charities Act in July 2005 there was no formal system of registration, nor any regulatory framework, for charities in New Zealand, although certain records of incorporated societies with charitable purposes and those charities incorporated as boards are held at the Companies Office and are accessible online. At present, while the Charities Commission as the centrepiece of a new framework has been put in place, there is some way to go before this system is fully operational.

Registration

Part II of the 2005 Act, dealing with registration, has not yet been implemented. Therefore, at present in New Zealand, instead of one process specifically for charities there are several, each dealing incidentally and in an unco-ordinated fashion with charities.

The Inland Revenue Department

In keeping with the essentially revenue-driven government approach to charities, the initial vetting and approval of charitable status has long been the responsibility of the Inland Revenue Department, which does not maintain a register of such organizations though it does keep a limited register of 'donee organizations'. The records of the Inland Revenue are not public due to secrecy provisions in the Tax Administration Act 1994, and information regarding tax rebates claimed and paid by Inland Revenue can only be obtained under the Official Information Act. In future the new registration duty vested in the Charity Commission will relieve the Inland Revenue of its power to determine the activities that constitute charitable purposes.

The Registrar of Incorporated Societies

Section 33 of the Incorporated Societies Act 1908 requires the Registrar of Incorporated Societies to keep a register of incorporated societies in which all incorporated charities are required to register. Section 28(1) of the Charitable Trusts Act 1957 requires the Registrar of Incorporated Societies to keep a register of boards. The Registrar is based in the Companies Office which is under the auspices of the Ministry of Economic Development. There is no requirement for the registration of either unincorporated associations or charitable trusts.

The Companies Office

Companies, including incorporated charities, must register with the Companies Office.

Regulatory role

There has never been a central regulatory body for charities in New Zealand. This may be due to an implicit understanding between government and the charitable sector that a self-regulatory approach from within the sector rather than an imposed state system was more appropriate in this society. However, as there was little or no monitoring of the activities of charitable organizations there was no means by which the public could identify and differentiate between legitimate charities. Further, the piecemeal regulatory environment was such that charitable organizations could find themselves having to deal with as many as five different government agencies on a regular basis. With the enactment of the Charities Act 2005, this is now to a large extent in the process of changing, though charities using government funding from different agencies will still have to deal with a number of different agencies.

The Inland Revenue Department

Such regulatory powers as existed in relation to charities were exercised by the Inland Revenue Department (though rarely, e.g. the Crown Forestry Rental Trust case) and this will continue to be the case unless and until appropriate regulatory functions are vested in the Charity Commission.

Organizations seeking tax exemptions on grounds of their charitable activity must first satisfy the Inland Revenue Department of their entitlement to 'charitable status'. If the Commissioner has reason to believe that the funds of a gift-exempt body are being applied for a purpose that is not charitable, benevolent, philanthropic or cultural, the Commissioner will inform the Minister.[35] All gift-exempt bodies have to keep sufficient records to enable the Commissioner of Inland Revenue to determine both the source of donations made to the organization and the application of its funds, whether in New Zealand or overseas.[36]

Charitable status

The Inland Revenue Department will only grant an organization 'charitable status' for income tax purposes if that organization satisfies four requirements:

1   it must be carried on exclusively for charitable purposes;
2   it must not be carried on for the private pecuniary profit of any individual;
3   it must have a provision in its rules requiring the assets of the organization to be transferred to another entity with charitable purposes if the organization ceases to exist; and
4   it must not have the power to amend its rules in such a way as to alter the exclusively charitable nature of the organization.

The Charities Commission

Part I of the Charities Act 2005, now in effect, established a new Autonomous Crown Entity, the Charities Commission, to implement and maintain a registration, reporting and monitoring system for charities. It is envisaged as having a light regulatory role, although in fact the responsible government Minister has considerably more power than is the case in England and Wales. The Commission will also be responsible for educating and assisting charities in relation to matters of good governance and management and for advising the government.

The High Court

The inherent jurisdiction of this court in relation to charitable trusts applies in New Zealand as in other common law countries. Part III of the Charitable Trusts Act 1957 sets out the court's powers in respect of *cy-près* schemes. In practice, however, and for the same reasons that prevail in other common law jurisdictions, the High Court no longer plays a prominent role in the regulatory framework for charities in New Zealand.

The Attorney General

The *parens patriae* functions of the Crown to protect and ensure the proper administration of charities devolves to the Attorney General in New Zealand as it does in other common law countries. The Attorney General may institute proceedings but must always be joined as a party to proceedings involving a charity. The Attorney General also has authority under section 58 of the Charitable Trusts Act 1957 to examine and inquire into all or any charities in New Zealand, including trusts for charitable purposes within the meaning of Part IV of the Act, and to examine and inquire into the nature and objects, administration, management and results thereof, and the value, condition, management, and application of the property and income belonging thereto. However, there is little evidence that the Attorney General has ever used the powers available under the inherent or statutory jurisdiction to exercise any substantial control over or scrutiny of charities. Reported cases involving the Attorney General show, almost without exception, that the proceedings were instigated privately rather than by the Attorney General. Inquiries[37] noted very few actions brought by the Attorney General against charities.

It is the duty of all trustees and persons acting or having any concern in the management or administration of any such charity into which any such examination or inquiry is being made, or of the property or income thereof, on request, to produce to the Attorney General or to the officer or person making the examination or inquiry all books, papers, writings and documents in relation to the charity or the property and income thereof, or to the administration, management, value, condition and application of that property and income, and to answer all questions and give all assistance in connection with the examination or inquiry which they are reasonably able to answer or give.

The Solicitor General's Office

Some functions of the administration of the Charitable Trusts Act 1957 are presently undertaken by the Solicitor General's Office.

Other agencies

A number of other agencies may have a regulatory role in relation to charities.

The Registrar of Incorporated Societies

The Registrar requires annual accounts to be completed only by those charities that are incorporated societies.[38] There is no requirement for these accounts to be audited. Incorporated Societies are also required to update constitutional records maintained by the Registrar of Incorporated Societies. Trust boards have no ongoing reporting obligations under the Charitable Trusts Act 1957, either to the Registrar or the Inland Revenue Department, other than to record constitutional changes on the public register. Trustees would be subject to the general law obligation to maintain accounts. In the future the Charities Commission will promulgate accounting requirements by regulation. This will be influenced by both Part II of the Review of the Financial Reporting Act 1993 and the introduction of International Financial Reporting Standards.

The Companies Office

Charitable companies are subject to the usual corporate reporting obligations under the Financial Reporting Act 1996 and the Companies Act 1993.

Regulating the fiscal environment [39]

In New Zealand, in keeping with its established revenue-driven approach to charities, responsibility for managing the tax environment as it relates to registered charities rests with the Inland Revenue Department. No specific accounting standard applies to the preparation of accounts of charities.[40] In June 2001 the Government released a discussion document entitled 'Tax and Charities' which attracted a record number of submissions (the most ever on a tax issue in New Zealand). The document canvassed various options for change related mainly to tax issues. It highlighted the lack of information about the charitable sector including who benefits, and how, from the tax assistance the government provides.

The Inland Revenue

This body has overall regulatory responsibility for matters relating to tax liability. It has no particular brief for charities as such. Its charitable status determining function, undertaken in response to applications for charitable exemption from tax liability, will transfer under the 2005 Act to the Charities Commission.

Tax

The legislative framework for taxes currently comprises the Income Tax Act 2004, the Tax Administration Act 1994 and the Estate and Gift Duties Act 1968. The Inland Revenue Department determines the eligibility of charities for exemption from income tax, gift duty, resident withholding tax on interest and dividends and fringe benefit tax. The tax provisions of the Charities Act 2005 are not likely to come into force until some time in 2007.

Certain income of charitable and other tax-exempt entities are exempt from income tax.[41] The exemption includes non-business income derived by a trust, society or institution established exclusively for charitable purposes and business income derived by such a charitable body, subject to certain exceptions. Fringe benefits tax does not apply to benefits provided by or on behalf of a charitable organization to its employees, except to the extent that such benefits are used, enjoyed or received principally in relation to, in the course of, or by virtue of, any employment that consists of any activity performed by the employees in the carrying on of a business by the charitable organization. Charities are also exempt from stamp and cheque duties under section 18 of the Stamp and Cheque Duties Act 1971. A gift creating a charitable trust, or establishing any society or institution exclusively for charitable purposes, or any gift in aid of any such trust, society or institution is not subject to gift duty nor, for most purposes, is conveyance duty payable on any instrument of conveyance establishing any such body.

Rates

Rates are not payable on any land used and occupied by or for the purposes of a charitable institution carried on for the free maintenance or relief of orphans, the aged, infirm, physically or mentally disabled, sick or needy, provided that it does not exceed 1.62 hectares in respect of any one such institution.

Donation incentives

For purposes of tax deductibility of donations, the New Zealand government has created the concept of 'donee organizations', the definition of which is a society, institution, association, organization or trust which is not carried on for the private pecuniary profit of any individual and the funds of which are, in the opinion of the Commissioner, applied wholly or principally to any charitable, benevolent, philanthropic or cultural purposes within New Zealand. Eligibility will qualify for a 33.3 per cent rebate on maximum donations by an individual of $1,890 per fiscal year.

Cy-près

Section 31 of the Charitable Trusts Act 1957 provides that where any property or income is given or held upon trust or to be applied for any charitable purpose, and it is impossible or impracticable or inexpedient to carry out that purpose, or the amount available is inadequate to carry out that purpose, or that purpose has been effected already, or that purpose is illegal or useless or uncertain, then (whether or not there is any general charitable intention) the property and income or any part or residue thereof or the proceeds of sale thereof shall be disposed of for some other charitable purpose, or a combination of such purposes, in the manner and subject to the provisions contained in Part III of the Act. Part IV of the Charitable Trusts Act 1957 makes similar provision for the establishment of schemes in respect of charitable funds raised by voluntary subscription where, again, it becomes impossible, impracticable or inexpedient to carry out the charitable purpose for which the money raised is held. In such cases, the legislation permits money or property to be disposed of for other charitable purposes.

These provisions essentially provide an alternative statutory procedure for dealing with the disposal of assets of defunct charities, a problem that in other jurisdictions would be addressed through application of the common law *cy-près* process. Although the legislation provides that the property, income or funds be disposed of for 'some other' charitable purpose there is a consistent line of judicial authority that a scheme should accord as closely as possible, in the changed circumstances, to the terms of the original trust, i.e. in accordance with the *cy-près* rule.[42]

Fundraising

New Zealand, quite remarkably, has not found it necessary to enact legislation directed specifically to the control of fundraising or collections.

The general law of contract and fair trading legislation governs the conduct of charitable fundraising.

In 1979, the Property Law and Equity Reform Committee recommended that every charity making a public appeal for funds be required to have its accounts audited, so that the auditor can advise the Attorney General of malpractice.

Lotteries

Any lotteries, prize competitions or games of chance conducted by societies are regulated by the Gaming and Lotteries Act 1977. This legislation adopts a lenient approach to the regulation of societies that conduct such activities for 'authorized purposes' which are defined in section 2 to mean any charitable, philanthropic, cultural or party political purpose or other purpose that is beneficial to the community or any section of it.

Trading

The Incorporated Societies Act 1908 provides that members can associate for any lawful purpose but not for pecuniary gain. A society may make profits from its activities (so long as they are not divided among or received by members) and providing the society does not become a trading operation or pursue profits to the exclusion of its other objects. The latitude thus permitted was well illustrated in *Auckland Medical Aid Trust* v. *Commissioner of Inland Revenue*,[43] where a trust, which derived almost all its income from providing abortions at a charge and virtually on demand, was found to be charitable.

In particular, section 5(c) of the Act provides that the members will not be deemed to be associating for pecuniary gain if the society itself is established for the protection or regulation of some trade, business, industry or calling in which the members are engaged or interested, if the society itself does not engage or take part in any such trade, business, industry or calling, or any part or branch thereof.

Income tax legislation exempts from tax any income derived directly or indirectly from any business carried on by or on behalf of or for the benefit of trustees in trust for charitable purposes within New Zealand, or derived directly or indirectly from any business carried on by or on behalf of or for the benefit of any society or institution established exclusively for such purposes and not carried on for the private pecuniary profit of any individual.[44]

Constraints on modern philanthropic activity

The constraints of the charity law framework in this jurisdiction are similar to those in England and Wales and other common law jurisdictions in terms of inhibiting the capacity of philanthropy to address the contemporary social inclusion agenda (see, further, chapter 8). There are, however, additional complications arising from the particular circumstances of the Maori.

Policy constraints: partnership with government

There is an argument that the Maori culture imperative would seem to be a dominant force in the partnership ethos cultivated by the New Zealand government and while this may or may not be in the long-term best interests of the Maori it does diminish the relative profile of all other socially disadvantaged groups. Ensuring that this ethos, and the new Charity Commission which has emerged from it, works to promote equity of opportunity in a context of ethnic diversity will test the viability of charity/government partnerships.

Government grants and contracts

Charities in New Zealand, as in England and Wales and elsewhere, are at increasing risk of compromising their purposes and their independence by the need to engage in the 'contract culture' (see, further, chapter 8).

Common law constraints

The primary common law characteristic of charity law in this jurisdiction is that it has been firmly revenue driven. The development of charitable purposes has been left to random and infrequent judicial determinations that have transferred from England and Wales principles that do not always best fit the patterns of social disadvantage in New Zealand.

Role of the courts

The High Court retains its traditional inherent jurisdiction over charities and ultimately it is a matter for the courts whether an entity is a 'charity' for tax purposes. As with other common law jurisdictions, the judiciary in New Zealand seldom have an opportunity to consider issues of principle. However when they do then, as in *Re Tennant*,[45] they sometimes demonstrate their capacity and willingness to broaden the law relating to charitable purposes. In that case the provision of a creamery to assist a small new rural community to become economically viable was found to be charitable.

The 'spirit and intendment' rule

In New Zealand this rule has generally been applied conservatively to restrict judicial discretion in relation to charitable purposes as was noted by Thomas J, in *Commissioner of Inland Revenue* v. *Medical Council of New Zealand*,[46] when he expressed the view that the 'spirit and intendment' rule should be used with more attention to contemporary circumstances than to case precedents.

Legal structures

In this jurisdiction, although the introduction of incorporated societies was well ahead of its time, the legislation governing legal structures for charities is now very dated. The restrictive effects of reliance upon such charitable forms as the trust and the unincorporated association in the highly professional, flexible and competitive modern market place are as for England and Wales and other common law jurisdictions (see, further, chapter 8). However, in jurisdictions such as New Zealand where some Indigenous people live with their extended family in closed communities and suffer embedded deprivation, these restrictions may be particularly obstructive.

Restrictions on advocacy/political activity

In this jurisdiction the restrictions on advocacy/political activity are very much as they are in England and Wales and the main case law precedents established there are followed in New Zealand (see, further, chapters 3 and 8). The accepted rationale for rejecting charitable status for an organization established for the primary purpose of lobbying against those who sought a change in the law was, as restated by Somers J in *Molloy* v. *Commissioner of Inland Revenue*,[47] due to the court having no way of knowing whether or not such a change would satisfy the public benefit test. Surprisingly, the relevant case law does not reveal the judiciary as being exercised with anything like a comparable volume of cases concerning issues of advocacy/political activity on behalf of its indigenous people as is the experience in such other common law nations as Australia and Canada.

Fiscal issues

In this jurisdiction there is a need to standardize the various tax assistance rules applying to New Zealand charities with overseas purposes.

Restrictions on business eligibility for charitable tax exemption   Under the Income Tax Act 2004, income derived directly or indirectly from a business will only be tax exempt if it was derived by or on behalf of or for the benefit of trustees in trust for charitable purposes within New Zealand, or derived directly or indirectly from any business carried on by or on behalf of or for the benefit of any society or institution established exclusively for such purposes and not carried on for the private pecuniary profit of any individual.

If the purposes are not limited to New Zealand the Commissioner may apportion the income between those purposes within New Zealand and those outside, and allow a partial exemption.

Restrictions on doneee eligibility for charitable tax exemption At present, the general rules that provide donors with rebates and deductions for their donations cover only charitable purposes within New Zealand. Specific parliamentary approval is required on a case-by-case basis for charities whose charitable purposes extend outside New Zealand. Over 40 organizations currently have such approval and these organizations are listed in the Income Tax Act 2004.

A set of criteria has been established for approving organizations seeking donor status with charitable purposes outside New Zealand. The funds have to be applied towards either: the relief of poverty, hunger, sickness or ravages of war or natural disaster; or the economy of developing countries (recognized as such by the United Nations); or raising the educational standards of a developing country.

The doctrine of cy-près In New Zealand the jurisdiction to settle *cy-près* schemes has always been exclusively judicial, which makes the process cumbersome, very expensive and time-consuming. Unlike most other common law countries, the *cy-près* powers have been subsumed into a statutory procedure which allows the court to administer the assets of charities. The lack of a forum, such as that provided by the Charity Commission in England and Wales, to swiftly and inexpensively apply the assets of a defunct charity to other charitable purposes has been a constraint on philanthropy in this jurisdiction.

Fundraising and trading etc. The lack of a regulatory framework for fundraising and the very dated statutory provisions relating to trading are not conducive to promoting public confidence in these methods of raising revenue for furthering charitable activities in the twenty-first century.

Public benefit matters

In New Zealand, as in England and Wales, there are other aspects of the public benefit test that operate to the detriment of philanthropic intervention on behalf of the socially disadvantaged.

Uneven application of the public benefit test There is no statutory presumption that gifts for the advancement of religion satisfy the 'public benefit' test. The New Zealand courts have, however, followed the UK courts in generally applying the judicial presumption that this purpose is beneficial to the public. Moreover, section 2 of the Charitable Trusts Act 1957 provides that charitable purpose means

> every purpose which in accordance with the law of New Zealand is charit-able; and, for the purposes of Parts I and II of this Act, includes every purpose that is religious or educational, whether or not it is charitable accord-ing to the law of New Zealand.

Therefore, in the context of Parts I and II of the Act, which deal with vesting of trust property and incorporation of trust boards respectively, 'religious purposes' do not need to satisfy common law requirements such as 'public benefit' in order to qualify as 'charitable purposes'.[48] The fact that the current application of the test in the context of the advancement of education permits some schools with charitable status to charge prohibitively expensive fees restricts the educational opportunities for many socially disadvantaged children.[49] This issue is equally relevant in relation to those hospitals and residential care facilities which by imposing service charges in effect discriminate against equal access by the socially disadvantaged.

Exclusion of matters clearly in the public benefit   There has been an obvious and long-standing fundamental difficulty in fitting the charity law framework to the needs of the Maori due to the fact that their communities are organized around blood relationships. A legislative initiative to resolve this difficulty has been a long time coming and it remains to be seen how the new provisions will work in practice.

Modern law constraints

The fact that the determination of charitable status has been the responsibility of the Inland Revenue Department has naturally inhibited any expansion in the range of charitable purposes.

Forum for developing charitable purposes

New Zealand has suffered the consequences of the same functional deficit in this area as all other common law jurisdictions, with the exception of England and Wales. The lack of a forum or body with the capacity to engage in an ongoing developmental role with the charitable sector, extending the range of charitable purposes and broadening the interpretation of matters constituting the public benefit, has constrained the effective use of philanthropy. This is perhaps most clearly illustrated by the enduring lack of fit between common law principles and the circumstances of the Maori. Although a Charity Commission has now been appointed, there is nothing specific in its brief to indicate that it might fill the present gap by assuming a developmental role as regards charitable purposes similar to that undertaken by the Commission in England and Wales.

Human rights, anti-terrorism and social justice legislation

New Zealand has in place a not untypical platform of social justice legislation including the Equal Pay Act 1972, the New Zealand Bill of Rights Act 1990, the Human Rights Act 1993 and the Employment Relations Act 2000. In January, the Human Rights Amendment Act 2001 came into effect. This restructured the Human Rights Commission and introduced additional safeguards against discrimination on grounds such as age, disability or sexual orientation in the policies and practices of government agencies. Under the Human Rights Amendment Act 2001, the primary functions of the Human Rights Commission are:

1   to advocate and promote respect for, and an understanding and appreciation of, human rights in New Zealand society; and
2   to encourage the maintenance and development of harmonious relations between individuals and among the diverse groups in New Zealand society.

It is in this context that the recent spate of anti-terrorism measures must be considered. In marked contrast to its traditional laissez-faire approach to fundraising for public benefit causes, the government has put or is now putting into place a comprehensive legislative framework to ensure rigorous regulation of possible opportunities for the use of funds for contrary purposes.

The Terrorism Suppression Act 2002   This legislation deals with the financing of terrorism and was subsequently amended by the Terrorism Suppression Amendment Act 2005, which criminalizes the financing of terrorist entities and complements existing terrorist financing offences. This has been reinforced by the Criminal Proceeds and Instruments Bill, which was introduced in Parliament in June 2005 to provide for the forfeiture of assets in relation to criminal activity such as money-laundering.

The Financial Action Task Force   In May 2005, the government funded the establishment of the Financial Action Task Force within the Ministry of Justice to ensure that all financial institutions meet standards for countering money-laundering and terrorist financing.

The Pacific Security Strategy   New Zealand's Pacific Security Co-ordinating Committee was established to consider a range of security issues for the Pacific Islands region. In September 2004, it was tasked with developing a Whole of Government Pacific Security Strategy.

The Border Security Act 2004   This act makes significant amendments to the Customs and Excise Act 1996 and the Immigration Act 1987 to permit, for example, the detaining of property at the border that is suspected to be the proceeds of crime.

The Crimes Act (United Nations Convention Against Corruption) Amendment Bill   The bill, due to be introduced in Parliament in 2006, will extend the definition of 'business' to include the provision of international aid.

The Financial Transactions Reporting Amendment Bill   This bill is to be introduced in Parliament in 2006 and will amend the Financial Transactions Reporting Act 1996 relating to wire transfers and cash couriers issues.

Charity law review and social inclusion

In June 2001 the government issued its discussion document *Tax and Charities*[50] and in October of that year the Minister for Finance announced a decision in principle to introduce registration, reporting and monitoring requirements for charities claiming tax-free status. In November 2001 the Working Party on Registration, Reporting and Monitoring of Charities was appointed to make recommendations on the type of registration, reporting and monitoring arrangements that should be introduced; to consider the issue of the public benefit test in relation to Maori organizations; to comment on possible improvements to the definition of 'charitable purpose'; and to consider the standardization of the various tax assistance rules applying to New Zealand charities with overseas purposes. The Working Party reported with its final recommendations on 31 May 2002.[51] On 5 March 2003 the details relating to the proposed Charities Commission were agreed and the Charities Act was approved by Parliament on 13 April 2005. Although this legislation will not come fully into effect for some time it is still possible to consider the probable implications of its provisions for the social inclusion agenda in New Zealand.

Proposed changes to definitional matters and legal structures

The Working Party recommended that legislative provisions be introduced to define 'charity' and 'charitable activities', and that there be a single body, a Charities Commission, responsible for the registration and monitoring of charities and for investigating complaints. The latter was in keeping with the recommendation of the 1989 Spencer Russell report,[52] the report of the Accountability of Charities and Sporting Bodies Working Party and the more recent Statement of Government Intentions. It was suggested that the Commission should also be responsible for the administration of the Charitable Trusts Act 1957, and for the 'defender of charities' role currently carried out by the Attorney General. It further recommended amendments to the Income Tax Act 2004 and Estate and Gift Duties Act 1968 to the effect that only charities registered with the Commission will be eligible for tax-exempt status. These recommendations, to some extent, have now been translated into legislative provisions as embodied in the Charities Act 2005.

Charitable purpose

While the Working Party's recommendations regarding 'charity' and 'charitable activities' have been acknowledged in the form of statutory provisions it cannot be said that these provisions add anything to the existing common law interpretation. No attempt has been made to statutorily extend the range of purposes.

Public benefit

The Working Party restricted its advice to the recommendation that the public benefit test be changed, so that in applying the public benefit test, an organization would not cease to be eligible for registered charity status simply because its purpose is to benefit a group of people connected by blood ties. The issues relating to the current uneven application of the test across the four *Pemsel* heads, which have so exercised other common law nations, did not in this jurisdiction attract any proposals for reform. Whether or not the linking of registration to a requirement that activities be demonstrably compatible with and clearly furthering an organization's declared charitable purposes will come to serve as a criterion for satisfying the public benefit test, thereby achieving the same end result, depends entirely upon the approach taken by the Charity Commission.

Legal structures

There are no provisions relating to actual or possible legal structures.

Proposed changes to the regulatory framework

From 1 July 2005 the Charities Commission was established as a new Crown entity. This will lead to a transfer to it of some responsibilities traditionally borne by the Inland Revenue Department. The Commission is required to have a good working relationship with Inland Revenue Department. While the two bodies are required to act in conjunction, there is no suggestion that the latter is required to take its lead from the Commission, as is the case in England and Wales. In fact, at this stage, the jurisdictional differences in the regulatory role assigned to the respective Commissions are striking. In particular the emphasis in England and Wales on investigatory powers to equip the Commission to ensure transparency and accountability, enable it to police standards of practice and prevent opportunities for abuse are noticeably underplayed in this jurisdiction. In New Zealand the Charities Commission would seem set to assume a role that primarily focuses on regulatory and monitoring functions with little educative and support responsibilities. As Dal Pont has pointed out:

> That it is chiefly a bureaucratic exercise is evidenced by the fact that of its over 150 sections almost half concern the operation of the Commission and

24 are about registration. Only six or so sections concern obligations outside of registration for charitable entities.[53]

The Charities Commission

Commissioners are appointed by the Crown, with a majority drawn from nominations made by the charitable sector, on a rotational basis. The administration of the Charitable Trusts Act 1957 is to be transferred to the Charities Commission. Decisions of the Commission may be challenged through the High Court (there is no provision for an independent Tribunal as in England and Wales). The Commission's core functions are in relation to the registration, support and supervision of charities of which the first two are seen as most important. It is anticipated that more functions may be added in time.

Registration   The Commission's key function is to establish and maintain a national register and to approve and register charities. The registration process will be voluntary and will not alter the legal status of charities. A charity that chooses not to register with the Commission will still be able to call itself a charity and solicit funds from the public but will not, however, qualify for tax-exempt status. The test for registration will be a legal one and organizations will be required to provide the Commission with documentation that not only sets out their aims and objectives but also describes the corresponding activities.

Registration automatically confers donee status (at least, at this stage, for charities with exclusively New Zealand purposes). All existing charities will be required to go through the proposed registration process which will have to be completed within two years. Organizations with income from public donations of over $100,000 in the previous year, excluding church collections and grants from grant-making bodies, will be required to supply a copy of their audited annual financial statements.

Once the Commission is satisfied that the organization is eligible, the charity would receive a registration number. Registration then acts as the gateway to the relevant tax exemptions including income tax, gift duty, resident withholding tax on interest and dividends and fringe benefit tax.

The Charities Act does not specify the amount of time from when the Commission's registry system goes live and when the registration process will need to be completed. That gap will be decided by the government once it has had a chance to consult with the Commission and get its views on how long the sector will need to adjust to the registration requirements and how long the Commission will need to process the applications it receives. At the earliest, the register went live in March 2006. At this stage it seems likely that entities will not have to register until well into 2006.

Support   The Charities Commission is to be a 'one-stop shop' for the legislative requirements of charities. It is required to provide an educative function for charities; for example by developing best practice, training resources and trust documentation templates. A key function will be its duty to provide advice and support to the sector and advice to government regarding the sector. It is required to report annually to the sector, and to government through the Minister of Finance, and to the Minister responsible for the Community and Voluntary Sector.

Regulatory role   The Charities Commission will exercise a supervisory role in relation to charities and the charitable sector. At this stage there is no indication of the precise powers and procedures available to the Commission whereby it may ensure that standards of transparency, good governance and accountability prevail in the sector. However, its monitoring, advice and support functions extend beyond financial matters to the activities of charitable organizations to ensure the activities of these entities are, and continue to be, charitable and accord with their stated objectives. They include collecting annual information from and monitoring the activities of registered charities.

It has the power to investigate the affairs of a registered charity, and any organization holding itself out as such. It encourages compliance through education and assistance. Where irregularities are detected it may use monetary or non-monetary sanctions, and can appoint a temporary managing trustee, or, in extreme circumstances, it can deregister a charity.

The Inland Revenue Department

This body will continue its administrative duties under the revenue legislation and retains the right to conduct an independent audit of charities to ensure they continue to be eligible for tax-exempt status (though, as with the role of the Attorney General, there is no evidence that this has been done on a regular basis with the exception of a few high-profile cases, e.g. Crown Forestry Rental Trust). It will also be responsible for assessing whether donations to a charitable entity are eligible for rebates and deductions (donee status). The information available to it through the registration and reporting regime will help the Inland Revenue in assessing risk. Protocols will be developed to govern the exchange of information between the Commission and the Inland Revenue Department.

The Maori and the public benefit test

The government's discussion document *The Taxation of Maori Organisations*[54] sets out the results of the review of the taxation regime as it applies to Maori organizations. The report contains proposals to amend the tax rules for Maori authorities, including the Maori Trustee, and to clarify how charity law applies to all organizations, especially *iwi*-based and *hapu*-based organizations and *marae*. It states the government's intention to relax the public benefit test so that blood ties among members of a Maori organization will not in future automatically prevent it from obtaining charitable status for tax purposes. In addition, *marae* situated on Maori reservations will qualify for charitable status for funds applied solely to the administration and maintenance of the *marae*.

Proposed changes to financial matters

The 2005 Act amends the Income Tax Act 2004, the Tax Administration Act 1994 and the Estate and Gift Duties Act 1968. These amendments do not effect substantive changes to financial matters but are largely technical adjustments to harmonize terminology with provisions in the 2005 Act.

Fundraising and trading

Curiously, the 2005 Act leaves untouched the law relating to fundraising and trading by charities.

Implications for social inclusion

It is striking that the Charities Act 2005 makes no concessions to the arguments advanced elsewhere in the common law world that the *Pemsel* classification of charitable purposes should be statutorily broadened to address contemporary social inclusion issues. As Dal Pont comments:[55]

> The challenge for government, to the extent that it plans to broaden the concept of charity, and thus broaden the availability of privileges (tax exemption, *sic*) is to target these in areas that are presently deficient and that should be encouraged in society . . . And yet it is curious that under the Charities Bill the targeting of areas for this purpose is aligned to a concept of charity that differs little or not at all in substance from that of nineteenth century England.

Strengths of reform proposals

The separation of the revenue collection function from the function of determining charitable status and the vesting of the latter in an agency that has a statutory duty to support and educate the charitable sector is undoubtedly an important strategic development. There are other reforms which in a more general sense will improve the fit between law and social need.

The simplification of the regulatory framework   The fact that the Commission is to act as a one-stop shop, obviating the necessity for a charity to comply with the requirements of several agencies, will save on administrative time and expense which can be directed instead to furthering charitable purposes.

The public benefit test and the Maori   Section 5(2) of the 2005 Act states that the existence of a blood relationship between the beneficiaries of the trust or members of the society or institution will not prevent a purpose from being charitable if it would otherwise satisfy the public benefit requirement. It also makes special provision for a *marae*[56] to be recognized as having a charitable purpose if the physical structure of the *marae* is situated on land that is a Maori reservation referred to in Te Ture Whenua Maori Act 1993 (Maori Land Act 1993) and the funds of the *marae* are not used for a purpose other than the administration and maintenance of the land and of the physical structure of the *marae*, and a purpose that is a charitable purpose other than under this paragraph. For the avoidance of any doubt, the provision concludes:

> if the purposes of a trust, society, or an institution include a non-charitable purpose (for example, advocacy) that is merely ancillary to a charitable purpose of the trust, society, or institution, the presence of that non-charitable purpose does not prevent the trustees of the trust, the society, or the institution from qualifying for registration as a charitable entity.

The activities test   A key criterion for registration, and for inclusion in the annual returns that determine continued registration, is evidence that the activities of an organization are in keeping with and demonstrably further its stated charitable purposes. This simple, clear and useful monitoring mechanism will also assist targeting by new charities and service selection by those in need.

Restrictions on advocacy/political activity   The specific provision enabling an organization to register as a charity even if it also has advocacy as a secondary or supplementary function as part of its charitable purpose is a step forward.

Weaknesses of reform proposals: charitable purposes

In New Zealand the decision has clearly been taken that the content if not the institutional framework of the common law legacy offers an appropriate and sufficient basis for the future of charity law in this jurisdiction. The absence of any provisions to correct either the well-recognized functional deficits attributable to this legacy or to address contemporary circumstances is most apparent in relation to charitable purposes which will continue to rest on the *Pemsel* classification.

The advancement of religion   The Charities Act 2005 would seem to leave unaltered the presumption that gifts and organizations for the advancement of religion or education satisfy the public benefit test; though this may be affected by the legislative caveat that registration requires evidence of objects-compliant activity.

No charitable purpose to address the causes of poverty   There is no provision to alter the focus on the effects rather than the causes of poverty.

No recognition for advocacy/political activity as a charitable purpose   The opportunity to statutorily clarify the law and firmly recognize advocacy/political activity as a charitable purpose in its own right has been pointedly rejected.

No charitable purpose to facilitate advancement of civil society   New Zealand, unlike England and Wales, has not found it necessary or desirable to make specific provision for organizations, gifts and activities that are conducive to promoting the growth of social capital and advancing civil society through purposes such as facilitating religious or racial harmony or equality and diversity, or civic responsibility or community development.

No charitable purpose to advance human rights, conflict resolution or reconciliation, etc.   Against the background of its extensive anti-terrorism legislative programme, the absence of any provisions acknowledging a need by the government to also address human rights concerns on either a national or international basis is striking.

No recognition for specific, contemporary, socially disadvantaged groups. Again, it has not been found necessary to single out particular socially disadvantaged groups as warranting charitable intervention. The particular groups that currently constitute the domestic social inclusion agenda in this jurisdiction (as identified in the report by the Human Rights Commission[57]) for reasons of youth, age, ill health, disability or financial hardship, etc., have not been statutorily acknowledged.

Weaknesses of reform proposals: other

Some other areas of weakness in the Charities Act 2005 as it relates to social inclusion may be briefly mentioned.

Partnership with government   There is no provision in the 2005 Act that clarifies, adds to or articulates the government's expressed policy of partnership with the community, voluntary and *iwi*/Maori organizations which it claims is symbolized by this legislation. The application of the public benefit test to the circumstances of the Maori and the appointment and composition of the Charity Commission needs to be balanced and contextualized if this legislation is to coherently represent the basis of a partnership.

Legal structures   The lack of provisions relating to facilitating the creation of new vehicles for charitable activity is particularly significant given the particular circumstances of the Maori. It is probable that endowed foundations, because they are free of fundraising concerns and have the capacity to make a sustained long-term commitment, would be more suitable than existing types of structure for charities aiming to regenerate impoverished communities.

Fiscal issues   The capacity of the 2005 Act to promote public trust and confidence in the charitable sector has been compromised by the lack of provisions to modernize the law relating to fundraising and trading. Moreover, the standing and relevance of the Charity Commission could have been considerably enhanced by vesting it with the powers of the High Court in respect of *cy-près* schemes.

Public benefit matters   The absence of any legislative intent to equip the Commission to address contemporaneous social inclusion issues through a strategic use of the public benefit test is clearly apparent. In that respect, government policy in New Zealand falls far short of the comparable approach in England and Wales where the Charity Commission has been positioned to fill that role by being vested with the powers and duties of the High Court.

Conclusion

The Charities Act 2005, on the face of it, has left charity law in New Zealand anchored to its common law legacy and largely unchanged in terms of its capacity to address contemporary social inclusion issues. While the establishment of a Charity Commission may indicate the beginning of a change process that will lead to significant adjustments in the legal framework for philanthropy, it also may not. The structures and processes have certainly been altered but the characteristic common law features of charity law in this jurisdiction remain firmly in place.

Chapter 12

Charity law and social inclusion in the United States

Introduction

The United States, an independent Constitution-based federal republic since 4 July 1776, with a strong democratic tradition, has a federal system of government, where authority is divided between the national government and the 51 states (including the District of Columbia) that together form the country. Each of these jurisdictions has independent responsibility for enacting legislation, providing a judicial system and for managing programmes of service provision.

Individual states legislate for the creation and operation of nonprofits and other legal entities (corporations, partnerships, trusts, etc.) provide their own rules for exemption from state taxes and issue related reporting requirements. While state laws governing nonprofits have broad similarities, they vary considerably in their details (although a growing number of states are adopting model nonprofit corporation acts, thus increasing uniformity across states).[1] Differences among state nonprofit regimes not only increase the overall complexity of the system but also allow nonprofits a certain degree of flexibility by allowing them to incorporate in a state with laws that fit the organization's needs.

The federal government provides a framework of law that sets model parameters for state legislation and it also exercises considerable influence through its discretion to fund programmes across states. The federal judicial system, based on the English common law, considers issues with a constitutional dimension and can thereby, to some extent, shape the laws and practice of all states.

This chapter begins with an overview of the country, a description of the charitable sector and the characteristics of its social inclusion agenda, followed by a brief historical outline of the legislative development of the law relating to charitable organizations. The template of functions (see, further, chapter 6) is then applied to identify and assess the characteristic features of the charity law environment in this jurisdiction, the key definitional matters, the legal structures for charities, registration and the regulatory framework and associated fiscal matters. This leads to an analysis of current legal constraints on the development of philanthropy. The chapter continues by examining the recommendations made in the report of the Panel on the Nonprofit Sector[2] and their significance for social inclusion issues. It concludes by reflecting on the distinctive characteristics of charity law in the US.

Charities and social inclusion

It has been said that:[3]

> America's voluntary spirit has shaped the history and character of our country since its inception. That great tradition of collaboration, generosity, and participation continues today in the form of public charities, private foundations, and religious congregations.

The country

Geographically, the US is the world's third-largest country (after Russia and Canada), comprising 50 states and the District of Columbia with a federal government. Its multicultural population of nearly 296 million consists mainly of white Caucasians (81.7 per cent), blacks (12.9 per cent), and Asians (4.2 per cent), with also a number of different indigenous communities[4] and a range of ethnic groups,[5] all of varying religious beliefs[6] and languages.[7] The free market economy of the US is the strongest, most advanced and technology-oriented in the world, characterized by steady growth, low unemployment[8] and low inflation.[9] In 2005 the US had a GDP of $12.37 trillion to which the continued growth of the services sector made the strongest contribution.

Socio-economic development and politics in the US have, since the end of the last millennium, been overshadowed by military preoccupations in Afghanistan and Iraq and by counter-terrorism strategies since the attacks of 11 September 2001.

The charitable sector

In terms of overall numbers and wealth, and relative to other nonprofits, charitable organizations are thriving in this jurisdiction.

Profile of the sector

The nonprofit sector in the US consists of public charities, private foundations and a range of other nonprofit entities. The first two are classified as tax-exempt under section 501(c)(3) of the Tax Code by the Internal Revenue Service and together constitute the charitable sector. According to the National Centre for Charitable Statistics, from 1964 to 2004 the US saw an increase: in the total of nonprofit organizations, from 1,084,897 to 1,397,263 (28.8 per cent); in public charities, from 535,888 to 822,817 (53.5 per cent); and in private foundations, from 58,774 to 102,881 (75 per cent); while all other non-profits declined in number from 490,235 to 471,565 (−3.8 per cent).[10] The greatest growth occurred in the 1980s and 1990s, with the total number doubling since 1977.

The Panel on the Nonprofit Sector suggests that charitable organizations fall into eight major categories:

1   arts, culture, and humanities, such as museums, symphonies and orchestras and community theatres;
2   education and research, such as private colleges and universities, independent elementary and secondary schools and non-commercial research institutions;
3   environment and animals, such as zoos, bird sanctuaries, wildlife organizations and land protection groups;
4   health services, such as hospitals, public clinics and nursing facilities;
5   human services, such as housing and shelter providers, organizers of sport and recreation programmes and youth programmes;
6   international and foreign affairs, such as overseas relief and development assistance organizations;
7   public and societal benefit, such as private and community foundations, civil rights organizations and civic, social, and fraternal organizations; and
8   religion, such as houses of worship and their related auxiliary services.

Finances and the sector

The charitable sector is wealthy. In 2000, the more than 1.4 million charitable organizations in the United States (excluding churches, which do not generally have to report their income and assets) had an estimated $939 billion in revenues and $2.07 trillion in assets.[11] In 2001, American private foundations and corporate donors made an estimated $2.46 billion in philanthropic grants, and public charities contributed an estimated $1.6 billion, for a total of approximately $4 billion in charitable contributions, both domestic and international. Charitable giving in the United States was 2.1 per cent of GNP in 2000, and has been at levels of 1.9–2.1 per cent of GDP since 1986[12] (compared with 0.63 per cent and 0.77 per cent in the UK). The pattern of charitable giving is interesting: religious organizations, 60 per cent; other, 13 per cent; education, health, and science, 13 per cent; human services, 9 per cent; arts, culture and humanities, 3 per cent; and social welfare, 2 per cent.[13]

Private foundations

The phenomenon of private foundations, while not exclusive to this jurisdiction, is, in terms of scale, a particular characteristic of the charitable sector. There is a history of personal fortune built on commerce being diverted to charity: Carnegie, A. (1835–1919), iron and steel manufacturing to libraries; Rockefeller, J. (1839–1937), oil production to education and sanitation; Getty, P. (1892–1976), industry to promoting the arts; Ford, H. (1863–1947), from car manufacturing to hospitals and support for 'good causes'; and Kellogg, W. (1860–1951), from cereals to community projects. Most recently and dramatically the Bill and Melinda Gates Foundation, which doubled its $30 billion assets in 2006 when it received the wealth of Warren Buffett, has added to this tradition. In 2005 alone, this foundation made charitable donations totalling $1.36 billion towards promoting health and education.

Support for the sector

The Panel on the Nonprofit Sector point out that most support for the sector comes from consumers of services and voluntary contributions: 38 per cent from dues, fees and other charges for goods and services; 17 per cent from individual contributions; and an additional 3 per cent from private foundations and corporate giving programmes. Government grants and contracts provide 31 per cent of the sector's revenues, and other sources, such as income from assets, supply the remaining 11 per cent.

The increase in the size of the charitable sector comes at a cost to the State. Evelyn Brody, a legal scholar, estimates that in 2000 the charitable deduction alone cost the US Treasury nearly $26 billion in forgone income tax.[14] That amount is expected to jump to $36 billion in 2005, according to the 2005 US Federal Budget.

Self-regulation of the charitable sector

The charitable sector has a long tradition of self-regulation. The first major effort to strengthen its performance in this area began in 1918, when a coalition of nonprofits established the National Charities Information Bureau to help the public learn about the ethical and stewardship practices of fundraising organizations. Since then associations have encouraged their members to meet standards, strengthen their systems of governance, ethical conduct and accountability while organizations have developed mandatory standards for their members and training programmes to improve ethics throughout the charitable community. In fact the Independent Sector recently adopted a Statement of Values and Code of Ethics for Nonprofit and Philanthropic Organizations which is also intended as guidance for nonprofits and foundations nationwide. As noted in a recent Johns Hopkins report:[15]

> The evidence at hand thus suggests that a substantial majority of nonprofit organisations, and certainly those belonging to the major national umbrella organisations, already have in place many of the ethics and accountability controls that the Senate Finance Committee staff has proposed to mandate by law.

The social inclusion agenda

There are considerable long-term social problems in this jurisdiction.

Poverty

The official poverty rate[16] in the US has increased for four consecutive years, from a 26-year low of 11.3 per cent in 2000 to 12.7 per cent in 2004. This means that 37 million people were below the official poverty thresholds in 2004. With 12 per cent of the population currently living below the poverty line, accompanied by falling family income in the lower income groups, there will be millions of socially disadvantaged families and communities requiring assistance from government and/or charity to keep them from destitution.

Health and social care

The ageing population is encountering rapidly rising medical costs, insurance costs and pension shortfalls which will bring many more into welfare dependency. There are also approximately 1 million people with HIV/AIDs in the US (and already 40,000 related deaths) in need of long-term health and social care. Now and for the foreseeable future there will be a role for charitable organizations in providing a lifeline for millions in the US 'for battered women, immigrants, homebound senior citizens, AIDS patients, the 43 million Americans without health insurance, and countless other constituencies who all too often fall through this nation's safety net'.[17]

The Native Americans

There are currently some 2,786,652 Native Americans in the United States of which a little over one-third live in three states: California (413,382), Arizona (294,137) and Oklahoma (279,559).[18] Their history of abuse and containment on reservations,[19] followed by a policy of enforced assimilation[20] through the use of boarding schools, and the outlawing of their language and culture, is not dissimilar to the history of indigenous people in Canada and Australia. Significantly, many have now achieved a measure of self-government. There are 563 federally recognized tribal governments in the United States each with the right to form their own government; to enforce laws, both civil and criminal; to tax; to establish membership; to license and regulate activities; to zone; and to exclude persons from tribal territories.

However, and again in keeping with indigenous people in Australia and Canada, a history of persecution followed by exploitation and then neglect has left Native Americans generally impoverished with a greatly weakened cultural identity, suffering from widespread unemployment, poor housing conditions and prone to many health problems including a high incidence of alcoholism, heart disease and diabetes. Although many tribes have established successful licensed casinos, the involvement in the gambling industry has been at a price and has brought with it the associated problems of addiction, and family and community conflict. The Native Americans have for many generations constituted one of the most socially disadvantaged minority groups in the US.

Multicultural issues/immigration etc.

The US has a long-standing reputation as the destination of choice for immigrants, coupled with a legal presumption that racial discrimination is contrary to public policy. It was in *United States* v. *Carolene Producte Co.*[21] that Stone J, in his famous footnote 4, declared that one of the grounds on which legislation could be subjected to 'more exacting judicial scrutiny' was if it was directed at particular religious, national or racial minorities or expressed prejudice against 'discrete and insular minorities'.[22] This approach has since been followed by the Internal Revenue Service (IRS) in a number of rulings which have upheld the charitable status of organizations that: set up to eliminate the discrimination that limited employment opportunities for qualified minority workers;[23] educated the public on the merits of racially integrated neighbourhoods;[24] investigated the causes of deterioration in a particular community and informed residents and city officials of possible corrective measures;[25] and a group that conducted investigations and research on discrimination against minority groups in housing and public accommodation.[26] However, it remains the case that racism, segregation of neighbourhoods and antagonism towards new immigrants remain significant social problems in this jurisdiction.

Need for a more inclusive agenda

The paradox presented by the experience of charity law and social inclusion in the most developed, powerful and democratic of the common law nations is unavoidable and perhaps most graphically illustrates the themes underpinning this book. Not only is it the world's richest country with perhaps the most avowedly patriotic population but it also displays alarming dysfunctional characteristics.

Despite all its advantages, the US has high levels of poverty, murder (especially of massacres by lone gunmen), State executions, military activity in other countries, corporate crime, imprisoned people, single parents, etc. It has low levels of voter participation, marriage durability and medical insurance for the poor. It has a large, relatively poor and marginalized indigenous community. Alongside such measures of social dysfunction we must set the evidence above of a wealthy, generous and thriving philanthropy; but one which devotes the smallest proportion of its resources, only 2 per cent, to social welfare. Does this imbalance between need and resources, between patriotic rhetoric and community pathology, have any implications for the charity law framework? Could the regulatory framework for the philanthropic environment be adjusted to create a better fit between the functions of charity law and the pattern of contemporary social need so as to facilitate a more effective channelling of resources?

Government policy

In the US, as Alexis de Tocqueville pointed out, society from its earliest days was accustomed to nonprofit organizations independently undertaking collective action on behalf of local communities.[27] The framing of the American

Constitution and its Bill of Rights sought to ensure, among other things, that the powers of government would be contained and could not unduly interfere with the independence of law-abiding individuals and communities. Consequently an established characteristic of this society is the manner in which such organizations spring up to carry out activities in concert with (and sometimes in opposition to) the State; both charities and government have long been viewed as complementary vehicles in the provision of public welfare. Certain services or utilities of a public benefit nature – such as universities, hospitals and community social services – were not necessarily seen as the responsibility of government and were often provided by nonprofit organizations. This approach was reflected in the tax system which both encouraged capitalism while rewarding charitable giving: a non-redistributive policy prevailed in relation to personal wealth (e.g. the absence of a 'death duties' tax facilitated the accumulation of family wealth through successive generations); but tax deductions were allowed for charitable donations (a positive enducement to help an impoverished neighbour). However, that tradition of independence from government interference and reliance on non-government organizations, coupled with the latter's eagerness to represent the needs of the grassroots in local communities etc., has become increasingly compromised in recent decades as the distinction between the public benefit roles of State and nonprofits grows less certain.

Charities assuming responsibility for government public service provision

During the 1980s, there was a widespread withdrawal of federal government spending in areas of general health and social care, community development and family support services. This occurred against a policy rhetoric articulated in the Reagan era as the government deliberately stepped aside to allow more room for the engagement of the armies of volunteers, organized by reputable nonprofit bodies, who could thereby make a vital contribution to building more responsible and caring communities.[28] Accordingly, the government shed much of its social service responsibilities, either by way of contracting with charitable organizations for service delivery or by simply privatizing services, resulting in nonprofits becoming major providers of various social welfare functions while also becoming increasingly dependent on the government for financial support. In 1996, the government provided roughly 36 per cent of all revenue for nonprofits; fees for services constituted another 54 per cent of revenues, with private contributions responsible for only 10 per cent. These figures may actually understate government support for the sector, since many health care, child care and other service organizations collect revenues by charging fees to clients who, in turn, are reimbursed or subsidized by the government. On the other hand, these figures do not take into account one of the most substantial forms of private contribution to charity: volunteer labour. There is some concern that by undertaking this role the independence of the nonprofit sector, and perhaps that of charities in particular, has become seriously compromised.[29]

Government assuming responsibility for charitable resources

During the 1990s, there were a considerable number of instances when nonprofit organizations (mainly hospitals and other health and social care facilities) were taken over or bought out by commercial businesses or where they simply converted from nonprofit to for-profit status. This conversion trend is a recent, growing and potentially very significant phenomenon.[30] It has been accompanied by heated controversy regarding the disposal of surplus assets.

In New York, the three-year litigation concerning the conversion of the Empire Blue Cross Blue Shield organization has just concluded in a novel fashion. The State has legislated to place the organization's assets in two specially created funds: the Public Asset Fund (95 per cent) and the Charitable Asset Fund (5 per cent). The legislation prescribes the specific health care services to which the funds are to be put, a three-year period of expenditure and the model of governance. As has been pointed out,[31] this statutory initiative enabling government to determine the future use of assets vested in a ceased charitable organization stands in complete contrast to the traditional *cy-près* approach whereby the assets would be transferred to a similar charitable organization without any government interference.[32] It does, however, bear some similarities to the strategy employed by the UK government in relation to the Lottery funds (see, further, chapter 8) and for the same reason: shortage of funds to meet the rising costs of public services, particularly health care, is forcing governments to look to charitable resources to make up the deficit wherever possible. Moreover, in New York it is clear that the State intends to use its newly created fund to leverage further funds from federal government and deploy the combined assets to meet salary costs for health care workers.

Arguably, this case provides an interesting example of charity and government experimenting with the possibilities of venture philanthropy, an experiment that may well be adopted in other states and jurisdictions.

Government, charities and preparations for a new regulatory framework

In this as in other common law jurisdiction, the blurring of the distinction between the public benefit responsibilities of government and the sector led to concerns regarding the functioning of the legal framework for charitable activity. Unlike other jurisdictions, however, and perhaps in recognition of the sector's traditionally independent role, the government simply passed the matter to the charitable sector for it to examine.

In September 2004, the Senate Finance Committee invited the Independent Sector[33] to assemble an independent group of leaders from the charitable sector to consider and recommend actions to strengthen governance, ethical conduct and accountability within public charities and private foundations. The Committee requested an interim report in February 2005 and a final report in the spring. The Independent Sector responded in October 2004, by announcing the creation of the Panel on the Nonprofit Sector.[34]

The Panel created two advisory groups: the Expert Advisory Group, drawn from academia, law and nonprofit oversight; and the Citizens Advisory Group, comprising leaders of America's business, educational, media, political, cultural and religious institutions. It also formed five Work Groups to examine key issues in governance and accountability:

1   governance and fiduciary responsibilities: composition, responsibilities, and compensation of boards of directors;
2   government oversight and self-regulation: enforcement of existing laws and systems of self-regulation;
3   legal framework: gaps in current laws and regulations governing charitable organizations;
4   transparency and financial accountability: improved reporting of financial and programme information; and
5   small organisations: impact of existing and proposed laws and reporting requirements on smaller charities and foundations.

History, current legislation and definitional matters

It is customary for US academics to trace the history of charity law in their country back to its roots in the common law of England[35] and it is generally acknowledged that the process of colonization included the transfer of that legacy to the US, albeit with some differences of emphasis:[36]

> Although it was clear from the start that the colonists would carry their charitable traditions with them from England to the New World, it was just as clear that circumstances in the colonies would lead to a particular American version of charity, one that would stress to an even greater extent than in England individual responsibility, the primacy of work and, eventually, high tolerance for blending charity and private enterprise.

Once the country gained independence, its primary source of legal authority ceased to be the laws of England but became vested instead in its Constitution which continues to evolve in accordance with the rulings of the Supreme Court.

The Constitution

In the US, all law – whether statutory, judicial or administrative – occurs within and can be tested against the overarching provisions of the Constitution together with its Bill of Rights.[37] There are certain constitutionally protected rights and principles that have a particular bearing on the charitable sector.

Right to form associations

While the Constitution has no explicit provision that guarantees the right to association, the US courts have interpreted the First Amendment to the Constitution as containing the implicit constitutional right to expressive association:

> Congress shall make no law respecting an establishment of religion, or prohibiting the free exercise thereof; or abridging the freedom of speech, or of the press; or the right of the people peaceably to assemble, and to petition the government for a redress of grievances.

The Supreme Court[38] has ruled that 'implicit in the right to engage in activities protected by the First Amendment' is a 'corresponding right to associate with others in pursuit of a wide variety of . . . religious . . . ends'. Further, in *NAACP* v. *Alabama ex rel. Patterson*,[39] it held that:

> [e]ffective advocacy of both public and private points of view, particularly controversial ones, is undeniably enhanced by group association. . . . It is beyond debate that freedom to engage in association for the advancement of beliefs and ideas is an inseparable aspect of the 'liberty' assured by the Due Process Clause of the Fourteenth Amendment, which embraces freedom of speech . . .

Because this right is grounded in freedom of speech, it is concerned primarily with 'expressive' association. It allows organizations to determine whom they will admit as members, insofar as those organizations have an expressive message that would be compromised otherwise.[40]

Right to privacy

Then there is the more general right to privacy, which confers on individuals and other entities the right to be protected from government intrusion. This gives rise to a legal presumption that the conduct of persons or businesses is a matter for self-regulation unless or until the law is infringed. Its effect can be seen, for example, in relation to the traditional independence of the charitable sector.

These and other rights and principles have formed a backdrop to the development of the law governing nonprofits, charitable organizations and the sector in this jurisdiction.

The common law

On gaining independence, many of the American colonies repealed all English statutes including the 1601 Act, and towards the end of the eighteenth century they rejected the doctrine of *cy-près* outright. Some suggest that this was because instances of royal prerogative were objectionable in the light of the separation of powers adopted by the colony and meddled with the right to dispose of private property.[41] *Cy-près* was reintroduced at the turn of the century. However, all states and the federal government retained, for the most part, a definition of charity rooted in the old common law which reflects a broad and open-ended notion of charitable purposes. This is illustrated by the following expression of that common law definition often quoted in the US courts:[42]

> A charity, in the legal sense, may be more fully defined as a gift, to be applied consistently with existing laws, for the benefit of an indefinite number of persons, either by bringing their minds or hearts under the influence of education or religion, by relieving their bodies from disease, suffering or constraint, by assisting them to establish themselves in life, or by erecting or maintaining public buildings or works or otherwise lessening the burdens of government.

The legislation

The legislative history of charity law in the US is entirely subsumed within the history of tax legislation. There has been no attempt to statutorily define 'charity' and as the term 'charitable' has been interpreted to incorporate the common law definition of charity it is generally assumed that this jurisdiction must, therefore, have been content to continue the common law interpretation (despite the litanies of typical charitable purposes that invariably appear in US statutes).[43] While each of the states have statutes governing charitable organizations, the federal government exerts substantial influence through its control of federal income tax and the related exemption for charitable nonprofits which, together with the following umbrella pieces of legislation and judicial decisions, bring a degree of commonality to law and practice across all states.

The Tariff Act 1894

This legislation provided tax exemption for nonprofit charitable, religious and educational organizations and tax deduction for corporate donations to charitable entities.[44]

Federal Income Tax Act 1913

This legislation, replacing the 1894 Act, introduced the current federal income tax regime and regulatory framework for charities as administered by the Internal Revenue Service. The provision that is now section 501 (c)(3) has been amended only five times since 1913 and the pertinent amendments for the general definition of 'charitable' were made in 1934 and 1954 – both codified aspects of the limitations on political activities that are now in the statute.

The Unrelated Business Income Tax Act 1950

This legislation, added to the IRS Code, removed the 'destination of income' test under which charities could claim tax exemption on commercial activities that were unrelated to their charitable purpose if they could show that the profits generated went to further those purposes. Whether or not such activities were related to an organization's purpose, the right to tax exemption would be lost if the commercial activity was disproportionate to charitable purpose activity.[45] The legislative intent was to prevent charities from using their privileged status to engage in unfair competition with commercial bodies.

The Internal Revenue Code 1954

This legislation saw the charitable tax exemption provisions brought together for the first time within section 501 of the Tax Code.

The Model Nonprofit Corporation Act 1964

This was the first federal attempt to introduce a model statute to govern nonprofits and versions of it are currently still in effect in Alabama, the District of Columbia, New Jersey, North Dakota, Texas, Virginia and Wisconsin.

The Tax Reform Act 1969

This legislation introduced an excise tax on the net investment income of private non-operating foundations to fund the exempt organizations' oversight function within the IRS. Those funds, to the disappointment of many, have never been designated for that purpose.

Uniform Management of Institutional Funds Act (UMIFA) Model Legislation 1972

This legislation was drawn up by the National Conference of Commissioners on Uniform State Laws to govern the management and expenditure of investment assets held by charitable organizations. It has been adopted in some form by most states and the District of Columbia but is generally not applicable to charitable trusts.

Title XX of the Social Security Amendments 1974

These provisions allowed states to use federal money to fund whatever social services they thought appropriate and generated a rapid expansion in the number of charities.

The Tax Reform Act 1986

This legislation placed significant restrictions on non-cash gifts to charity and led to a drop in giving. The restrictions were partially repealed by Congress in 1990 and fully repealed in 1993.

The Revised Model Nonprofit Corporation Act 1987

This legislation, based loosely on California law, sets out basic parameters for the structure and composition of boards. It requires that:

> a director shall discharge his or her duties as a director, including his or her duties as a member of a committee (1) in good faith; (2) with the care an ordinarily prudent person in a like position would exercise under similar circumstances; and (3) in a manner the director reasonably believes to be in the best interests of the corporation.

It has been adopted in whole or in modified form by 22 states[46] for regulation of tax-exempt entities, including charitable organizations.

The Welfare Reform Act 1996

This legislation facilitated the rise of faith-based organizations in the role of providers of publicly funded services as the federal government reached out to organizations through the Charitable Choice clause in the 1996 Act, enabling them to assist in the welfare reform effort.

The Uniform Supervision of Trustees for Charitable Purposes Act 1996

This legislation requires all charitable trustees (and, although this is less clear, corporate directors) to register with the state Attorney General's office (so that it is at least aware of the charities under its jurisdiction). It also empowers the Attorney General to investigate potential wrongdoing, among other things by calling witnesses and demanding the production of relevant documents.

The Workforce Investment Act 1998

This was designed to make the business sector at the local level a more engaged player in helping low-skilled workers integrate into the workplace.

Sarbanes-Oxley Act 2002

This Act imposes new obligations and penalties on corporate officers and directors of publicly traded companies, and mandates increased disclosure by corporations to the Securities and Exchange Commission. For example, publicly traded companies must have an independent audit committee and chief executive officers must certify financial statements. Penalties for non-compliance include imprisonment and fines. Two specific provisions apply to all entities (including nonprofits): prohibitions on destruction of litigation-related documents and on retaliation against whistleblowers who identify specific types of financial wrongdoing. Although intended to address primarily the pervading corporate crisis resulting from scandals involving Enron, Arthur Andersen and several other large corporations, it is clear that the federal corporate accountability provisions laws of the Sarbanes-Oxley Act will be extended to charities and other nonprofits (e.g. New York is expected to shortly apply it to all nonprofits).

The American Jobs Creation Act 2004

This legislation limits the deductions taxpayers can claim for donations of motor vehicles to charitable organizations.

The Panel on the Nonprofit Sector Reform Proposals 2005

In 2005, having conducted its examination of the environment for nonprofit organizations, the Panel published its *Report to Congress and the Nonprofit Sector on Governance, Transparency, and Accountability* with specific recommendations for new legislation to strengthen governance, transparency and accountability.

Definitional matters

As legislatively stated 'the term charitable is used . . . in its generally accepted legal sense' which is understood as importing the common law interpretation.[47] A major Supreme Court case, *Bob Jones University* v. *United States*,[48] added a 'public policy' limitation to the meaning of charitable in the Internal Revenue Code, declaring that educational organizations that practice racial discrimination in their admissions policies are not permitted to be exempt from tax under section 501(c)(3).

Charitable intent

The presence or absence of charitable intent has never been as determinative of charitable status in this jurisdiction as elsewhere in the common law world. From an early stage it was accepted that the utility of a gift could compensate for an absence of altruism. In *Fire Insurance Patrol* v. *Boyd*,[49] for example, the fact that the provision of a fire patrol by an insurance company was commercially motivated did not negate its benefit to the public and its eligibility for charitable status.

Public benefit

Most states do not distinguish between mutual benefit and public benefit nonprofits. A charitable organization, however, must not confer a private benefit that is not incidental to its charitable purposes, or have the purpose of so doing. Where other types of nonprofit organizations benefit the private, social or economic interests of their members, charitable organizations must benefit the broad public interest and Congress has therefore provided, with very limited exceptions, that only those charities organized under section 501(c)(3) are eligible to receive tax-deductible contributions. The law in the US has been at pains to make and police a distinction drawn between 'public charities' and 'private foundations' in order to copper-fasten the requirement that the purposes and activities of the former are absolutely committed to public benefit; where there is doubt, then the latter is the default assignation.[50]

In this jurisdiction there is a legal presumption, though not in legislative form as in Ireland, that religious organizations *per se* satisfy the public benefit test. Under the First Amendment of the Constitution, Congress is forbidden to enact a law 'respecting an establishment of religion or prohibiting the free exercise thereof'. Given the history of the founding of the US, it is clear that interference in any way with religious practice is frowned upon and that religion receives special deference in American law. Religious charitable trusts enjoy the same privileges as religious corporations.

Exclusively charitable

In the US, as in England and Wales and other common law jurisdictions, an organization's resources must be devoted exclusively to charitable purposes if it is to come within the meaning of section 501 (c)(3) of the IRS Code and related regulations.[51] To do so it must in effect pass the operational test applied by the IRS which interprets 'exclusively' to mean 'primarily' or 'substantially'.[52]

Independent

The independence of charities, a characteristic derived from trust law, is as important and as threatened by the contract culture in this jurisdiction as in all others that share the common law legacy.

Non-governmental

The laws of the various states and the federal government permit nonprofit organizations to bid on public procurements. Some procurement systems allow specially qualified nonprofit organizations to apply for and obtain special status that permits them to have preferences in bidding or to make unsolicited proposals to the public agencies.

Nonprofit distributing

A charitable organization's founding articles, in conjunction with applicable law, must prohibit it from ever distributing its net earnings to members, directors or other insiders (even upon dissolution). For an organization to be charitable, no part of its net earnings can inure to the benefit of insiders in the organisation. However, as illustrated by *United Cancer Council v. Commissioner*,[53] this imperative is now interpreted somewhat liberally.

In this jurisdiction, more so than in other common law nations, the shift of charities towards the commercial profit-making world came early, has been decisive and is now well established. As has been said:[54]

> In recent times, as the trends towards social entrepreneurship and venture philanthropy have accelerated and as the bounds between for-profit and nonprofit have blurred our vague, ill-discussed, ill-defined legal definition of charity has been too amorphous to lend structure to the difficult task of sorting out what is and is not charitable in the eyes of the law.

Charitable purposes

Since 1959, when the IRS regulations (ancillary to the 1954 Tax Code) were issued, the following broad description of such purposes has been adhered to:[55]

> Relief of the poor and distressed or of the underprivileged; advancement of education or science; erection or maintenance of public buildings or monuments, or works lessening of the burdens of Government; and promotion of social welfare by organisations designed to accomplish any of the above purposes, or (i) to lessen neighbourhood tensions; (ii) to eliminate prejudice and discrimination; (iii) to defend human and civil rights secured by law; or (iv) to combat community deterioration and juvenile delinquency.

The absence of any reference to religion, the broad phrasing of the terms 'lessening . . . the burdens of Government' and 'promotion of social welfare' and the specifying of amorphous matters such as 'to lessen neighbourhood tensions' possibly distances the US interpretation of charitable purposes a little from the mainstream common law interpretation as *per Pemsel* etc.

Legal structures for charities

In this as in other common law jurisdictions, charitable activity is organized within entities structured as either an unincorporated association, a trust or as a corporate body. A distinctive feature of the development of charity law in the US is the early reliance upon the charitable corporation. This is partially attributable to the rejection, on independence, of the 1601 Act and other English legislation. Thereafter the charitable trust fell into relative disuse as it was assumed that the equitable powers for enforcing a charity in trust form derived from that statute. Although this conception of equitable powers was later overturned,[56] corporations for charitable purposes nevertheless flourished to become the dominant legal form.[57] Consequently, the most common legal vehicle for charitable activities in the United States is now the nonprofit corporation. The chief alternative to the nonprofit corporation is the trust. While corporations are created pursuant to statute, the law of trusts is largely a creation of the common law (though many states have, to varying extents, passed statutes codifying trust law).[58] Finally, in addition to the nonprofit corporation and the trust, groups of individuals can form unincorporated associations governed only by their mutual agreement, and requiring no registration with the State.

Types of structure

In this jurisdiction, a charitable organization is any tax-exempt organization recognized as such by the IRS under section 501(c)(3) of the Internal Revenue Code (IRC). A 'charitable organization' can be either a public charity or a private foundation: a distinction which originated in the Tax Code but has since become a part of the basic structural framework for charitable organizations in the United States; some 48 states have now passed laws adopting this distinction.

Regulatory framework

The activities of charitable organizations are governed by regulatory powers applied at federal and state levels: the Internal Revenue Service is the only body with a central registration/regulatory function; while all states have regulatory powers located in the offices of the Secretary of State and the Attorney General.[59]

Registering charities

As the IRS is the only government body with responsibility for oversight of the nation's charitable sector it maintains the register of all tax-exempt or nonprofit organizations, of which public benefit organizations (the term usually used to describe 'charities' or 'charitable organizations' in this jurisdiction) receive the highest level of tax benefits (including tax-preferred donations).[60] Under the Revised Model Nonprofit Corporation Act 1987 an organization either self-declares that it is a public benefit organization or is deemed to be one under state law if it is an IRC section 501 (c)(3) organization. In addition, some states have enacted the Uniform Supervision of Trustees for Charitable Purposes Act 1996, which requires charitable trusts to register with the Attorney General's office. Publication of the charter or articles of incorporation or trust deeds of any such registered body is generally not required under the laws of individual states, although they all have electronic databases of the incorporated nonprofit organizations in their jurisdictions.

Charitable status

Determination of charitable status and registration as such is undertaken solely for the purpose of establishing eligibility for tax exemption and is the responsibility of the IRS. Foreign organizations can also apply to the IRS for recognition as charitable or social welfare organizations under section 501(c)(3)–(4) of the Internal Revenue Code.

Whether a body qualifies as a public benefit organisation is a decision made in accordance with section 501 (c)(3) – 1 (d)(2) of the Internal Revenue Code. In applying this test, the IRS interprets 'charity' in its 'generally accepted legal sense' and it will apply an 'activities test' to establish whether an organization's activities conform with its purposes, both of which must be charitable. When determining charitable status, the IRS will also determine whether the organization is a 'public charity' or a 'private foundation'.[61]

Public charities   This type of charitable organization receives at least one-third of its finances from a broad segment of the general public. Public charities include schools, hospitals, churches and any other charities that receive their financial support from a broad group of donors or patrons.

Section 509 of the Internal Revenue Code and associated regulations also identify two other types of public charities termed 'publicly supported' organizations, because the funding requirements stipulated in the Code and regulations are aimed at ensuring that only organizations with widespread financial support from the general public will qualify. One type qualifies as publicly supported because it normally receives at least one-third of its basic financial support in the form of contributions and grants from the general public, from governmental entities, from certain other organizations that themselves qualify as publicly supported organizations, or from any combination of the foregoing.[62] The other qualifies under section 509 (a)(3) if it satisfies two tests: not more than one-third of its basic financial support may be investment income or certain income from commercial activities unrelated to the organization's charitable purposes; and at least one-third of its basic financial support must come in the form of a combination of contributions, membership dues and income generated from the performance of the organization's charitable purposes.

A community foundation is a tax-exempt organization that generally holds a number of permanent funds created by many separate donors, all dedicated to the long-term charitable benefit of a specific community or region. This institution is generally recognized as a public charity, is not subject to the more stringent rules that apply to private foundations, and has been a prominent feature on the charity landscape in this jurisdiction since the forming of the Cleveland trust company in 1914. Typically, a community foundation provides grants and other services to assist other charitable organizations in meeting local needs, and also offers services to help donors establish endowed funds for specific charitable purposes. They may be incorporated. A new and proliferating form of foundation is the 'pooled funds' or 'mutual foundation' which are commercial community foundations that provide more flexibility than a private family foundation. The past two decades have seen substantial growth in community development corporations which concentrate all grant-making on community development projects. There are currently approximately 4,000 community development corporations in the US investing in their neighbourhoods and being managed by local residents.

Private foundations   This type of charitable organization is a grant-making institution that does not conduct direct charitable activity, is typically established by a single individual, family, or company and receives more than two-thirds of its support from its founders or from investment income earned by an endowment. Private foundations[63] are subject to substantially more restrictive rules than public charities (e.g. they are not permitted to engage in any political activities what-soever, either directly or indirectly).[64] They are also required to distribute a spe-cific amount of their income each year. The 'distributable amount' is defined as 5 per cent of the aggregate fair market value of the foundation's assets in excess of indebtedness incurred with respect to the assets, and their donors receive less favourable tax treatment for contributions. If a public charity fails to meet its 'public support test' of receiving at least one-third of its income from the public in the form of contributions and grants, it is generally reclassified as a private foundation.

A corporate foundation, also known as a company-sponsored foundation, is a private foundation that receives its primary funding from a profit-making busi-ness. The foundation is a separate, legal charitable organization even though it often maintains close ties with the founding company, and it must abide by the same rules and regulations as other private foundations.[65]

Regulating charities

Individual states each have responsibility for ensuring that nonprofit organiza-tions act in compliance with the law but only the IRS exercises a central regula-tory authority. It applies varying degrees of regulation for different classes of charity, with differences based not on formal legal features but on features that indicate a greater possibility for abuse. Because private foundations are suscep-tible to donor control they attract a variety of special rules which aim, in one manner or another, to enhance their public accountability and curb their poten-tial to confer personal benefits on persons and institutions closely associated with them.

The regulatory role of the states

All states impose record keeping, audit, and annual reporting requirements on incorporated nonprofit organizations based within their jurisdictions. The legal requirements are generally quite specific and more rigorous rules are imposed on public benefit organizations. Since 1975, 48 states and the District of Columbia have passed laws imposing the restrictions on private foundations as stated in Chapter 42 of the Internal Revenue Code.[66]

In most states the primary responsibility for enforcing these laws and investigat-ing complaints of fraud or abuse of tax-exempt status is borne by the Attorney General. State charity regulators monitor adherence to charitable solicitation laws, investigate complaints of fraud or abuse of tax-exempt status, and maintain lists of registered nonprofit organizations.

The regulatory role of the Internal Revenue Service

In keeping with the essentially revenue-driven government approach to charities, the initial vetting and determination of charitable status and subsequent audit responsibilities have long been the responsibility of the Internal Revenue Service as exercised through its Exempt Organizations Branch.

Education and support   The Exempt Organizations Branch works closely with organizations that seek and obtain tax-exempt status, providing services and advice and generally assisting them to better serve the public. They also issue regulations (which require public notice and comment procedures) and rulings (which do not), thus giving not only informal but also formal advice on a regular basis. Litigation about aspects of tax-exempt status is more frequent in the US then in other countries and the resulting judgments provide all nonprofit organizations with information about how courts view the IRS oversight of the public benefit sector.

Supervision   All private foundations and many public charities[67] are required to file annual information returns[68] with the Internal Revenue Service that include information about the organization's finances and operations. The Generally Accepted Accounting Principles (GAAP) regime applied by the Financial Accounting Standards Board (FASB) sets out the relevant standards; in particular FAS 116 and 117 impose special rules for fund accounting and income reporting in relation to nonprofit organizations. The annual information return serves as the primary document providing information about the organization's finances, governance, operations and programmes for federal regulators, the public and many state charity officials. At the federal level, the Tax Exempt and Government Entities Division of the IRS reviews applications for tax-exempt status, audits a sample of the information returns (the Forms 990) filed annually by nonprofits, and enforces the requirements imposed by the tax code on charitable organizations. It is also authorized to impose fines and other penalties and, as a last resort, it can revoke tax-exempt status.

The courts

Unlike other common law jurisdictions, there is a significant level of litigation in the United States, both about tax and non-tax aspects of charitable status. For example, where an application for incorporation is rejected, or where the organization is in fact operating in an illegal manner, the Attorney General can petition the courts to revoke the corporate charter.

The Attorney General

In this as in all common law jurisdictions, the Attorney General has almost exclusive rights to sue to enforce the terms of a charitable trust, whether or not incorporated. This official has ongoing rights to intervene in the public interest, but these are circumscribed by the terms of the donor's initial disposition.[69] In many states, however, the Attorney General has exercised little or no oversight over the charitable sector, leaving regulation of the sector entirely to the Internal Revenue Service.

The state Attorney General is empowered to supervise and regulate charities and must oversee their liquidation and dissolution, whether voluntary or involuntary. Charities are responsible for filing reports with the Attorney General on a regular basis and these are open to the public. Some states have enacted the Uniform Supervision of Trustees for Charitable Purposes Act 1996, which assigns certain responsibilities to the Attorney General's office.

Incorporating authority

A public benefit organization can become incorporated, without the intervention of the Secretary of State, so long as its governing documents do not disclose any illegal or violent purposes or any that are otherwise against public policy, its name is not confusing, redundant, etc. The various states maintain registers of nonprofit corporations including corporate charities with the appropriate government body. There is considerable variation in state reporting requirements for charitable corporations with only 25 states requiring charitable corporations to report on the status of the corporation to state officials at certain intervals.

Regulating the fiscal environment

In theory, the state Attorney General or other specified state authority is charged with regulatory responsibility for charitable organizations and their fiscal environment[70] but in practice this has generally been exercised at federal level by the IRS as it applies the Tax Code.[71] However, as has been pointed out:[72]

> Over the past 20 years, funding for Internal Revenue Service oversight of exempt organisations has remained essentially constant while the sector has nearly doubled in size and become even more complex. Funding of oversight at the state level varies substantially among states, but all lack sufficient resources to provide adequate oversight of the charitable sector.[73]

Tax

Public benefit organizations (both charitable and social welfare), like numerous other kinds of nonprofit organization, must apply to the Internal Revenue Service to be recognized as tax-exempt, with the exception of churches, which are generally presumed to be tax-exempt. An organization that qualifies as a public charity under section 501 (c)(3) is exempt from all income tax for federal purposes and generally will also qualify for exemption from state income taxes as many states 'piggyback' their exemptions and returns on the federal determination.

While VAT is uncommon in the United States, most states do impose some sort of sales (turnover) tax. There is wide variety in the nature of exemptions granted for charitable purposes. As in other areas, the law is generally designed to provide benefits to nonprofits without giving them an unfair advantage when they engage in business similar to that conducted by for-profit companies. States commonly provide property tax exemptions for certain charitable organizations.

Certain limited exemptions exist under federal law for liability in relation to customs, duties and excise taxes for particular types of charities (e.g. certain educational institutions). Public charities can, however, be subject to excise taxes in certain situations. Most importantly, if they engage in 'excess benefit transactions' such as paying a president too high a salary, public charities will incur an excise tax.

Donation incentives

Tax incentives for charitable giving in the United States have been part of the tax code since the eighteenth century, and are significant in size, amounting to nearly $17 billion in tax expenditures.[74] As has been pointed out:

> The key feature of U.S. tax incentives for giving is that they directly benefit the donor. Donors who itemise deductions (in practice those who own homes and are thereby able to qualify for the mortgage interest deduction) are able to deduct the full charitable value of their contributions from their taxable income.[75]

Indeed, the US has 'the world's most generous tax concessions'[76] for philanthropy and 'no other nation grants subsidies at such a high level or across so many types of activities'.[77]

Although non-charitable organizations and social welfare organizations qualify for tax exemption only charitable organizations can receive tax-deductible donations. Generally, contributions to domestic 501(c)(3) charitable organizations are deductible.[78] Corporations can deduct contributions of up to 10 per cent of their income each year. An individual can generally deduct contributions to public charities of up to 50 per cent of income; there is a lower limit of 30 per cent on contributions to private foundations. In addition, contributions of property other than cash are generally valued not at their current value, but at their 'basis' (usually the cost at which the donor acquired them). Contributions of property to public charities may also be valued at basis if their use is not related to a charitable purpose or if they have been held for a year or less. Bequests to charitable organizations are also deductible, and are not subject to the same rules and percentage limits that govern other contributions.[79]

The American Jobs Creation Act 2004 will have an effect on individuals and corporations with regard to charitable contributions: sections 883 and 884 will require increased reporting for non-cash charitable contributions and will limit the deductions allowed for charitable contributions of vehicles under section 170 of the Internal Revenue Code 2. The changes seek to prevent individual and corporate taxpayers from taking excessively generous deductions for their donations.

Cy-près

The doctrine of *cy-près* applies in the US as it does in other common law jurisdictions.[80] Frequent use of *cy-près* is found where there are unconstitutional or illegal conditions in a trust, such as provisions that would violate law and public policy against racial discrimination. Generally, contention arises in relation to whether an organization to which charitable assets were to be diverted had purposes that were close enough to those of the dissolving corporation.[81]

Fundraising

Fundraising is regulated at state level. The regulations tend to be complex and inadequate due in part to First Amendment concerns. The National Association of State Charities Officials and the National Association of Attorneys General have developed a Uniform Registration Statement.[82] The Supreme Court has held that charitable solicitations cannot be banned solely because a high percentage of the revenues go to fundraising costs rather than to the organization's charitable purposes.[83]

Trading

Treasury Regulation section 1.501(c)(3)–1(e), as amended in 1990, clearly permits charities to engage in commercial activities subject to the usual common law caveat that the organization is not established or operated for the primary purpose of carrying on an unrelated trade or business, a caveat that seeks to eliminate a perceived source of unfair competition with commercial enterprises. Those that engage in such activities run certain risks: if the trade or business is not in furtherance of its exempt purpose and becomes predominant, they can lose their charitable status and entitlement to tax exemption.[84] In addition, it is 'the purpose towards which an organisation's activities are directed, and not the nature of the activities themselves, [that are] ultimately dispositive of the organisation's right to be classified as a section 501(c)(3) organisation'.[85]

Constraints on modern philanthropic activity

The charity law framework in this federal jurisdiction functions within a complex legal environment where the Constitution and its Bill of Rights, social justice, human rights and anti-terrorism legislation and the pressures resulting from government withdrawal from areas of social welfare provision all play a part.

Policy constraints: partnership with government

In the US, unlike the situation in other common law jurisdictions, there is no explicit formal partnership in effect between government and the nonprofit sector. The reality is, however, that very similar arrangements are in place following two decades of government transfer and privatization of health and social care services. The result is a system in which nonprofits are now major providers of various social welfare functions and (at least in certain fields such as education and child care) have become increasingly dependent on the government for financial support.

Government grants and contracts

In 1996, the government provided roughly 36 per cent of all revenue for nonprofits; fees for services constituted another 54 per cent of revenues, with private contributions responsible for only 10 per cent. These figures may actually understate government support for the sector, since many health care, child care and other service organizations collect revenues by charging fees to clients who, in turn, are reimbursed or subsidised by the government.[86] On the other hand, these figures do not take into account one of the most substantial forms of private contribution to charity: volunteer labour. This trend toward reliance upon ever greater levels of government financial support has not affected all charitable organizations equally; religious organizations depend overwhelmingly on private donations for their support, and in fact receive more than half of all private contributions annually.[87]

Undoubtedly, however, the traditional independence of charities in the US and their capacity to assertively address and represent the interests of minority groups is becoming steadily more compromised as the sector is drawn into working to the government's agenda.

Native Americans

The success of casinos in indigenous communities demonstrates the viability of commercial ventures in that context and suggests their potential to support more broadly based community development. The failure to extend and diversify from that base would seem to indicate an absence of modern philanthropic models involving partnership arrangements between charity, government and business.

As in other common law jurisdictions (notably Canada, New Zealand and Australia) there may also be constraints emanating from the blood-link basis of relationships in indigenous communities which by breaching the 'public' component of the public benefit test could compromise eligibility for charitable status.

Common law constraints

The primary common law characteristic of charity law in this jurisdiction is that it remains firmly dominated by the revenue-driven functions of the IRS.

Role of the courts and the Attorney General

In theory the Attorney General has an inherent jurisdiction to supervise, protect and control charities. However, in practice it is unusual for this officer to play any direct regulatory role.[88] In this most litigious of common law nations, the courts have a relatively greater volume of charity law cases to process but there is little evidence that as a result charitable purposes in this jurisdiction are being judicially developed in a manner that makes them better fitted to address contemporary social circumstances than elsewhere in the common law world.

The 'spirit and intendment' rule

This common law rule applies in the US, but again there is little evidence of its currently being employed to creatively extend charitable purposes to fit patterns of contemporary social need.[89]

Legal structures

In this jurisdiction, the dominant structure for charitable activities is the non-profit corporation to which the chief alternative is the trust. Both operate within an essentially common law context in which the dominant principles (and rules regarding the role of the Attorney General, the use of *cy-près*, etc.) are rooted in the law relating to trusts. Arguably, this tension between corporate form and trust principles does not assist philanthropic functionality. Moreover, while the clear legal distinction drawn between public charities and private foundations is, in this context, both understandable and necessary it also serves to highlight the fact that in the US a significant proportion of philanthropic resources are tied up in the latter, perhaps in perpetuity, for purposes that do not necessarily translate into improvements to the contemporary circumstances of the socially disadvantaged.

Restrictions on advocacy/political activity

The usual constraints apply also in this jurisdiction (see, further, chapter 3); they were added to the Tax Code in 1934 and require tax-exempt charities to comply with the common law restriction on the political activities of charities. Charitable organizations under section 501(c)(3) of the Code, which are eligible for tax-deductible contributions, must not have any substantial part of their activities devoted to influencing legislation;[90] social welfare organizations – which are not eligible for those tax-deductible contributions but are still exempt from income tax – can engage in unlimited lobbying activity, so long as it is related to their social welfare purpose.[91] This is a real constraint at a time when democratic principles require that voices of dissent be heard.

Fiscal issues

'American tax policies regulating philanthropy promote inequality' says Bob Reich,[92] and he may well be right. This is compounded by other problems.

Differentials in level of donee entitlement to charitable tax exemption

Because the level of a donee's tax exemption corresponds to their tax bracket, the wealthier the donee the higher their level of tax exemption and vice versa for poor people – i.e. it costs poor people more than rich people to make the same donation.

Differentials in level of community benefit from charitable tax exemption privileges

The wealthier the donee the higher their level of tax exemption and therefore the higher the level of public subsidy for the donee's chosen charitable purpose. Given that in this jurisdiction a significant proportion of local community 'public services' (e.g. schools, universities, child care facilities and hospitals) are in fact non-government facilities, the outcome is often that wealthy communities can channel tax-exempt privileges towards building and maintaining such facilities far better than can poorer communities: an inequitable distribution of resources directly subsidized by a diversion of tax dollars that would otherwise be available to fund government services. This must accentuate existing social inequality.[93]

Restrictions on donee eligibility for charitable tax exemption

Under section 170 of the Internal Revenue Code a tax deduction has generally been permitted for charitable contributions, but the recently introduced American Jobs Creation Act 2004 will now negatively affect this entitlement for both individuals and corporations. The changes seek to prevent individual and corporate taxpayers from taking excessively generous deductions for their donations by requiring increased donor reporting. The intended effect of limiting donor tax deduction entitlement may also reduce the incentive to donate property to charitable organizations.

The doctrine of cy-près

The doctrine of *cy-près* is applied somewhat more conservatively in the US than in other common law jurisdictions. Commentators have frequently criticized current *cy-près* decisions, saying the courts are too restrictive in reforming trusts which in turn must hinder the process of redirecting charitable resources.

The public/private differentiation between charitable organizations

This differentiation, on the basis of the degree of public financial support, while logical, does lead to considerable complexity in relation to compliance with various IRS tax rules. This complexity is accentuated by overlapping federal and state laws. Because of a lack of state-level enforcement, there has been a steady strengthening of the powers of the IRS in recent decades through the transfer to it of tax mechanisms for enforcing duties that previously belonged to the states. This lack of a clear basis for attributing responsibility between state and federal levels and for co-ordinating state systems of fiscal rules must act as a constraint on national philanthropic activity.

Public benefit matters

In the US there are other aspects of the public benefit test that operate to inhibit effective philanthropic intervention on behalf of the socially excluded.

Redistribution via charitable organizations does not favour the poor   The outcome of the present system is that only 2 per cent of charitable resources end up being channelled towards the poor via social welfare organizations. Moreover, the remaining 98 per cent of non-social welfare recipients benefit additionally from the tax subsidy that would otherwise have been available to the government for funding services for the poor.

Uneven application of the public benefit test   The activities of and gifts to religious organizations are exempted from the public benefit test; indeed the particular deference to religion is evident in regulatory law and practice as it applies to charities. As a result, religious corporations have a long history and their exemption from taxes has been held not to violate the Constitution.[94] As has been pointed out 'the largest piece of America's charitable pie is going to the sustenance of religious groups – for their facilities, their operating costs, and their clergy salaries'.[95] Given that 60 per cent of annual donations in this jurisdiction go to fund religious organizations (excluding their service provision), which are not always acceptable to the more socially marginalized groups, there is arguably every good reason to fully apply the public benefit test.

Modern law constraints

The fact that the determination of charitable status occurs within a tax-driven regulatory environment dominated by the Internal Revenue Service is the single most significant constraint.

Lack of coherence in charity law administration

The division of responsibilities between federal and state levels regarding charities is not very clear and supervision is inadequately resourced, with the IRS generally being left to safeguard standards through administration of the Tax Code. The difference in statute law between states and in the type of government body assigned lead responsibility for charitable organizations tends to generate a certain amount of opportunistic forum shopping.

Lack of an appropriate forum for developing charitable purposes

Typically, in this common law jurisdiction as in all others except England and Wales, there is no forum to counterbalance the tax-driven priorities of the government agency assigned responsibility for charity and charitable organizations, a situation that has attracted comment from US academics.[96] The IRS, by all accounts overstretched as regards its core functions, lacks the motivation, authority and, in a wider sense, the capacity, to independently set precedents capable of introducing real change to the range of established charitable purposes etc.

Although the courts in the US have more opportunities than their counterparts in other common law jurisdictions to consider issues affecting charities, the constraints of cost, time and adverse publicity combine to ensure that they still do so relatively infrequently and necessarily in a random manner. Consequently, in this jurisdiction, there is no forum capable of proactively advancing the judicial development of charitable purposes.

Overseas aid

In the United States, international grants are made by private foundations, corporate foundations, corporate matching gift programmes and an array of public charities, including community foundations, donor-advised funds, operating organizations that provide cash grants and in-kind services, and others. In addition, many religious congregations and organizations provide cash grants for activities abroad, although their activities are not as closely monitored as those of public charities and private foundations. In general both public charities and private foundations are permitted to make gifts to foreign organizations, consistent with their US charitable purposes (under section 501 (c)(3) so long as the foreign charity is a US 501 (c)(3) equivalent or the US donor 'exercises expenditure responsibility'.

However, the domestic organisation must have real discretion in how to use the funds; if it is found to be merely a conduit for donations to a foreign charity, then donations will not be tax-deductible.

Domestic organizations must also ensure that money given to a foreign organization will, in fact, be used for their charitable purposes. In this regard, public charities are subject to a fairly flexible standard: they must maintain sufficient discretion and control to ensure that the funds are properly used. Private foundations must comply with more stringent requirements.

In the wake of 9/11, the Treasury Department has issued non-binding guidelines suggesting procedures that international grantmakers should follow in order to minimize the possibility of charitable grants being diverted to terrorist organizations.[97] These include gathering a great deal of information about potential grantee organizations and then comparing that information against US lists of suspected terrorists and terrorist organizations to verify that there are no connections. The US organizations should also see to it that a recipient organization implements procedures to minimize the risk of their funds being diverted. While grantmakers have criticized these rules for requiring more information than is reasonably obtainable in many countries, and for failing to recognize that not all international grants pose the same risks of diversion,[98] it is not yet clear what steps along these lines charitable organizations should take. The resulting uncertainty has the potential to discourage grantmakers from making grants, particularly to obscure charities in high-risk areas.

Only a fraction of annual grants made by US charities goes to international activities, perhaps 15–18 per cent, including grants to US-based intermediaries that make sub-grants or directly implement programmes abroad. On the basis of geographical distribution, the largest proportion of US overseas grants (12 per cent) goes to England.

Human rights, social justice and anti-terrorism legislation

This, the most advanced democracy in the common law world, has in place much the same set of laws governing these matters as other such nations. This legislation is most often enacted at state level and functions in a rights environment framed by the Constitution and its Bill of Rights.

Human rights   The US Constitution, its Bill of Rights, together with the 13th 14th and 15th Amendments, may be considered to provide a body of provisions equivalent to the European Convention on Human Rights with nationwide application. In the past they have served the nation well in the fight against slavery, racial discrimination and segregation and as the principal means of safeguarding political, religious and other freedoms. At present, particularly since 9/11 and the ensuing global war against terror, human rights in this jurisdiction have been under continual threat. The litany of human rights infringements is considerable: invasions of privacy, intrusive inspections and questionable detentions under the USA Patriot Act; there is the well documented practice of 'extraordinary rendition', as well as allegations of torture at prisons in Iraq, Afghanistan and Guantánamo Bay. Despite the Supreme Court ruling in *Hamdan* v. *Rumsfeld et al.* on 29 June 2006, that the military commissions established to try Guantánamo Bay detainees violate both US law and the Geneva Conventions, the now 4-year-long detention without trial of some 450 persons (including teenagers) continues.

Social justice   While the laws of this jurisdiction address much the same domestic social justice concerns (equity, equality and non-discriminatory practices, etc.) as elsewhere, there are nonetheless some paradoxes.

The US does not treat health care as a fundamental human right and provides publicly funded medicine only to people falling into certain limited categories. This has resulted in a wide gap in the quality of treatment between those who can afford health insurance, or who have it provided as an employee benefit, and those who do not. As of 2004 the United States had the highest percentage of people in prison of any nation in the world and racial minorities, notably blacks and

Hispanics, are over-represented. Unlike other developed nations, the US also: imposes capital punishment; does not provide universal right to abortion; and does not recognize same-sex marriages.

Anti-terrorism   The three principal directive measures taken by the US government, following the 9/11 terrorist attacks on the World Trade Center and the Pentagon, were: Executive Order 13224, Blocking Property and Prohibiting Transactions with Persons Who Commit, Threaten To Commit, or Support Terrorism (23 September 2001); the USA Patriot Act, Uniting and Strengthening America by Providing Appropriate Tools Required to Intercept and Obstruct Terrorism (24 October 2001); and the Treasury Department's Anti-Terrorist Financing Guidelines: Voluntary Best Practices for US-Based Charities (November 2002).

In a progress report issued in 2003, exactly two years after the attacks, the Treasury Department reported that 173 nations had now joined the United States in implementing orders to freeze terrorist assets, more than 100 countries had introduced new legislation to fight terrorist financing, and 84 countries had established Financial Intelligence Units to share information. The report noted that during the previous two years the United States and its international partners had taken action against 23 charities 'involved in the funding of terror'; 315 individuals and organizations had been officially listed as terrorists; $136.7 million in assets had been frozen, including $36.6 million in the United States; and 'countless millions in additional funds [have been] prevented from flowing to terrorists by disruption of terrorist financing networks, deterrence of donors' and other international efforts.[99]

All this has had an impact upon the US philanthropic community. Public charities engaged in international activities are affected because all financial transactions, including technical assistance and humanitarian relief, are covered by the three measures. There is now considerable uncertainty regarding the information that US charities are required to seek about potential foreign recipients before making grants and about estimating the risk of funds being diverted for terrorist use. Few doubt the unmistakable message that the government views nonprofits, particularly private foundations, as a possible source of funding for terrorists and that charities constitute a weak link in the fight against terrorism.

Charity law review and social inclusion

The US is currently engaged in the most comprehensive review of the governance, regulations and operations of the charitable community undertaken for three decades. The review, unlike all others presently underway in common law nations, conforms to the traditional model by focusing pretty much exclusively on improving monitoring and control systems while reducing opportunities for abuse.

Proposed changes to definitional matters and legal structures

In June and July 2004, the US Senate Finance Committee conducted hearings on *Keeping Bad Things from Happening to Good Charities* and a round-table discussion on oversight and reform, and then released a discussion draft of possible solutions.[100] The Committee followed with additional hearings in April and June 2005. In testimony before the Committee, IRS Commissioner Mark Everson identified a number of issues:

- misuse of charitable entities, such as donor-advised funds and Type III supporting organizations, so they benefit the donor rather than the receiving organization or the public;
- abusive credit counselling organizations, many of which may have been set up not to assist debtors but to enrich the organizations' for-profit partners;
- overstated charitable deductions by taxpayers, most often involving non-cash contributions;
- widely varying methods for determining the compensation of executives; and
- inconsistent and limited disclosure of governance practices.[101]

The US House Ways and Means Committee, under the leadership of Chairman Bill Thomas, also began an examination of the charitable community in 2004. The Committee is examining the legal history of the tax-exempt sector; its size, scope and impact on the economy; the need for congressional oversight; and what the IRS is doing to improve compliance with the law. Taken together, the examinations underway by Congress, the IRS and the sector itself constitute a significant review of the charity law framework. Unfortunately there is no indication that this review will consider either matters of definition or the necessity for adjustments to the regulatory framework to ensure that it is better equipped to address contemporary social inclusion issues.

Proposed changes to the regulatory framework

The primary and repeated recommendation made by the Panel on the Nonprofit Sector in its report is that Congress should authorize additional resources to the IRS for overall tax enforcement and for improved oversight of charitable organizations. The focus is very much on methods of improving the quality of financial information available on charitable organizations. At this stage there is no indication that any of the following matters will arise for consideration: alternative legal structures; advocacy/political activity; application of the public benefit test; a possible Charity Commission type body; a statutory broadening of the *Pemsel* classification of charitable purposes to address contemporary social inclusion issues such as the causes of poverty, the circumstances of Native Americans, promotion of civil society, partnership with government, international aid, human rights, etc. Other than the fact that all charities are likely to be subjected to greater levels of surveillance, which may well further inhibit their freedom of action, there would not seem to be any particular implications arising from this review process for social inclusion.

Conclusion

The United States is the most advanced and powerful of the democratic common law nations but it also has some of the most intractable social problems. It is the lead protagonist, using the most sophisticated and expensive weaponry ever developed, in some of the more marginalized and impoverished nations on earth. It has the wealthiest charitable sector sandwiched between a 12 per cent rate of national poverty and the world's largest concentration of billionaires. Given its history of coping with slavery, racial discrimination and the integration of immigrants, it has much to contribute to our understanding of social inclusion and yet it currently finds itself at the centre of a growing rift between developed western democracies and the Islamic nations, or some of them. Arguably, philanthropy in the US functions in a manner that does not address these dichotomies either at home or abroad and may even exacerbate them.

The current charity law reform process offers an opportunity to consider the current misfit between the law and the particular pattern of social need in the US, and to give strategic and focused consideration to improving the functions of that law in relation to specific areas of need. At the least, ways could be found to increase the current 2 per cent level of contributions to social welfare charities and to reverse the current inequitable distribution of tax-exempt privileges between rich and poor donees that can amplify relative community disadvantage. At best, the capacity of American charities to mediate and offer ameliorative assistance, in situations where socially disadvantaged communities and nations are becoming polarized and alienated, could be strengthened and the challenge presented by contemporary philothropic initiatives such as the Bill and Melinda Gates Foundation could be embraced. Any such change would require a different approach to that currently adopted by the government.

Chapter 13

Charity law and social inclusion in Canada

Introduction

Canada is a not an untypical common law country: its institutions and laws, including the law relating to charities, derive to a considerable extent from those of England and Wales; it contains the remnants of an indigenous people and culture that never fully recovered from the impact of colonization; its development owes much to successive waves of immigrants; and though it is now accustomed to independence and sustaining a pluralist civil society it has yet to wholly work through its particular colonial legacy. Charity law forms a part of that legacy.

This chapter begins with an overview of the country, its primary socioeconomic indicators, a profile of the charitable sector and the characteristics of its social inclusion agenda. This is followed by a brief historical outline of charity law in Canada as developed through its legislative milestones. The template of functions (see, further, chapter 6) is then applied to identify and assess the characteristic features of the charity law environment in this jurisdiction, the key definitional matters, the legal structures for charities, registration and the regulatory framework and associated fiscal matters. This leads to an analysis of current legal constraints on the development of philanthropy. The chapter continues by examining the protracted charity law review process, considers the recommendations made in the Joint Regulatory Table report[1] and their significance for social inclusion issues. It concludes by reflecting on the distinctive characteristics of charity law in Canada.

Charities and social inclusion

As pointed out in the Johns Hopkins report, 'because of its long tradition of relying on nonprofit and voluntary organisations to address the needs and interests of its population, Canada has one of the largest and most vibrant nonprofit and voluntary sectors in the world'.[2]

The country

Canada is a federal country with ten provinces, three territories, and a federal government. It is the second-largest country in the world (after Russia) of almost 10 million square kilometres with a total population of approximately 33 million, including a number of different indigenous communities[3] and a range of ethnic groups[4] with varied religious beliefs.[5]

Since the Second World War, Canada has been transformed from a largely agricultural economy into one that is now primarily industrial and urban with a particularly strong service sector. Although politically distanced from the US, it shares with its neighbour the common characteristics of an affluent, high-tech industrial society. In 2004 Canada had a strong GDP of $1.023 trillion, of which exports (85 per cent to the US) accounted for roughly a third and with a growth rate of 2.4 per cent. The unemployment rate then stood at 7 per cent.

The charitable sector

Although 'our information on the sector is quite poor'[6] there is still more than sufficient to conclude that charities make a significant contribution to the social and economic fabric of Canada. The Johns Hopkins report, for example, states that:[7]

> The nonprofit and voluntary sector is an economic force in Canada. It accounts for 6.8 percent of the nation's gross domestic product (GDP) and, when the value of volunteer work is incorporated, contributes 8.5 percent of the GDP. If one sets aside the one percent of organisations that are hospitals, universities, and colleges, the remaining organisations contribute 4.0 percent of the nation's GDP. Nonprofit and voluntary organisations employ 12 percent of Canada's economically active population, and provide 13 percent of its non-agricultural employment. Excluding the one-third of paid employees working for hospitals, colleges, and universities, the sector still employs nine percent of the economically active population and provides 10 percent of the non-agricultural employment. The entire nonprofit and voluntary sector engages nearly as many full-time equivalent workers as all branches of manufacturing in the country. Canada's nonprofit and voluntary sector is the second largest in the world when expressed as a share of the economically active population. It relies more on the efforts of paid employees than sectors in other countries. However, the absolute amount of volunteer effort exceeds both the average for developed countries and the overall international average, although it trails that of countries such as Sweden, Norway, the United Kingdom, and the United States. Service activities are a more dominant feature of nonprofit and voluntary organisational activity in Canada than is the case elsewhere. About 74 percent of all Canadian nonprofit and voluntary sector workers (both paid and volunteer) are engaged in the delivery of direct services such as education, health, and housing (compared to

64 percent internationally). Health organisations employ a much larger per-centage of workers in Canada than is the case in other countries. Overall, there are fewer individuals involved with organisations supporting expressive activities (e.g., arts, culture, religion, sports, recreation).

Canadian nonprofit and voluntary organisations receive more revenue from government than do those in other countries. This pattern is primarily attributable to the influence of hospitals, universities, and colleges. When these organisations are set aside, fees are the dominant source of revenue, followed by government payments. Government funding is particularly prominent in the fields of health, education, and social services, reflecting the special form that the welfare state has taken in Canada.

It has been estimated[8] that Canada's voluntary sector consists of approximately 175,000 organizations of which close to 81,000 are charities (80 per cent with an annual income of less than $250,000 per year) the income of which is to a large extent derived from service contracts. The sector employs approximately 1.3 million people or roughly 9 per cent of the national workforce, pays more than $40 billion annually in salaries and benefits and contributes approximately $90 billion per year to the Canadian economy.[9]

The retreat of the State as public service provider has resulted in funding shortages for a sector that has been accustomed to relying on government for 60 per cent of its funding, while also generating greater demands for its services and increased expectations as to its capacity to make good the public service shortfall.[10]

The social inclusion agenda

In this jurisdiction the social inclusion agenda comprises an interesting mix: some complex cultural divisions arising from its particular experience of colonialism; and some social issues not untypical of most modern western nations.

The First Nation people

The 'First Nation', indigenous or Aboriginal peoples of Canada were formally recognized in section 35 of the Constitution Act 1982 as comprising the Indian, Métis and Inuit communities.[11] The Inuit are the indigenous people of Nunavut,[12] a newly created territory of some 2 million square kilometres occupying almost one-fifth of the land mass of Canada with a population of a mere 26,745, of which 82 per cent are Inuit living in 28 villages.[13] In keeping with the experience of other common law countries, Canadian history also records abuse suffered by its First Nation people at the hands of the non-indigenous population.[14] This section of the population, with a socio-economic profile that includes higher than average rates of suicide, unemployment, homelessness, health care problems and family breakdown and with some communities suffering trans-generational embedded poverty, now represents a significant challenge to the government's social inclusion agenda. As observed by Stone J in *Native Communications Society of BC* v. *Minister of National Revenue*:[15]

> the State has assumed a special responsibility for the welfare of the Indian people. Unlike the vast majority of their fellow citizens they are rather a people set apart for particular assistance and protection in many aspects of their lives.

There is little indication from charity case law that issues affecting the circumstances of indigenous people are reaching the courts or that they are treated in an enlightened manner on the rare occasions when they do (though a significant body of other case law related to aboriginal issues has been developed over the past ten years, including at the Supreme Court of Canada level). In the above case the court recognized 'the special legal position in Canadian society occupied by the Indian people', but any hopes that this might lead to further helpful judicial determinations on behalf of indigenous people have not been realized.[16] In this post-colonial common law jurisdiction, the challenge for philanthropic intervention is in working with government bodies to find the leverage necessary to strengthen community capacity and assist community leaders to move indigenous people and communities from State dependency to a position of more autonomy.

The Anglo/French cultural divide

In tandem with the work of reconciling the cultures of its indigenous and non-indigenous people, this jurisdiction has also had to reconcile the French and English aspects of its colonial legacy and their respective legal systems. The tensions in the latter context reached a point where it seemed that the alienated Québécois would establish a separate constitutional identity within Canada. This movement stalled after the failure to secure a majority in the 1995 referendum but the reconciliation work necessary to build a truly civil society continues.

Poverty

Canada, an affluent and high-tech society, also has a considerable poverty problem,[17] evidenced by the fact that 'despite consecutive years of economic growth more than one million children, or almost one child in six, still live in poverty'.[18] This picture is reinforced by a research finding that:[19] 'Poverty increased throughout Canada in the early 1990s, but more so in metropolitan areas. Between 1990 and 1995, poor populations in metropolitan areas grew by 33.8 per cent, compared to 18.2 per cent outside metropolitan areas.' Due to the low wage levels 'for many Canadian families, having a job isn't a ticket out of poverty, but simply admission into the ranks of the working poor'.[20] These ranks are likely to consist of lone parents, people with disabilities, post-1990 immigrants, Aboriginal people and single people aged 45–59.

Health and social care

Canada has suffered a decade and more of public service retrenchment that has seen drastic cuts in health care and education services. The government is now faced with a considerable challenge if it is to ensure equity of access to such services for poorer sectors of the population.

Multicultural issues/immigration etc.

Canadian society is a diverse ethnic and cultural mix. It has one of the highest proportions of immigrants to total resident population of any country in the world: approximately 17 per cent compared to 10 per cent for the USA and less for European countries. In the last decade or two, the assimilation of waves of immigrants from non-European countries has broadened the diversity and increased cultural tensions.[21] Although, as the Ontario Court of Appeal noted in a 1990 case involving a charity that limited scholarships to white, Protestant, British subjects, racial discrimination 'is patently at variance with the democratic principles governing our pluralistic society in which equality rights are constitutionally guaranteed and in which the multicultural heritage of Canadians is to be preserved and enhanced'.[22] In practice this provincial law decision is now largely forgotten though the judicial approach is reflected in that adopted by Revenue Canada in relation to organizations established to eliminate racial discrimination or foster positive race relations within Canada.[23]

Need for a more inclusive agenda

The challenges now facing the government have been succinctly summarized as:[24]

• Rising income inequality – government taxes and transfers are doing less than in the past to even income distribution.
• A labour market polarised by globalisation into high-paid knowledge work and low-paid service work affects health and other forms of wellbeing.
• People may be poor even when employed. There is rising participation in employment, but also growth of precarious work paying inadequate wages.
• An ageing society and increased lone-parent and two-earner households leave families unable to provide children and vulnerable adults the care provided in the past.
• Difficulties in achieving social inclusion for immigrants and visible minorities and barriers to economic and social integration.
• Challenges to the advancement of Aboriginal peoples.

Government policy

In Canada, as in other common law countries, the process of shaping a new regulatory framework for charities and charitable activity is set within a government policy to consolidate its partnership with the voluntary sector. In this jurisdiction, the seeds for partnership were sown in 1995 when twelve national umbrella organizations covering most parts of the voluntary sector came together as the Voluntary Sector Roundtable to enhance the relationship between the sector and the government, to strengthen the sector's capacity, and to improve the legal and regulatory framework governing the sector.

Government, charities and preparations for a new regulatory framework

The work of the Voluntary Sector Roundtable led to the creation of the Voluntary Sector Initiative and then to its development of an *Accord Between the Government of Canada and the Voluntary Sector* which was reached by the Joint Accord Table (composed equally of voluntary-sector members and public servants) and signed in 2001. At the signing Prime Minister Jean Chrétien explained:[25]

> Today, more than ever before, Canada depends on the combined strength of its private, public and voluntary sectors. While each of these contributes to our quality of life and deserves recognition, we are showcasing today the special value of the voluntary sector. A sector that engages Canadians across the country in the life of their communities, providing services and giving voice to shared concerns. A sector that is, in short, essential to our collective well being.

History, definitional matters and legal framework

Although the Statute of Charitable Uses 1601 may never have had any direct application to this jurisdiction, nevertheless the history of Canadian charity law can in effect be traced back to the 1601 Act. It has subsequently largely evolved within the common law tradition with a form and content not dissimilar to other nations such as Ireland, Australia and New Zealand, all of which share the same heritage (see, further chapters 1 and 2).

Historical outline

As has been observed:[26]

> Canada has a long tradition of relying on nonprofit and voluntary organisations to address the needs and interests of its highly diverse population. This reliance had its beginnings in the voluntary activity of Canada's Aboriginal peoples, was formalised by the first French and English settlers, and grew with the arrival of immigrants from around the world. In the 20th century, the Canadian state built on these foundations by turning to nonprofit and voluntary organisations to deliver state-funded services.

The common law

Canada is a bijural jurisdiction in which, according to section 8.1 of the Interpretation Act 1985, 'both the common law and the civil law are equally authoritative and recognized sources of the law of property and civil rights in Canada'. However, although the civil law system remains in Quebec, the common law prevails at the federal level and is central to the nation-wide decision-making processes of Revenue Canada as governed by the Income Tax Act 1985. Charity law in this jurisdiction is therefore rooted in the common law and in Lord Macnaghten's classification of charitable purposes in *Pemsel*.[27] This source has been approved many times by Canadian courts, including the Supreme Court,[28] though arguably it may need to be tested again in the light of the Interpretation Act 2001.[29] Although the courts rely on the common law definition, their interpretation of 'charity' is somewhat narrower than in other common law jurisdictions.[30]

The legislation

The federal government, three territories and ten provinces that comprise the governing framework of Canada all have varying levels of jurisdiction over not-for-profit organizations and charities. Of primary importance to the law governing charities at all levels is the Income Tax Act 1985, but neither it nor any other legislation provides a definition of 'charity' or of 'charitable purposes'. However, for a charitable entity to qualify for tax-exempt status it must be a 'registered charity' with Revenue Canada which, under the 1985 Act, is defined as 'a charitable organisation, private foundation or public foundation' (see, further, p. 353). The following pieces of legislation provide the main federal milestones in the evolution of modern charity law in Canada.

- *The Constitution Act 1867*
  Section 92(7) of this Act directed that the jurisdiction for 'the establishment, maintenance and management of hospitals, asylums, charities and eleemosynary institutions' was to be a matter for provincial rather than federal legislature.
- *The War Charities Act 1917*
  This legislation was enacted to control fraudulent fundraising and encourage efficiency in charities supporting the war effort. It was the first federal legislation to govern charitable organizations.
- *An Act to Amend the Income Tax Act 1950*[31]
  This statute laid the foundations for the present differentiation between legal structures for charities by dividing them into charitable organizations, charitable trusts and charitable corporations.
- *The Income Tax Act Reforms 1972*
  Following the report of the Carter Commission[32] the federal government made some minor amendments[33] to the Income Tax Act 1950.

- *The Income Tax Act Reforms 1976*
  Following the issue of its Green Paper entitled *The Tax Treatment of Charities*,[34] the federal government introduced legislation[35] in a major reform of the federal tax regime applicable to charities. In addition to measures dealing with disbursement quotas, the statute introduced the present distinction between operating charities (charitable organizations) and granting charities (foundations), the latter being further divided into public and private foundations.

- *An Act to Amend the Income Tax Act and Related Statutes 1984*[36]
  Following its discussion paper entitled *Charities and the Canadian Tax System*,[37] the federal government introduced legislation dealing with the definition of charity, the political activities of charities, the possibility of extending tax-exempt status to 'citizen interest groups', the federal registration procedures and other matters.

- *A Better Tax Administration in Support of Charities 1990*[38]
  Following its review of the tax regime in the late 1980s, the federal government in 1990 published the above discussion paper which dealt with: the definitionof'relatedbusiness';disclosureconcerningfundraisingcosts;theforeign activities of charitable organizations; political activities; public disclosure requirements; and the annual filing requirement.

- *The Voluntary Sector Reform Proposals 1999*
  In 1999, having examined the environment for nonprofit organizations, the Voluntary Sector Roundtable issued two reports. The first, *Building on Strength: Improving Governance and Accountability in Canada's Voluntary Sector*, was from the Panel on Accountability and Governance in the Voluntary Sector, chaired by Ed Broadbent (the 'Broadbent Panel').[39] The second was the Report of the Joint Tables, *Working Together – A Government of Canada/Voluntary Sector Joint Initiative*, which made recommendations to improve the regulatory framework. This group consisted of leaders from the sector and key federal government (the 'Joint Tables report').[40]

In June 2000, a year after the issue of the Broadbent and Joint Tables reports, the Voluntary Sector Initiative was launched and the Joint Regulatory Table was then formed to address the issue of improving the legislative and regulatory environment in which the sector operates. In the following year the Government of Canada and the voluntary sector signed the Accord, designed to enhance the relationship between both parties and strengthen the capacity of the voluntary sector[41]. The Joint Regulatory Table continued the work on regulatory issues that had begun with its *Working Together* report and in 2003 issued its recommendations for an improved regulatory system in *Strengthening Canada's Charitable Sector: Regulatory Reform* (see, further, p. 368 *et seq.*).

Other federal legislation with an important if indirect bearing on charities included:

- *The Canada Corporations Act 1970*

This identified the terms and conditions for incorporating non-profit organizations.

- *The Competition Act 1985*
  This prohibited deceptive fundraising practices.
- *The Personal Information Protection and Electronic Documents Act 2000*
  This statute specifically prohibited the sale of donor, membership and other fundraising lists without the active consent of individuals on such lists.

Finally, it should be noted that in 2001 the federal government passed the *Federal Law – Civil Law Harmonization Act, No. 1*[42] and section 8.2 of the *Interpretation Act,*[43] which requires provincial law to be applied when interpreting a federal statute involving the law of property and civil rights.[44]

Definitional matters

In the words of Revenue Canada:

> as the Act (the Income Tax Act 1985, *sic*) does not define what is charitable, we look to the common law for both a definition of charity in its legal sense as well as the principles to guide us in applying that definition.[45]

Charitable intent

In Canada, as in England and Wales (see, also, chapters 3 and 8), the judiciary when determining charitable status will look to the intention of the testator. The presence or absence of altruism in the donor's intention will then be crucial to the judicial determination. This approach was illustrated in *Canada Trust Co.* v. *Ontario Human Rights Commission,*[46] which concerned a trust that provided scholarships on a restricted basis – to students who were needy, white, of British parentage or nationality, and Christian of the Protestant persuasion. The court, in considering whether the class restriction was contrary to public policy, sought evidence as to the testator's motivation and concluded that he had intended to be discriminatory.

This approach was reinforced in the report by Ontario Law Reform Commission which suggests that donor motivation is all-important.[47] Where a donor attaches 'malevolently discriminatory provisions' then the motivation is likely to be not altruism but racism, sexism or bigotry and therefore contrary to public policy. However, this provincial decision has little bearing on the federal registration process.

Public benefit

The public benefit test has an uneven application across the four *Pemsel* heads. As with other common law countries, there is a presumption in favour of charities that advance religion (and education). This presumption has given rise to some controversy in the light of the Canadian Charter of Rights and Freedoms.

Exclusively charitable

In Canada, a registered charity – whether a charitable organization, private foundation or public foundation – must be exclusively charitable in its purposes and activities. It is an organization 'whether incorporated or not, (a) all the resources of which are devoted to charitable activities'.[48]

The 'exclusively charitable' requirement, a long-established common law principle, is the main regulatory standard in the 1985 Act and is reinforced through the disbursement quotas.

As noted by Iacobucci J. in *Vancouver Society of Immigrant and Visible Minority Women* v. *M.N.R.*,[49] the question whether an organization is constituted exclusively for charitable purposes cannot be determined solely by reference to its stated purposes, but must also take into account the activities in which the organization is currently engaged. This 'activities test' is a significant characteristic of charity law in Canada.

Independent

In this jurisdiction importance is attached to the necessity of a charity maintaining a sense of distance between itself and those who may seek to influence the use of its resources. In particular, successive amendments have been made to the 1985 Act to protect a charity from being controlled by a donor of group of donors. In that event it will be deemed to have become a private foundation. However, government funding, being a very significant source of revenue for a limited number of charities (see, further, the National Survey of Nonprofit Voluntary Organizations report), also threatens to compromise their capacity to act independently.

Non-governmental

The dividing line between the public benefit service provision of government bodies and that of charities is somewhat uncertain. As noted in the Johns Hopkins report: 'current government funding practices appear to be turning many non-profit and voluntary organisations into cost-efficient extensions of government'.[50] This is evidenced by the fact that more than half (51 per cent) of all non-profit and voluntary sector revenue in Canada comes from government.[51] As that funding becomes more short-term, more competitive and less predictable, with support being targeted to government-prioritized programmes and projects, charities are finding it correspondingly more difficult to retain their independence from government.

This trend became more pronounced with the introduction of amendments to sections 110.1 and 118.1 of the Income Tax Act which expand the list of 'qualified donees' as defined in subsection 149.1(1) to include municipal or public bodies performing a function of government in Canada. The amendments became necessary after the Quebec Court of Appeal in *Tawich Development*

Corporation v. *Deputy Minister of Revenue of Quebec*[52] held that an entity could not attain the status of a municipality by exercising municipal functions, but only by statute, letters patent or order.

Nonprofit distributing

It had been widely believed (following *Alberta Institute of Mental Retardation* v. *The Queen*)[53] that a charity does not compromise its status as such by making a profit, providing that the profit does not accrue to individuals or shareholders[54] but is directed solely towards furthering its tax-exempt purpose – the so-called 'destination of funds' test. However, this test has since been specifically repudiated as good law in Canada.[55]

Charitable purposes

These are as first identified in the 1601 Act, later classified in *Pemsel* (see, further, chapter 3) and subsequently extended under the fourth head through use of the 'spirit and intendment' rule.[56] An interesting example of the latter occurred in *Everywoman's Health Centre Society* v. *Canada*,[57] concerning a society established to provide 'necessary medical services for women for the benefit of the community as a whole' and carrying on 'educational activities incidental to the above' in the form of a free-standing abortion clinic, which was found to be eligible for registration as a charity. The court held that:

> [the] Society's purposes and activities at this point in time [i.e. the operation of the clinic] are beneficial to the community within the spirit and intendment, if not the letter, of the preamble to the Statue of Elizabeth and ... the Society is a charitable organisation within the evolving meaning of charity at common law.

However, generally the fourth *Pemsel* head has been narrowly interpreted by the courts in this jurisdiction with the result, as pointed out in the Johns Hopkins report, that it:[58]

> excludes many organisations that are widely seen as providing public benefits (e.g., environmental organisations, rights groups, organisations providing services to ethnocultural groups). While Canadian charity laws are based on the same legal precedents as those in the United Kingdom and the United States, these countries have taken a broader view of the definition of charitable purpose.

Legal structures for charities

Most registered charities are incorporated. They can be incorporated under the laws of the provinces, which they mostly are, or they can be incorporated under federal law. Federal regulation, through the Income Tax Act 1985, is more pervasive than provincial regulation.

Types of structure

The Income Tax Act distinguishes first between non-profit organizations and charities. It then further distinguishes between charities that are registered as charitable organizations, public foundations or private foundations.

Charitable organizations   These are organizations that dedicate their resources to carrying out 'charitable activities'. They are primarily service-provider entities and are not permitted to make grants totalling more than 50 per cent of their income in any one year. They may take the form of a trust, unincorporated association or corporation. Registered charitable organizations can be incorporated under the incorporation statutes of any of the individual Canadian provinces or territories. It is also possible to incorporate under a federal statute, the Canada Corporations Act, as a 'nonshare capital' corporation, which permits the organization to operate in all Canadian jurisdictions.

Foundations   There are specific statutory rules affecting foundations in Canada, which distinguish between private and public foundations, in addition to registered charities. Under the Income Tax Act, a registered charity is a 'public foundation' if:

- it is constituted and operated exclusively for charitable purposes;
- it is a corporation or a trust; and
- it gives more than 50 per cent of its income annually to qualified donees. (This provision disqualifies a grant-making charity from being a charitable organization and applies equally to public and private foundations.)

A registered charity is a 'private foundation' if:

- it is constituted and operated exclusively for charitable purposes;
- it is a corporation or trust; and
- it is not a 'charitable organization' or a 'public foundation'.

Although, as has been pointed out: 'The more important distinction is that a public foundation and charitable organisation must receive more than 50% of its capital from unrelated sources and and 50% of its directors must be at arm's length from each other.'[59]
The Income Tax Act imposes greater restrictions on private foundations than charitable organizations or public foundations. In Canada the term 'private foundation' generally means a family foundation. The fastest-growing sector of philanthropy in Canada is community foundations, which recorded 83.2 per cent growth in assets between 1994 and 1997.[60]

The July 2005 amendments to the Income Tax Act 1985

The above definitions of charitable organizations and public foundations (as *per* subsection 149.1(1) of the Act) were amended in July 2005 by consolidating legislation that replaced the 'contribution' test with a new 'control' test. The rationale for amending the definitions was to permit such charities to receive large gifts from donors without concern that they may be deemed to be private foundations.

Regulatory framework

In Canada, the regulatory framework for charities is revenue-driven and therefore dominated by tax legislation. The Constitution provides that taxation is to be a federal matter which enables the federal government, in effect, to determine the grounds for charitable tax exemption. This it has done in the Income Tax Act 1985. The Canada Customs and Revenue Agency (Revenue Canada, as it became known in late 1999), is the federal authority responsible for regulating charities under the Income Tax Act and for registering and revoking charitable tax-exempt status. The Constitution Act 1867, however, makes provincial governments responsible for establishing, maintaining and managing charities operating in and for the provinces (the 1867 Act, together with the Quebec Act 1774, guarantees Quebec the right to apply the civil law of gift to charitable donations) while Parliament has given the same jurisdiction to the territories. The majority of provinces, with the primary exception of Ontario, do not single out nor do they regularly supervise charities.

This bifurcated approach to regulating charities places a clear and firm priority on establishing revenue collection as the governing function, to be addressed by a coherent body of tax legislation administered in a standardized fashion by a central government agency. It leaves to the legislatures of provinces and territories the lesser functions of charity support, supervision and the development of charitable purposes.

Registering charities

The responsibility for determining charitable status and registering charities is vested by the Income Tax Act 1985 in the Minister of Revenue and transferred through ancillary regulations to the director of the Charities Division (now the Charities Directorate) of the Canada Customs and Revenue Agency (Revenue Canada). In this jurisdiction, tax-exempt status does not wholly equate with charitable status: all non-profits are equally tax-exempt; if not registered as a charity, a non-profit organization would still be tax-exempt.

Registration

The Income Tax Act 1985 provides for the registration of charities.[61] Under section 248(1) a registered charity means:

(1)   a charitable organisation, private foundation or public foundation, within the meanings assigned by subsection 149.1(1), that is resident in Canada and was either created or established in Canada,

(2)   that has applied to the Minister in prescribed form for registration and that is at that time registered as a charitable organisation, private foundation or public foundation.

In determining whether an organization is registerable as a charity, Revenue Canada will examine its purposes and activities: both must be charitable and all of the organization's resources must be devoted exclusively to those activities (subject to the 10 per cent rule in respect of political activities). It must also maintain proper records and is required to disburse a certain amount on its charitable activities each year (the 'disbursement quota'). Generally, a charity must spend for charitable purposes at least 80 per cent of an amount equal to the 'receipted' income received in the immediately preceding taxation year.[62] Approximately 4,000 organizations apply for charitable registration each year of which 3,000 are approved and about 2,500 charities are deregistered.[63]

Transparency   Since the introduction of the 1998 amendment to the Income Tax Act, Revenue Canada may, at the request of any individual, release information regarding a registered charity's governing documents, the names of its directors and any warnings, conditions or revocation relating to its registration, including the reasons.[64] Every charity must file an annual Registered Charity Information Return with Revenue Canada and while much of that information is available to the public, the results of any audit conducted by that agency regarding the affairs of a charity are confidential. Certain religious charities are exempted from the public reporting requirement regarding financial information.

Regulating charities

Revenue Canada is the central regulatory body for charities and its Charities Division conducts between 500 and 600 audits each year. Under the Income Tax Act, each of the subdivisions of 'registered charity' – charitable organizations, public foundations and private foundations – are separately regulated. The only regulatory sanction effectively available to Revenue Canada is deregistration, which can be imposed for failures such as not meeting disbursement quotas, improper record-keeping and infringement of rules relating to business activities.[65]

The courts and the Attorney General

In Canada the opportunities for judicial consideration of matters of principle and purpose in charity law arise so infrequently that the courts have long since lost their power to adjust the law to fit contemporary social circumstances. On the rare occasions when such opportunities do occur, it is largely by way of appeal (an expensive and lengthy process) to the federal Court of Appeal from a Revenue Canada decision to: deny an application for registration as a charity; remove such registration; or designate an organization (as a charitable organization, public foundation or private foundation) with a status disputed by that organization. As noted in the *Strengthening Canada* report:[66]

> Perhaps the most striking thing about the number of appeals that have been launched from the Charities Directorate's decisions is that only 28 charity cases in total have ever gone to court. And of these 28 cases, nearly half have produced judgments that were brief, dealt with procedural issues, or otherwise did not produce precedents in charity law.

The role of the Attorney General has become nominal and is now largely of procedural interest only.

The Solicitor General

The new Charities Registration (Security Information) Act gives the Minister the power to jointly sign a certificate with the Solicitor General, and if the certificate is upheld as reasonable by a judge of the Federal Court, it disqualifies an organization from registration.

Regulating the fiscal environment

The Income Tax Act 1985 regulates the fiscal environment for charities.[67] Not only does it provide a federal power for determination of their charitable status but that power also provides for their supervision, requires annual income tax returns and allows for the deductability of donations to charities. In addition, the provinces also have a role in regulating charities, in particular overseeing their fiduciary relationships, ensuring that there is no fraud, etc.[68]

The Canada Customs and Revenue Agency (Revenue Canada)

Revenue Canada has regulatory responsibility for all matters relating to tax liability and, in the absence of any body with functions similar to the Charity Commission in England and Wales, it effectively governs charities through the federal powers provided by the Income Tax Act.

Tax and rates

Two major benefits result from acquiring charitable status: exemption from income tax under Division H of Part 1 of the Income Tax Act (which is largely available to all non-profits); and the ability to issue donation receipts to both corporate and individual donors. Of the latter, as Iacobucci, J. has noted, this additional benefit is 'designed to encourage the funding of activities which are generally regarded as being of special benefit to society' and is potentially 'a major determinant' of the success of a charitable organization.[69]

In Canada there are no death duties and no gift taxes (though there is a deemed disposition on death which triggers capital gains taxes and therefore is a form of death duty; further, a gift is a disposition so the donor will pay taxes on the transfer if there is any capital gain). In relation to the federal Goods and Services Tax (GST), all registered charities are entitled to a rebate of one-half of the GST, regardless of revenue source. Some charities are entitled to larger rebates (primarily hospitals and universities).

Donation incentives

Under the Canadian tax credit system for individuals,[70] a donor is entitled to claim the full fair market value of any gift made to a qualified donee for tax relief. In 2002, the federal level of relief for an individual consisted of a tax credit of 16 per cent[71] of the value of the gift up to CD$200 of annual gifting and 29 per cent of the value in excess of this amount. The true value of the tax credit is much higher since it also comprises an addition for applicable surtaxes and for provincial taxes. The net result is that the individual tax credit is equivalent to a full deduction, aside and apart from the first CD$200. The rules for corporate donors are the same except that corporations get a deduction, not a tax credit.

Foundation disbursements

In addition, all charities must now disburse an additional amount equivalent to 3.5 per cent (4.5 per cent before the introduction of the 2005 amendments) of investment assets. Private foundations must also disburse 100 per cent of investment and all gifts received from other charities, less specified gifts. The disbursement quota for a public foundation and a charitable organization is the same as that for a private foundation (as detailed above) except that they must spend 80 per cent of all amounts received from other registered charities during its immediately preceding year, less any 'specified gifts'.

Cy-près

Canadian courts apply the doctrine of *cy-près* to alter the purposes or to dispose of the assets of charitable trusts (see, also, chapter 3). Should the charity become defunct, its assets must be available to be redirected by a *cy-près* scheme to the same purposes.

Fundraising

There are no federal fundraising guidelines and generally a light regulatory regime prevails at provincial and territorial level, though Alberta has a Charitable

Fundraising Act. Fundraising legislation governs the manner of fundraising, required registration and record-keeping, etc. for charities and other non-profits that solicit funds or otherwise raise funds from the general public of more than CD$25,000.

Trading

Charitable organizations and public foundations are permitted to conduct 'related business activities' while private foundations are prohibited from carrying on any business activities. The Canadian courts previously held that any activity was a related business activity if the profits were used in the charitable activities of that organization, and this approach was endorsed in *Alberta Institute of Mental Retardation* v. *The Queen*.[72] In its comments on this case, the Quebec Law Reform Commission criticized the criteria relied upon by the court and suggested, more simply, that 'a business is unrelated unless the business directly advances the charitable purposes of the charity or is ancillary or incidental to the advancement of those purposes'.[73] As noted earlier, the Federal Court of Appeal has now clearly stated that the 'destination of funds' theory is not the law in Canada.[74] There are, however, cases where a charity in Canada has established a wholly owned subsidiary to carry on business activities.

Constraints on modern philanthropic activity

Philanthropy in Canada occurs against a complex background. The charity law framework is itself subject to the overarching principles of the Constitution, the Charter of Rights and Freedoms, the Canadian Human Rights Act and to the cross-cutting provisions of various statutes such as the Canada Corporations Act 1970 and the Personal Information Protection and Electronic Documents Act 2000. It must respond to its colonial legacy as represented by the needs of indigenous people and to the aspirations of the Québécois. It needs to address the cultural isolation experienced by the waves of recent non-European immigrants. There are also the difficulties presented by a domestic social inclusion agenda not untypical of other modern western nations which require the needs of those suffering, for example, from poverty, disability, age and gender discrimination to be acknowledged and attended to. The response must then be co-ordinated in a coherent fashion across multi-level tiers of government. It is unsurprising that the effort to achieve this, using the provisions of a 400-year-old statute as the principal tool, have not been wholly successful.

Policy constraints: partnership with government

As in England and Wales, Ireland and New Zealand, the task of shaping a modern legal environment for philanthropy is being undertaken in the context of a partnership arrangement between government and the voluntary sector. While the advantages of partnership to the former are clear, it is not without difficulties for the latter.

National umbrella organizations

In recent years, many charities have coalesced in groups or consortia under the aegis of umbrella organizations formed to support, educate, represent their interests and raise the public profile of the sector. The strategic importance of these umbrella organizations is apparent in the pivotal role they play in negotiating on behalf of their membership with government bodies. However, they can only acquire and retain charitable status if they also give effect to charitable purposes, i.e. deliver charitable programmes. Their capacity to perform a strategic role is in effect compromised by the requirement that they also perform as a charity.[75]

Government grants and contracts

Charities in Canada as elsewhere risk compromising their obligation to remain independent by becoming increasingly reliant upon the grants and service-delivery contracts provided by government bodies.

First Nation people

In Canada as in New Zealand there is a policy to positively discriminate in public service provision to favour indigenous people.[76] This has been reinforced by the courts and by Revenue Canada, which have determined that purposes and activities restricted to the needs of Aboriginal peoples of Canada are charitable and meet the public benefit test. However, the policy itself is insufficient to overcome the common law obstacles associated with nexus of relationship that can impede philanthropic intervention on behalf of small groups and local communities.

International aid

That Canadian charities may contribute to the alleviation of distress in other jurisdictions has been accepted since at least *Lewis* v. *Doerle*,[77] where a trust – to promote, aid and protect citizens of the US of African descent, in the enjoyment of their civil rights as provided by the US constitution – was held charitable. It is clear also that the charitable status of such an organization is not dependent upon it also contributing to the public benefit within its home jurisdiction,[78] unlike the equivalent position in England and Wales where in some circumstances this is open to doubt.[79] The constraint represented by the ruling in *McGovern*,[80] however, does operate to restrain charities in Canada, as in England and Wales, from engaging elsewhere in activities that could expose them within the jurisdiction to the accusation that they are seeking to change laws or policies (see, also, chapters 6 and 8).

Common law constraints

The characteristics of the common law legacy operate to constrain Canadian charitable activity in much the same way as in England and Wales (see, also, chapter 8).

The 'spirit and intendment' rule

In Canada, more so than in other common law jurisdictions (excepting England and Wales, where it no longer has much relevance), this rule has generally been applied conservatively, restricting the potential to creatively develop charitable purposes to meet contemporary circumstances. Judicial disdain was typified by the attitude of Southey J in *Re Laidlaw Foundation*,[81] when the court in Ontario held all purposes beneficial to the community (in this case, amateur sport) as being within the spirit and intendment rule but he added that it is 'highly artificial and of no real value . . . to pay lip-service to the preamble of a statute passed in the reign of Elizabeth 1'. However, in a notable exception, the court in *Re Vancouver Regional Free Net Association and Minister of National Revenue*[82] utilized the rule to confirm the charitable status of an organization established to provide free community access to the Internet, the rationale being that the service could be viewed as a contemporary equivalent to the 'highways' declared charitable in the Preamble.

Legal structures

In Canada there is the customary reliance upon the common law structures of trusts, unincorporated associations and corporations (construed, in this jurisdiction, as different species of the genre 'charitable organization') and clear statutory recognition is given to public and private foundations as having an equal legal standing (all are incorporated entities, trusts or statutory creations). The former are subject to the same limitations in this jurisdiction as elsewhere (see, for example, chapter 8).

Restrictions on advocacy/political activity

In Canada, as in other common law jurisdictions, the restriction on political activities continues to inhibit effective lobbying by charitable organizations on behalf of the socially disadvantaged. Such prohibited activities are deemed to include communicating to the public that the law, policy or decision of any level of government in Canada or a foreign country should be retained, opposed, or changed. The Income Tax Act does, however, allow limited amounts of political activity. It permits an organization to carry out such activities provided that:[83]

- it devotes part of its resources to political activities;
- those political activities are ancillary and incidental to its charitable activities; and

- those political activities do not include the direct or indirect support of, or opposition to, any political party or candidate for public office.

The traditional common law restriction is reinforced by a Canadian novelty – the so-called '10 per cent rule' – which, in effect, operationalizes the requirement in the Income Tax Act that an if organization devotes 'substantially all' of its resources to charitable purposes and only a small part is directed towards non-partisan political activities of an 'ancillary and incidental' nature, then it may retain its charitable status.[84] The effect of this restriction has been illustrated in a number of cases. For example, in *Re Co-operative College of Canada and Saskatchewan Human Rights Commission*[85] the college had an object 'to protect the interests of co-operatives and credit unions by appropriate action in making representations to legislative, administrative, judicial and other bodies'. The aim of changing the law to favour credit unions was held to be political and therefore vitiated the organization's claim to be exclusively charitable.[86] In *NDG Neighbourhood Association* v. *Minister of National Revenue*,[87] the Notre Dame de Grace Neighbourhood Association, an organization devoted to the interests of the urban poor and dealing with social issues in the community, accessibility to community resources, development of educational facilities and services to the disadvantaged, was held not to be charitable, again on the grounds of political activity. The emphasis on lobbying and on defending people's rights made the organization too political for these activities to be incidental and ancillary. Because, as was judicially stated, the organization 'not only has activities beyond education but . . . it is in effect an activist organisation',[88] it failed to qualify as a charity. Again it may be that, despite its stated purposes and its various activities, a charity is in fact pursuing a political agenda. This was found to be the case in *Alliance for Life* v. *M.N.R.*,[89] where the Federal Court of Appeal upheld the decision of Revenue Canada to deregister an organization on the basis that its educational activities were in fact efforts to promote its political views on pro-life issues in order to influence public attitudes.

Determining whether activities amount to charitable education or political advocacy is a difficult and very uncertain matter accompanied by the dire penalty of loss of charitable status.[90] This risk acts as a considerable restraint on the advocacy activities of organizations and on funding by donors, particularly the larger foundations, as the consequences of becoming embroiled in such a dispute are so serious. In particular, the fact that advocacy or campaigns to raise public awareness may be interpreted as political activity can have grievous consequences for the socially disadvantaged.[91] This situation is further compounded by a perception[92] that Revenue Canada applies these ill-defined advocacy rules in an inconsistent, arbitrary or discriminatory manner.[93] The Broadbent report gave some consideration to this matter and recommended that the government should:[94]

> Reaffirm and maintain the legitimacy of space for non-partisan political advocacy. While partisan activities should continue to be forbidden, the right to bearing a public witness on an issue affecting the very purpose of a charitable organisation should be affirmed. The rules governing advocacy

activity need to be clarified in ways that can be better understood, that militate against arbitrary application and that cohere with the values of a healthy civil society.

This recommendation was subsequently endorsed by the Joint Tables Report. Arguably, the restrictions may also impede the right to freedom of expression as upheld in section 2(b) of the Charter of Rights and Freedoms.[95]

Fiscal issues

In this jurisdiction, the government's commitment to the revenue-driven approach as a basis for regulating charities is very evident.

Revenue Canada's tax compliance role   The federal role of this agency is limited to helping charities comply with the Income Tax Act. The Voluntary Sector Initiative has, however, broadened its remit in respect of educating and providing support to the sector.

Revenue Canada sanctions   The traditional concern to regulate charities so that opportunities for tax avoidance are minimized has been evidenced by the blunt powers vested in Revenue Canada. The lack of intermediate sanctions available to this agency has forced charities to adopt a conservative role, avoiding entrepreneurial initiatives, rather than risk exposure to the deregistration sanction.[96] However, as previously noted, intermediate sanctions came into law in 2005.

First Nations and qualified donee status   In *Tawich Development Corporation* v. *Deputy Minister of Revenue of Quebec*[97] the court held that merely exercising municipal functions was not sufficient to attribute to a body the status of a municipality. This status could only be achieved as a result of statute, letters patent or order. In response, Revenue Canada drafted amendments to the Income Tax Act to include 'public bodies performing a function of government' within the category of qualified donees. However, to qualify for such recognition, a band must be considered to be a public body performing a function of government. This imputes a requirement that it has either been acknowledged as performing such a function within by-laws passed under subsections 81 and 83 of the Indian Act, or it has reached an 'advanced stage of development' as formerly required under the Indian Act.[98] Although the introduction of amendments to sections 110.1 and 118.1 of the 1985 Act have been interpreted generously by Revenue Canada, the constraint that a band, as a political body, is not always able to obtain the status of a qualified donee, would seem to impose an avoidable burden upon one of Canada's most socially disadvantaged minority groups.

The doctrine of cy-près   The fact that in Canada the jurisdiction to settle *cy-près* schemes remains exclusively judicial makes the process cumbersome, expensive and time-consuming.

Fundraising, trading, etc.   The lack of an adequate regulatory system governing accounting and fundraising in the various provinces does not promote public confidence and may well act as a constraint to these methods of raising revenue for charitable activities.

Overseas charitable intervention   Intervention outside the jurisdiction by Canadian registered charities is limited to either making a donation to a 'qualified donee' or to carrying out charitable activities directly itself. The provisions of the Income Tax Act 1985, preventing such a charity from simply sending funds or other resources to an intermediary charity based in the foreign jurisdiction, constitute an unnecessary constraint on prompt action in circumstances where urgent relief is required. While this can to some extent be circumvented by the recipient overseas charity contracting as an agent of the one registered in Canada, and thus placing the latter in a position to technically comply with the 'own activities' test, it is nonetheless a hindrance.

Public benefit matters

In addition to the above-mentioned definitional aspects of the public benefit test there are others that are particularly counter-productive in the context of Canada's social inclusion agenda.

Uneven application of the public benefit test   As with other common law countries, there is an uneven application of the public benefit test across the four *Pemsel* heads coupled with a non-statutory presumption that it will be satisfied in relation to gifts to religious and educational organizations.

The First Nation people and the advancement of education   In Canada, as in New Zealand and Australia, there can be difficulty in marrying the traditional common law interpretation of 'education' with modern methods of communication and skill development to achieve charitable status for organizations engaged in developmental roles with indigenous communities. For example, in *Native Communications Society of B.C. v. Minister of National Revenue*[99] the central issue was whether the provision of an outreach multimedia communications service to link up dispersed indigenous communities could be defined as charitable. The Minister's decision to refuse charitable status, on the ground that such activities could not be construed as advancing education, was overturned by the Federal Court of Appeal, which found the activities charitable under the fourth *Pemsel* head. The more recent *Vancouver Society of Immigrant and Visible Minority Women v. M.N.R.*[100] did not concern Canada's indigenous people but did concern an issue with direct bearing on their circumstances. In that case the court held that a society with objects of providing educational forums and workshops to immigrant women to help them find employment, and carrying on incidental and ancillary political activities and raising funds for these purposes, was held not to be eligible for registration as a charity on the basis that the objects of the organization were not exclusively charitable. This decision was a considerable setback for the potentially strategic role that charities could conceivably play in facilitating the social inclusion of minority groups. The, perhaps enduring, significance of this Supreme Court judgment, however, lies in the finding made by Iacobucci J. that the definition of 'educational' could encompass the workshops, seminars, etc. which the society provided. He further held that providing information and advice for a narrowly defined purpose, such as attaining employment, was also advancing education. This judicial view may in the long run have important ramifications for the role of charities in the context of political activities. Both cases illustrate the present constraints imposed on philanthropic intervention by archaic common law precedents that prevent a broader interpretation of education capable of addressing the contemporary needs of indigenous communities.

The First Nation people and the 'poor relations' rule In Canada, as in New Zealand, the blood-link is a characteristic of indigenous communities and gives rise to the ancillary issue as to whether this constitutes a personal nexus that compromises the 'public' component of the public benefit test, and therefore the capacity of indigenous communities to establish organizations with charitable status or that of charities to work with such communities. The guidance issued by Revenue Canada indicates that this rule is operative:[101]

> An organisation cannot qualify for registration with purposes established to assist Aboriginal Peoples of Canada if it further restricts its beneficiaries to a limited class of eligible persons, also known as 'a class within a class'. For example, limiting beneficiaries to a particular nation that excludes members of other nations does not meet the necessary element of public benefit.

This approach, in contrast to that adopted in New Zealand, must significantly inhibit the development of community-based philanthropic initiatives.

Modern law constraints

In Canada, as in most other common law countries, the main constraints on the development of more relevant and effective methods of philanthropic intervention stem from the fact that the regulatory framework conforms to the archetypal revenue-driven model.

Lack of coherence in charity law administration

Under section 92(7) of the Constitution Act 1882, the provinces have been given the authority to make laws regarding the 'establishment, maintenance, and management of charities in and for the Province'. Federal supervision is focused on ensuring that charities registered with Revenue Canada comply with the requirements of the Income Tax Act 1985 in order to receive related tax-exempt benefits. Provincial supervision ranges from virtually no regulation to imposing a

significant supervisory regime. Some provinces, notably Ontario, have sophisticated systems for registering and supervising charities, ensuring that charitable
assets are used only for charitable purposes. Other provinces and municipalities
have introduced fundraising legislation. There is no co-ordinating mechanism
between federal and provincial levels regarding charities, no opportunity to
develop a consistent approach in their interpretation of the law and considerable
uncertainty in some instances (e.g. in relation to nation-wide umbrella organizations) as to which level of supervision is appropriate.

There is also disparity between the provinces regarding the department vested
with responsibility for charities. The office of the Attorney General is sometimes
so designated while at other times it is the Minister of Finance, the Minister of
Government Services or some other minister. As has been pointed out 'this means
that charity regulation does not get on the agenda of federal-provincial ministers
because no such gathering brings together the disparate ministers responsible for
the issue'.[102]

This multi-level regulatory approach is a constraint on charities as they have to
negotiate tiers of rules, and on the general public who are uncertain where regulatory responsibility lies. More serious, however, is the likelihood that its effects are
also felt by the socially disadvantaged who may be confused as to where to look for
authoritative information and thus inhibited from seeking assistance.

Lack of an appropriate forum for developing charitable purposes

In Canada, any liberal development of philanthropic purposes, methods or structures is at the discretion of Revenue Canada and would logically be counter to its
main function. As has been said:[103]

> In the entire history of the Charities Directorate involvement with charities,
> there has not been a single reported legal decision in which CCRA (Revenue
> Canada, *sic*) has intervened or litigated to preserve a gift to charity. The cases
> are legion in which CCRA has litigated to deny that the transfer of property
> to a charity was a gift.

Moreover, this agency is required to follow judicially established precedents
which, as fewer and fewer charitable issues appear before the courts, tend to be
very dated and not always applicable to contemporary circumstances. The first
level of appeal from a Revenue Canada decision is to the federal Court of Appeal
which is prohibitively expensive for most charities and where matters are determined through judicial reliance on established precedents, which serves mainly to
perpetuate an archaic interpretation of charity. As in other common law jurisdictions, the lack of an alternative and more accessible forum, such as the Charity
Commission in England and Wales, has resulted in a certain ossifying of the law
which has had a constraining effect on practice.[104] In the field of race relations,
for example, the decision of the British courts in *Re Strakosch*[105] that 'appeasing
racial feeling within the community' was a political purpose and therefore

non-charitable, was followed by and remained binding on Revenue Canada until renounced by it in 2003.[106]

Human rights, anti-terrorism and social justice legislation

As a modern liberal democracy, Canada has in place much the same set of laws addressing much the same domestic social justice concerns (equity, equality and non-discriminatory practices, etc.) as other such nations. These are most often legislated for at provincial and territorial level though some, like the Employment Equity Act 1995, are the subject of federal legislation. This body of legislative provision is set within the governing principles to be found in the British North America Act 1867 and the Constitution Act 1982.

Constitution rights   Section 2(a) of the Charter of Rights and Freedoms guarantees the right to freedom of religion and conscience. Its relevance to a charity depends on the extent to which the latter can be defined as engaged in 'public' purposes. Any organization exercising statutory powers would be subject to the Charter,[107] as would any public or quasi-public institution 'insofar as they act in furtherance of a specific governmental program or policy'. Where the purposes of an organization breach the fundamental legal principles of the Charter, it cannot be said to be acting in the public benefit and therefore cannot claim or retain charitable status. For example, in *Wren*[108] a discriminatory restrictive covenant prejudiced against Jews was struck down. However, many charitable organizations and their activities represent positive discrimination as they undoubtedly intend to benefit some to the exclusion of others. Again, in *Canada Trust Co.* v. *Ontario Human Rights Commission*[109] the Ontario Court of Appeal, overturning the decision of the court at first instance, found that the Leonard Foundation was not a charitable trust as the blatantly discriminatory basis upon which it operated was contrary to public policy.

The uncertainty regarding such an interpretation of discrimination may unduly constrain well-intentioned charitable organizations and require legislative clarification. As has been noted, 'the difficulty will be to define the difference or point of balance between discrimination that is prohibited on the grounds of public policy and discrimination that is permitted because it advances a legitimate interest of a legitimate community'.[110]

Human rights   The Canadian Bill of Rights 1960 followed by the Canadian Human Rights Act 1985 gave rise to provincial and territorial human rights legislation that prohibits, among other things, discrimination because of race, religion or creed, colour, nationality, ancestry and place of origin.[111] The International Centre for Human Rights and Democratic Development Act 1985, established that Centre to initiate, encourage and support co-operation between Canada and other countries in the promotion, development and strengthening of democratic and human rights institutions and programmes that give effect to the rights and freedoms enshrined in the International Bill of Human Rights.

Nonetheless, in *Toronto Volgograd Committee* v. *M.N.R.*,[112] an organization devoted to promoting peace and understanding between Toronto and Volgograd in the USSR through education, public awareness, exchanges and meetings was denied charitable status because its activities and objects were viewed by the court as 'no more than propaganda', being 'education for a political cause, by the creation of a climate of opinion'. It would seem, in this instance, that modern legislative intent failed to prevail against established charity law precedents.

Anti-terrorism   The events of 9/11, followed by UN Security Council Resolution 1373 (see, further, chapter 6), prompted Canada and many other modern western nations to introduce anti-terrorism legislation and measures to prevent the international flow of charity money to fund terrorism. The Anti-Terrorism Act 2001 was such a response. Part 6 of that Act also created the new Charities Registration (Security Information) Act 2001 which in section 2(2)(b) authorizes the scrutiny of financial data on organizations for the purpose of 'determining eligibility to become or remain a registered charity'. However, as has been pointed out:

> the focus should not be solely on the destination of the money ... it is important to realise that donors to charities that misuse their funds for terrorist or other purposes may be victims who have been failed by the regulatory regime in Canada rather than being villains 'funding', 'facilitating' or 'contributing to' terrorism.[113]

The use of these powers, accompanied by the suspicion that some charities may be tainted by association as a consequence of their humanitarian involvement in countries with regimes inimical to government policy, may well deter funders and obstruct overseas charitable activity.

Other legislation such as the Foreign Missions Amendment Act 2002 and the Public Safety Act 2004 has reinforced the tough Canadian legislative response to the threat of terrorism and illustrates a more general contemporary trend in which the contrast between government reluctance to invest in regulatory frameworks that would facilitate good causes as opposed to an enthusiasm for investing in those that might prevent bad ones has become very striking.

Charity law review and social inclusion

The Ontario Law Reform Commission has the distinction of completing the first of the many charity law reviews conducted by common law jurisdictions. Its *Report on the Law of Charities*[114] was a challenging and philosophical study that stimulated a debate on the necessity to transform traditional charity law into an appropriate legal framework for contemporary philanthropy that has continued ever since across the common law world. Subsequently the Supreme Court of Canada suggested that the definition of charity in Canada should be broadened,[115] commentators have agreed[116] and a review of the not-for-profit and charity sector in Canada also suggested broadening the definition.[117]

Proposed changes to definitional matters and legal structures

In May 2003 the Joint Regulatory Table issued its report *Strengthening Canada's Charitable Sector: Regulatory Reform*. In March 2004, the federal government announced that it accepted 69 of the table's 75 recommendations. The bill was introduced and approved in 2005 and the recommendations (minus the six the government did not accept) are now in effect.

The report of the Joint Regulatory Table cannot, however, be seen as an extension of the work done by the Ontario Law Reform Commission as it did not have a broad mandate to review and suggest changes to the law of charities. It had six issues referred to it (by agreement between government and the sector) and was responsible for two action items – amendments to the annual reporting form and changes in the rules related to business activities. Although the *Strengthening Canada* report did not deal solely and specifically with charity law, as the majority of its recommendations have now been translated into legislation it must form the basis for the following consideration of the possible future federal alignment of charity law and social inclusion in Canada.

Charitable purpose

The Joint Regulatory Table notes that 'charity' is not legislatively defined, but other than explaining the *Pemsel* classification it goes no further than to suggest that 'policy guidelines should be developed on the nature and extent of the regulator's authority to identify new charitable purposes that flow from the application of the common law to organisations under the Income Tax Act'.[118]

Public benefit

The Ontario Law Reform Commission, in its *Report on the Law of Charities*, proposes that 'charity' should be defined as the altruistic provision to others of 'the means of pursuing a common or universal good'.[119] This is not pursued in the Joint Regulatory Table report.

Legal structures

The Joint Regulatory Table does not question the adequacy of existing structures for charities and makes no proposals for change.

Changes to the regulatory framework

The Joint Regulatory Table recommended that government and the sector should undertake a thorough review of regulatory issues affecting those not-for-profit organizations that are not charities.[120] It suggested that four fundamental principles should guide federal regulatory reform:

1   the regulatory framework that governs charities should facilitate public trust in the work of charities in Canada;
2   the regulatory framework should uphold the integrity of the provisions in the Income Tax Act that govern charities;
3   the regulatory framework should ensure fair application of the law and transparency in regulatory decision-making processes and;
4   the regulatory process should be as simple, non-duplicative and cost-effective as possible.

Primary regulatory body

The Joint Regulatory Table was specifically prohibited from making any recommendations in respect of the primary regulatory body. Instead it was confined to examining various models and to a discussion of the benefits and disadvantages of each. Their report does, however, state that the present system needs to be furthered developed.

Regulatory functions   Building on the work of the 1999 Joint Tables process, the report suggests four possible federal regulatory models for charities that could be considered:

1   an enhanced Charities Directorate that would continue to operate within Revenue Canada;
2   a complementary agency that would work alongside Revenue Canada;
3   a hybrid model that would split regulatory functions between two institutional bodies; and
4   an independent commission.

Each model would be assessed in terms of its ability to: ensure public confidence in voluntary organizations; maintain the integrity of the tax system; and ensure a supportive and enabling environment for voluntary organizations. It also notes that there would be benefit in exploring opportunities to develop a better co-ordinated system of regulation with the provinces and territories.

Support functions   The Joint Regulatory Table report acknowledged a need to provide charities with a broad education/support or 'nurturing' service but considered that this should not fall to Revenue Canada except insofar as support and education are needed on issues of registration and compliance with the Income Tax Act. The report considered that a different body from within the sector should provide guidance to voluntary organizations. It also recommended that a ministerial advisory group be established with broad representation from the voluntary sector, national umbrella organizations, lawyers and other allied professionals.[121] This recommendation resulted in the Charities Advisory Committee being established to provide a forum for ongoing discussion of regulatory issues.

In fact it has gone further and established the Charities Advisory Committee as well as a Technical Issues Committee.

Registration

The Joint Regulatory Table report suggests that new procedures be put in place to operationalize principles of transparency and accessibility in relation to the register, subject to the need to protect the privacy rights of charities. Also, new appeal provisions became law in May 2005 under section 172.

The role of the courts

The Joint Regulatory Table report suggests that to save time and money a new forum for reviewing Revenue Canada decisions should be established within Revenue Canada that would provide an expeditious process confined to reviewing the relevant file and reconsidering the decision. In addition, accepting that more cases should be brought before the courts so that the decisions can clarify charity law in complex or novel cases, the report recommends access to the Tax Court of Canada for a *de novo* hearing before referral to the federal Court of Appeal. Any such appeal process should be eligible for assistance with costs from a revenue fund to be established for that purpose. However, the government did not accept the recommendations regarding the Tax Court and the appeal fund.

Proposed changes to fiscal matters

Fundraising, trading, etc.

There are no proposals in the Joint Regulatory Table report relating to fundraising because the topic was outside the Table's authority, in part (at least) because fundraising is considered to be within the constitutional authority of the provinces. However, the Uniform Law Commission has recently drafted a model bill for consideration by all of the provinces and territories.

Implications for social inclusion

The underpinning premise in *Strengthening Canada* is that the future regulatory regime for charities should remain governed by the provisions of the Income Tax Act. This perspective dictates the approach taken by the Joint Regulatory Table and the contents of its report. There is no consideration given to how its proposals will play out for the end-user.

Strengths of proposals

The proposals of the Joint Regulatory Table concentrate on efficiency improvements to the mechanics of the existing regulatory system. Some of these will impact on social inclusion issues.

Charitable purposes   The recognition given to the need to further develop charitable purposes in line with contemporary need is important. The proposal to do so by increasing access to the courts and through a new case review process, had they been accepted by the government, would have improved the existing situation.

Education/support for the charitable sector   Again, the acknowledgement that charities need ongoing education and support and that this should be provided at 'arm's length' from Revenue Canada, is a step towards making the system more sensitive and responsive to emerging social needs. The suggestion that the sector should be responsible for education, primarily through umbrella organizations, has since been progressed.

Weaknesses of reform proposals

The report of the Joint Regulatory Table is not the product of needs-led research: it makes no pretence of approaching the subject from a perspective of unmet social need; it does not identify let alone prioritize the distinctively Canadian areas of social disadvantage; and consequently it does not deal with any necessity to adjust the charity law framework accordingly. To fault it for non-delivery on matters treated as outside its terms of reference may, therefore, be seen as unfair criticism. However, charity law has to relate to social disadvantage, and this system like any other must have functions and processes tailored to deal with its particular input if outcomes are to be effective. This report does not go far enough. There are some particular shortcomings.

Charitable purposes   The assumption that extending the range of charitable purposes can be accomplished through a combination of the existing registration process, greater access to the courts and through a new case review process, to be conducted by Revenue Canada on an in-house basis, is unwarranted. This may increase the frequency with which issues present but they will still present at random and the response of the system is open to being compromised by making the new case review component an in-house function of Revenue Canada. A more strategic approach to developing charitable purposes is needed, through a new forum dedicated to that task, separate and independent from the revenue-driven function. It would seem, however, that establishing a body with functions similar to those of the UK Charity Commission is barred by the Constitution.

Advocacy/political activity   In a nation comprised of so many disparate social groupings it is particularly important that existing restrictions on advocacy/ political activity, by charities seeking to represent the interests of those who perceive themselves as alienated, are removed.

Indigenous issues   The 'public' aspect of the public benefit test may well need legislative adjustment if the test is to accommodate the circumstances of Canada's First Nation people. Specific measures may need to be introduced if charities are to more effectively address the needs of ethnocultural groups, e.g. through small, localized community development schemes.[122]

Public benefit issues   There are many areas in which the existing common law approach to matters of public benefit is not accommodating contemporary issues. The prevention of poverty is one such issue, given that so many Canadian citizens are employed but are on or below the poverty level and outside the welfare benefits system. The advancement of human rights, conflict resolution/ reconciliation, the promotion of religious/racial harmony and equality/diversity are also activities that might merit specific legislative recognition as being for the public benefit and therefore warranting charitable status.

Partnership with government   The difficulty highlighted in the Johns Hopkins report,[123] whereby government funding policies threaten to transform some charities into government agencies (the scale of this problem is difficult to estimate, it could be that it is confined to a specific group of 'quangos'), has not been acknowledged in the Joint Regulatory Table report. This issue may require legislative provisions to introduce new structures for charities (particularly for 'umbrella organizations') if they are to retain their independence and be in a position to form authentic partnerships with government.

Fiscal issues   Again, legislative measures may need to be introduced to counter existing restrictions on matters such as the use of *cy-près* schemes to vary objects and redirect assets (this may have to be province-based rather than federal legislation) and on the channelling of funds to overseas charities.

Conclusion

Given that charity law reform has been in the air for some time now and that the current federal review process has been underway for the past four years, there are few indications that the government is preparing to make any significant changes to charity law and none that it intends to do so in ways that may have positive implications for the contemporary social inclusion agenda in Canada. If the report of the Joint Regulatory Table could be understood as a preliminary ground-clearing exercise, now awaiting a government initiative to move the process into a new stage involving a strategic and focused consideration of the functions of charity law in relation to specific areas of social need, then perhaps there are grounds for optimism and for deferring comment. However, progress to date reveals little awareness of the current misfit between the law and the particular pattern of social need in Canada or willingness to engage in a more fundamental rethink of the federal institutional framework for philanthropy. If anything, what is currently emerging most clearly is government retrenchment; a falling back to a defensive position with a focus on anti-terrorism legislation accompanied by an emphasis on measures that provide for the closer scrutiny of charities finances rather than facilitate their effectiveness.

Conclusion

Altruism, the cornerstone of the 'gift relationship', is a necessary but insufficient basis for the future development of philanthropy. In a modern context of fundamental rights, there are very few circumstances in which a 'gift' is of itself a legitimate response to deprivation. We are all diminished by poverty and by unresolved issues of social inclusion. We are all endangered by the possibility of alienation undermining our efforts to build and sustain civil society. The developed nations that share the common law heritage have come to recognize the importance of the utility component that Titmus acknowledged could accompany altruism. It is in all our interests to ensure that a new regulatory framework for philanthropy strategically addresses poverty and social inclusion on community, national and international levels. The 'gift relationship' must become less of a one-way transaction and more of an 'exchange relationship' that allows donor and recipient to work in partnership.

The modern role of philanthropy is governed by a traditional charity law framework which is no longer wholly appropriate as a means for channelling philanthropic resources in a way that effectively addresses poverty and issues of social inclusion. The reasons for this are largely to be found in certain aspects of the common law heritage that continue to provide a shared context for charity law in many modern western societies. *Charity Law and Social Inclusion* has identified a set of themes, drawn from the developmental history of charity law and evident in the jurisdictions studied and in current national law reform processes, which are largely derived from and are representative of the more problematic aspects of that shared heritage. It is suggested that these themes will need to be addressed by governments if they are to construct a regulatory environment that will facilitate appropriate and effective philanthropic intervention on social inclusion issues in the twenty-first century.

Partnership with government

History records that the close relationship between charity and government in public benefit provision has always been a feature of the development of charity law in a common law context. All jurisdictions studied, with the exception of the US, revealed recent government declarations of intent to further develop partnership arrangements with the voluntary and community sector (or nonprofit, or third sector) as a means of addressing social inclusion, developing social cohesion and consolidating civil society. Whether explicitly stated or not, a revised charity law framework was viewed as a specification of the terms of reference for the new government/charity partnership that would provide an expedient way of progressing this policy.

The public/private balance

As the State retracts in all developed common law countries, accompanied by government policy to promote the partnership ethos, there is every reason to believe that the boundary between the responsibilities of government and charity will become increasingly uncertain and that the predations of commerce will force both to give up ground. In England and Wales the piecemeal break-up of public services seems likely to result in much the same distribution of public benefit service provision between government, business and non-profits as in the US. Recent developments in both jurisdictions indicate a steady convergence. In England and Wales a decision[1] of the Commission, which may in due course be followed by other common law nations, has signalled a readiness to move further down this road by permitting government to delegate the delivery of public services to charities. In the US, a state legislative initiative[2] indicates a new government willingness to utilize charitable resources to fund the delivery of public services. The conversion rate of non-profits to commercial entities in the latter jurisdiction[3] is particularly revealing and may be anticipated in England and Wales as a follow-up to privatization.

This trend provides cause for concern in relation to the ability of charities to maintain their independence. On the other hand, it has to be acknowledged that the problems of poverty and social inclusion are of such an embedded and complex nature that they can only be realistically addressed through partnership arrangements that allow strategic interdisciplinary and multi-sector approaches to be instituted and sustained. Any such partnership must also, of course, include representatives of those whose need is to be addressed: they are the stakeholders best placed to gauge the need, judge what will work and for whom the outcomes have most significance.

The survey on jurisdictions noted that while partnership arrangements were overtly and explicitly pursued as declared government policy, it was also very often the case that governments were pursuing the same policy in more covert ways.

Government funding   The same pattern of government funding of charities, whether by direct grant aid or through contracts for service provision, was the norm in all jurisdictions studied. This trend shows every indication of increasing and carries considerable risks for the charitable sector both because of the preferential basis upon which some types of charity attract such funds and because of the resulting inhibiting effect on their freedom to dissent from government policies. As the locus for determining public benefit moves more within government control, so there is a risk of a proportionate diminution in the probability of charities independently championing the cause of dissident socially marginalized groups.

The National Lottery   This has now become a well-established social institution widely used by governments to channel charitable funds towards public service provision: it is a convenient milch cow that enables responsibility for public utility maintenance to be transferred to charities, thereby avoiding or defraying equivalent government expenditure. In the UK, the creation of the New Opportunities Fund as a separate and more directly controlled body than the Community Fund, working to government priorities, is seen by some as further evidence of takeover by stealth.[4]

Community foundations[5]   This type of charitable trust, used to support local community causes, was first established in the US in 1914, emerged in the UK in the 1980s and has since become widespread in over 35 countries. As Anheier and Leat explain:

> community foundations are rooted in, and emphasise building, local communities; they encourage and provide vehicles for corporate giving; they are governed locally; they encourage citizen-donor involvement and 'democratise' giving by enabling smaller donors to create what are, in effect, their own mini-foundations (e.g. donor-advised funds) within an established infrastructure; and they seek to work with rather than apart from local government and businesses.[6]

In England and Wales the government has been involved in funding the start-up costs of community foundations and has played an active role in guiding their investment in social infrastructure for local communities.

Restrictions on advocacy/political activity

The constraints on political activity by charities are deeply rooted in the common law and were evident in the contemporary law and practice of all jurisdictions studied. They present a real obstacle for the many charities that view campaigning for change in laws affecting the interests of the socially disadvantaged as a moral obligation. While some common law jurisdictions now adopt a more permissive approach (such as the US, where charities are permitted to be politically active but limits are placed upon the amount of funds and resources which can be so used), most others continue to deny charitable status to an organization established to challenge government policy, to campaign for a change in the law or even to advocate for the retention of current policy or law.[7] Given that effective intervention on social inclusion issues will necessarily involve assertive advocacy and lobbying for change in law and policy, it is of considerable importance that obstacles such as the ruling in *McGovern* v. *A-G.*[8] are removed and charities legally freed up to undertake that role.

In England and Wales the outcome of the charity law review indicated a new government willingness to relax the application of this constraint in certain circumstances. It is, however, difficult to see how those common law nations that have chosen to leave the traditional constraint intact will be in a position to follow in the future, as they have in the past, the related case law precedents emerging from this jurisdiction.

Human rights and anti-terrorism

The caution displayed by all developed nations in their approach to endorsing the European Convention, or in formulating a national equivalent, provides an interesting contrast to the speed with which they introduced rafts of anti-terrorism legislation. While these are clearly not concerns specific to common law countries, they were prevalent in all surveyed and constituted a theme with a bearing on the relationship between charity law and social inclusion.

Restrictions on rights

The charity law review processes commenced with much optimism. They occurred against a background of recent national commitments to human rights legislation and emerging case law which endorsed legal rights of great importance for charities such as the rights to freedom of association, of expression and from discrimination together with important guiding principles such as 'necessity', 'proportionality' and 'equality of arms'. The reform of charity law seemed set to broaden the scope of public benefit and enable a new philanthropy to address a greater range of contemporary social problems.

Instead, across the common law jurisdictions, charity law reform shows every sign of succumbing to a growing international security imperative. This is demonstrated particularly clearly in the contrast between expectation and outcome of the New Zealand process. There is a broad danger that reform processes intended to liberalize charities may well relapse into the traditional focus on strengthening powers for their inspection and supervision.

The experience in England and Wales, in Scotland and in Northern Ireland, has been somewhat different. On the one hand the process has resulted in what may turn out to be far-reaching reforms which, in conjunction with human rights legislation, have the potential to revolutionize some aspects of charity law, at least within the UK. On the other hand, the introduction of tough anti-terrorism provisions is likely to restrict the scope of some human rights and the freedom of action of charities. In the UK jurisdictions as elsewhere, the efforts of charities to progress social inclusion for ethnic minorities are being constrained by new government anti-terrorism measures, which by causing further alienation may exacerbate rather than reduce issues of national and international security. What is needed instead is a proportionate and discriminating legislative response, that is human rights-compliant, to the real but limited threat presented by the link between charities and terrorism, that does not impede the vital link between charities and the socially marginalized.

Surveillance of funds

Heightened government awareness of the threat posed by terrorism has also translated into new measures for inspecting and tracking the funds of charities and other non-government organizations. Again, this tends to constrain freedom of action and cause defensiveness in organizations that now more than ever should be encouraged to develop more innovative social inclusion strategies.

International aid, development and relationships

Such activity, while by no means confined to that undertaken by the developed common law nations, demonstrated their commitment to promote social inclusion on an international scale, was a strong dimension of the role of their charities and emerged as a definite theme in the survey.

Aid and development

In all jurisdictions studied, charities contributed to the immediate alleviation of poverty, natural disaster and other forms of distress in undeveloped nations. This form of charitable activity, replicating the traditional supplicant/benefactor dynamic, would seem to be open to the same criticism levelled at that relationship: it is clearly necessary, useful and legitimate within its own terms; it provides an opportunity to demonstrate altruism and it generates social capital; but as it deals with effects rather than causes, it leaves intact the social conditions that required the intervention to prompt further such intervention in the future; and it gives rise to the suspicion that those with the resources wish to achieve palliative care. This interpretation is substantiated by UN reports that the poor in sub-Saharan Africa and elsewhere are getting poorer.

Increasingly charities in the nations studied, as elsewhere, are also turning to longer-term methods of intervention. Contributing to building the socio-economic infrastructure is viewed as remedying the social conditions that prevent underdeveloped nations from becoming more self-sufficient and as being more cost-effective in the long run. This new approach has brought with it a need for new legal structures for the charities concerned and a keener awareness of other constraints.

Constraints

The survey revealed that some charities continue to be impeded by the rule that the public benefit test requires some 'benefit' to accrue to the 'public' of the jurisdiction in which the charity is based.[9] Also, charities in common law nations can be further inhibited by the decision in *McGovern* v. *A-G*.[10] Their involvement in countries where government policies are inimical to democratic norms may necessitate negotiating terms of engagement. This in turn may mean exposure to the challenge that they are engaging in political activity – which could threaten their charitable status. Moreover, the threat posed by international terrorism is prompting governments to constrain the discretion of international charities by requiring that they avoid making resource inputs to those countries. Ironically, while the international role of charities as mediators and resource providers has never been more necessary to the disadvantaged and alienated it has also never been more constrained by the governments of the western world.

Comity of nations

Arguably, the work of international charities has the potential to make an import-ant contribution to the task of building a new comity of nations and for that reason alone should be facilitated.

Issues relating to indigenous people/multicultural matters

Unsurprisingly, the legacy of colonialism is a feature of charitable activity in some of the common law nations studied, as it is in the many that were not. *Charity Law and Social Inclusion* has found that while issues of social inclusion in developed nations were most starkly demonstrated in the contemporary circumstances of the remnants of their first inhabitants, not dissimilar issues were also present in the circumstances of their latest arrivals.

Indigenous people

Cultural estrangement was the most obvious characteristic of the relationship between indigenous and non-indigenous people in countries such as Australia, Canada and to a lesser extent New Zealand, as vividly illustrated by enduring myths regarding the cause of aboriginal health and social decline.[11] In Australia the relationship has deteriorated to the point where it could be fairly said that its Indigenous population now regard themselves as alienated from the rest of Australian society. Given the duration of philanthropic involvement, there is an urgent need for a new approach if philanthropy is to have a more meaningful and sustainable impact upon such chronic embedded deprivation. It has been claimed that only where there is significant community involvement in management and decision-making has there been any real progress on health and education in Native American communities.[12] This would indicate that a partnership approach, rather than the traditional one-way supplicant/benefactor transaction, is the better way forward. It also clearly requires the removal of obstacles in existing charity law, such as any interpretation of 'public' that debars access to charitable resources on the grounds that prospective recipients are linked by kinship.

Immigrants etc.

The cultural estrangement experienced by immigrants, refugees, migrant labour and/or asylum seekers as they establish ethnic enclaves in the cities of the common law nations studied and elsewhere, is redolent of that suffered by indigenous people. Again, the gap of mutual misunderstanding and the drift towards alienation requires a new approach, and very probably this should entail a similar involvement of the disadvantaged in the planning and management of any proposed philanthropic intervention.

Fiscal issues, particularly tax orientation

Finances lie at the heart of charity law. Regulating finance-related matters, particularly the tax liability of organizations engaged in public benefit activity, remains the primary goal of charity law in all the common law nations. How this is achieved was a major theme in the survey.

Revenue driven

The persistence of the deep-rooted tax orientation approach to charities is evident in the revenue-driven policy of many governments. In all jurisdictions surveyed, eligibility for tax exemption requires that charities be subject to the government body vested with responsibility for the collection of tax revenues.

Where, as in Canada, official recognition of an organization's charitable activities is provided only to ascertain their eligibility for tax exemption, then the ancillary registration and regulatory functions are performed exclusively by the relevant tax collection agency, which thereby determines charitable status. Where, as in England and Wales, there is an additional body with responsibility for such ancillary functions then it rather than the taxing authority determines charitable status. Some jurisdictions, such as Ireland, have in place a different type of government body, quite separate and independent of the tax authority, without regulatory powers but with varying responsibilities for the support, supervision and development of charities.

Where the primary legal function of a government body is to police the collection of State revenues this has not proven conducive to it willingly facilitating any avoidance of liability, even on the grounds of charitable activity. This is particularly the case in relation to new and innovative methods of philanthropic intervention, such as the use of venture capital in a community development approach to poverty relief, or in relation to new forms of social disadvantage such as the current phenomenon of migrant labour or asylum seekers.

The doctrine of cy-près

The *cy-près* mechanism is a potentially very powerful tool for applying the assets of a defunct charity to address contemporary social inclusion issues. In the post-colonial context of common law nations, it has been instrumental in facilitating the redistribution of property (often now prime real estate) formerly held on trust for the Crown for use instead by contemporary charities.[13] However, its usefulness has been constrained by the survival of two accompanying common law caveats: that the donor should have a 'general charitable intent'; and that any variation of a charity's objects or redistribution of its assets should be done so as to achieve a result 'as close as possible' to the objects of the original gift. Also, traditionally, it has only been available when the original use was rendered impossible or impracticable rather than simply ineffective, and it has been a jurisdiction exercised by the High Court unless statutorily transferred.

If *cy-près* is to fulfil its potential in the common law jurisdictions then the constraining rules would need to be removed or amended and a new balance struck between respecting a donor's intentions and meeting contemporary social needs. Such a development could only be helped by vesting jurisdiction in an independent government agency, similar to the Charity Commission in England and Wales, which would have the power, the willingness and the creativity to design innovative large-scale *cy-près* schemes. Failure to modernize *cy-près* will see this common law process displaced by a statutory procedure as decision-making in this context moves from the charitable sector to government (as in New York).

Trading etc,

Given the need for many contemporary charities to compete in the market place, the constraints generally imposed by the 'primary purposes' rule and in relation to profit distribution etc. can have a disproportionately inhibitive effect and greatly restrict their competitive ability. There is much to be said for a more discriminatory policy that encourages charities to generate a commercial capacity in marginalized communities and foster non-profit trading arrangements with producers in developing countries (e.g. the Fairtrade Foundation). Arguably, this is the case regardless of whether it is a charity running a business or a business running a charity.

However, too often the trading role of charities is insufficient to offset the damage caused by the simultaneous involvement of their governments in protectionist policies for domestic producers, the politics of international trade and in loan repayment arrangements that do so much to perpetuate the conditions of deprivation in those same countries.

Roles of the court and the Attorney General

The common law is judge-made law and as such charity law has always been dependent upon judicial decision-making for its development while the *parens patriae* jurisdiction, as vested in the office of Attorney General, was traditionally equally significant as a source of authority for the protection of charities. The survey was therefore attentive to the role currently played by these two institutions.

The courts

In all jurisdictions studied, with the exception of England and Wales, decision-making by the revenue-driven tax authority has gradually superseded that of the High Court as the primary influence in shaping the development of charity law. The expense of proceedings, their random nature and the accompanying adverse publicity have combined to steadily reduce recourse to the courts. As a consequence the law has gradually atrophied in those nations, resulting in its becoming increasingly inaccessible and irrelevant to the socially disadvantaged whose circumstances comprise the modern social inclusion agenda.

In recent years the courts in some jurisdictions have utilized the 'spirit and intendment' rule to ground decisions that have creatively extended the interpretation of charitable purposes in relation to the needs of the socially disadvantaged.[14]

In England and Wales the Charity Commission, as opposed to the tax authority, being vested with the powers of the High Court, has been able to strategically promote the development of charitable purposes.

The Attorney General

In no common law country has there been any indication of a willingness to revive the use of *parens patriae* powers in the context of the law relating to charities (unlike the enthusiasm with which those powers have been utilized in the UK and elsewhere in the context of the law relating to children). Arguably, the strong parallels – centring on the gaps in the statutory framework which left the subjects inadequately protected from contemporary forms of neglect and abuse – would have equally justified resorting to the powers of that ancient jurisdiction. In theory, the Attorney General is well placed in all common law jurisdictions to initiate protective intervention which (as happened in relation to child care law) could then have led to a broadening of the principles and tightening of practice in respect of fitting the law to appropriately accommodate contemporary issues. The neutering of the role of Attorney General in this context has, perhaps, been a matter of some significance for charity law in all common law jurisdictions.

Forum for developing charitable purposes

Whether an independent body has been established and empowered to determine status, develop charitable purposes and influence the eligibility criteria for charitable exemption applied by the tax authority is clearly crucial in the context of fitting the charity law framework to current patterns of social need. Again, this was a primary theme in the survey of common law jurisdictions.

All jurisdictions, with the exception of England and Wales, lacked such a body. While both New Zealand and Ireland have similarly named commissions, in neither case is that body vested with the powers necessary for it to act as a forum for developing charitable purposes. In the post-9/11 political climate, the constraints imposed by the lack of such a forum greatly reduces the opportunities available for the development of charitable purposes.

In England and Wales, the Charity Commissioners are strategically positioned and legislatively empowered to hold a singular role in relation to the Inland Revenue and the courts. The Commission is equipped with the powers, responsibilities and resources to provide the charity support functions necessary to further develop charitable purposes in line with pressures from the social inclusion agenda. In particular, the crucial statutory responsibility to maintain and review the Register of Charities is vested in the Commission which means that it rather than the Inland Revenue acts as the gatekeeper of charitable status, with powers to extend the range of charitable activity to fit with contemporary social circumstances. It is also armed with sufficient regulatory powers to review, closely inspect and supervise the continuing relevance of traditional charitable purposes and resources for modern manifestations of social need and in addition may do so through the creation of *cy-près* schemes.

The proactive mode of intervention developed by the Commission enables it to engage strategically and frequently with charities and the sector, thereby shaping practice in a way no longer available to the High Court and not required of the Inland Revenue.

Legal structures

In some common law nations, but most tenaciously in England and Wales, the trust has continued to serve as the primary legal structure for charities. Its limitations are now widely acknowledged and there is a new willingness to experiment with forms of incorporation. In other such nations – including Australia, New Zealand, the US and Canada – as noted in this study, reliance is placed upon incorporated bodies rather than trusts. The associated difficulties in applying common law principles in a statutory law context are recognized, as is the need to experiment with forms of incorporation that provide for a better meshing of trust principles with company law. In short, there is now a readiness to develop the structures necessary to facilitate the new methods of philanthropic intervention required to address contemporary social inclusion issues. These are needed if the necessary partnerships – co-ordinating the involvement of not-for-profit organizations, government bodies and end-users – are to be established. The survey therefore regarded legal structures as an important theme.

Incorporated charities

The governments in both England and Wales and Ireland are proposing new forms of incorporation for use specifically and exclusively by charities: the Charitable Incorporated Organization and the Charitable Designated Activity Company respectively. Both will provide: a more appropriate alternative to the company limited by guarantee; for members and managers to be insulated from the financial liabilities of the company; for it to agree contracts, hold land titles, sue and be sued; and for simpler registration and reporting requirements than is now the case. It is envisaged that new charities and many existing ones will opt for this incorporated structure in a development that acknowledges the shortcomings of the trust/foundation as an attractive structure for entrepreneurs and the cumbersome nature of the current dual registration and reporting requirements that burden charities which are also companies limited by guarantee.

Foundations

Most UK charities take the form of a foundation (or trust as it is most usually referred to) but this is not necessarily the case in other jurisdictions, where charities most often take the form of corporations. In the US and Australia, for example, the trust model is not so prevalent and the latter jurisdiction at least has failed to emulate the UK example and integrate trust concepts into the corporate form.

Endowed philanthropic foundations With its financial base secured by an endowment, such a foundation is uniquely free from the fundraising concerns that drive the management of other charities. This gives them an independence and capacity for strategic long-term intervention that often attracts pioneering social entrepreneurs. The modern endowed charitable foundation, which can effectively bridge the public/private divide, would seem to offer a particularly appropriate vehicle for targeting resources, pioneering strategies, leveraging in resources and sustaining intervention on behalf of the socially marginalized. Some – such as the Joseph Rowntree Foundation, the Esmee Fairburn Foundation and the Barrow Cadbury Trust – are research-led organizations capable of shaping government policy in the UK in a manner previously only available to non-charitable endowed foundations such as the Joseph Rowntree Reform Trust (philanthropic but not charitable).

In recent years a new model has emerged: the endowed charitable foundation established by a wealthy private individual dedicated to pursuing its own programme of intervention in respect of a specific area of social need (e.g. Bill Gates and AIDS in Africa).

Public benefit issues

The survey revealed that only in England and Wales was the government preparing to introduce quite radical changes to the central concept of public benefit. Other jurisdictions settled for a cautious extension to the existing four *Pemsel* heads, although this was coupled with general recognition that in determining public benefit the 'activities test' should be applied.

Charitable purposes

The more basic structural flaws in charity law as developed among the nations sharing the common law tradition remain largely intact. These include:

- no charitable purpose to address the causes of poverty;
- no removal of the restrictions on advocacy/political activity; and
- no removal of the legal presumption favouring religion.

In no jurisdiction, other than England and Wales, was there any indication of a legislative intent to extend the definition of charitable purposes to include such matters of central importance to contemporary issues of social inclusion as:

- the advancement of human rights, conflict resolution or reconciliation, etc;
- the advancement of civil society;
- promoting the welfare of specific socially disadvantaged groups and indigenous people; and
- promoting multicultural relationships, on a community, national and international basis.

Notes

Acknowledgements

1 Director, Centre of Philanthropy and Nonprofit Studies, Queensland University of Technology, Brisbane, Australia.
2 See Picarda, H., *The Law and Practice Relating to Charities'* (3rd edn) Butterworths, London, 1999.
3 See, Dal Pont, G., *Charity Law in Australia and New Zealand*, Oxford University Press, Melbourne, 2000.
4 Deputy Director of Education, Law Society, Dublin, Ireland.
5 See Anheier, H. and Leat, D., *Creative Philanthropy: Toward a New Philanthropy for the 21st Century*, Routledge, London and New York, 2006
6 Principal Research Associate at the International Bureau of Fiscal Documentation.
7 Director, Centre for Voluntary Sector Research, Sheffield Hallam University, Sheffield, England.
8 Executive Director of The Muttart Foundation, one of Canada's largest private foundations and until recently the voluntary-sector co-chair of the Joint Regulatory Table.
9 Principal, Benefic Lawyers, Vancouver, Canada.
10 Principal, Benefic Lawyers, Vancouver, Canada.
11 General Manager, Pacific Leprosy Foundation.
12 Executive Director, National Center on Philanthropy and the Law, New York University School of Law.

Introduction

1 With the notable exception of Barbados.

I The gift relationship: charity and the law

1 See, Titmus, R., *The Gift Relationship: From Human Blood to Social Policy*, Allen and Unwin, London, 1970.
2 Ibid.
3 See, for example, Frank, R., 'Motivation, Cognition and Charitable Giving' in Schneewind, J. B. (edn), *Giving: Western Ideas of Philanthropy*, Indiana University Press, Bloomington, 1996. Also, see: Banks, J., and Tanner, S., *The State of Donation: Household Gifts to Charity*, 1974–96, Institute for Fiscal Studies, London, 1997; Cheal, D., *The Gift Economy*, Cambridge University Press, Cambridge, 1988; and Halfpenny, P., and Lowe, D., *Individual Giving and Volunteering in Britain*, (7th edn), Charities Aid Foundation, Kent, 1994.
4 See, Gerwirth, A., 'Private Philanthropy and Positive Rights' in Paul, E., Miller, F.,

Paul, J., and Ahrens, J., eds, *Beneficience, Philanthropy and the Public Good*, Basil Blackwell, Oxford, 1987, p. 78.

5 *Income Tax Special Purposes Commissioners* v. *Pemsel* [1891] AC 531.

6 This rule refers to the common law practice of extending by analogy a recognition of charitable purpose to those activities which, although not enumerated in the Preamble to the Statute of Charitable Uses 1601, are judicially viewed as being so close to those listed that they can be construed as coming within the intention of that legislation.

7 See, for example, Gurin, M. G. and Van Til, J., 'Philanthropy in its Historical Context', in Van Til, V. *et al.* (eds), *Critical Issues in American Philanthropy, Strengthening Theory and Practice*, Jossey-Bass Publishers, San Francisco, 1990, where a distinction is drawn between charity (person-to-person alleviation of need) and philanthropy (strategic approach to social problems).

8 Christianity was not unique in this respect: Buddhism teaches the love of mankind as the highest form of righteousness; Islam requires a tithe of one-tenth of income to be given to those in need; and the Jewish religion urges its followers to assist the poor and practise charity.

9 See *Report of the Committee on the Law and Practice relating to Charitable Trusts* (Cmnd. 8710), HMSO, London, 1952, para. 36.

10 A 'chantry' (from the 'Chanting of the Mass') was a religious service founded and endowed by a benefactor for the repose of the soul of one or more persons. It was an important institution of the mediaeval Church and very popular in the fourteenth and fifteenth centuries. See Wood-Leigh, K., *Church Life under Edward III*, 1934, p. 91; cited in Brady, J., *Religion and the Law of Charities in Ireland*, Northern Ireland Legal Quarterly, Belfast, 1975, p. 12.

11 See Westlake, *The Parish Gilds of Mediaeval England*, 1919, where mention is made that 'the gild of the Blessed Virgin Mary in the parish church of St Botolph at Boston founded in 1260 gave a yearly distribution of bread and herrings to the poor in alms for the souls of its benefactors'; cited in Brady, *Religion and the Law of Charities in Ireland*, p. 14.

12 See King Edward's code promulgated at Andover (*c.* 963). Also, see the laws of the West Saxon King Ine (688–94) which directed that 'Church-scot is to be given by Martinmass; if anyone does not discharge it, he is liable to 60 shillings and to render the church-scott twelve-fold', as cited in Brady, *Religion and the Law of Charities in Ireland*, p. 6.

13 See, Whitelock (edn), *English Historical Documents 500–1042*, at p 365; as cited in Brady, *Religion and the Law of Charities in Ireland*.

14 See, Brady, *Religion and the Law of Charities in Ireland*, p. 6.

15 See McIntosh, M., 'Poverty, Charity and Coercion', *Journal of Interdisciplinary History*, 35(3), 2005, pp. 457–79, esp. p. 467 where she also refers to the punishment of the 'undeserving' poor.

16 Lord Northington's remark being apt: 'it is indifferent to the donors in what species of charity they give their money: not service to the poor, but vanity is their motive.' See *Attorney-General* v. *Tyndall* (1764) Amb.614, p. 713.

17 See, for example, *Giving Time, Getting Involved – A Strategy Report by the Working Group on the Active Community* (the Warner report), Home Office, London, 1999.

18 See *Income Tax Special Purposes Commissioners* v. *Pemsel*, op. cit., where Macnaghten L.J. said of 'charity' that 'of all words in the English language bearing a popular as well as a legal signification I am not sure that there is one which more unmistakably has a technical meaning . . .' (p. 581).

19 In England and Wales a limited definition was provided in the Recreational Charities Act 1958 and will be available in the forthcoming charities legislation.

20 Also known the Statute of Elizabeth; 43 Eliz 1, c. 4. The Preamble lists charitable purposes; e.g. 'relief of aged impotent and poore people' and 'marriages of poore maides'.

21 See, *Income Tax Special Purposes Commissioners* v. *Pemsel* op. cit., where Macnaghten L.J. first classified charitable purposes as follows:

> Charity in its legal sense comprises four principal divisions: trusts for the relief of poverty; trusts for the advancement of education; trusts for the advancement of religion; and trusts for other purposes beneficial to the community not falling under any of the preceding heads.

22 See Picarda, H., *The Law and Practice Relating to Charities* (3rd edn), Butterworths, London, 1999.

23 A parental jurisdiction inherently vested in the monarch, exercised by the Chancellor, delegated to the Court of Chancery and then administered by the High Court and the Attorney General. See Seymour, J., '*Parens Patriae* and Wardship Powers: Their Nature and Origins', *Oxford Journal of Legal Studies*, 14(2), 1994.

24 See the leading Irish case of *Re Cranston* [1898] IR 431. Also, see the comments of Lord Sterndale MR in *Re Tetley* [1923] 1 Ch 258, p. 266. See, further, chap. 2.

25 See *Hoare* v. *Osborne* (1866) LR 1 Eq, 585 *per* Kindersley VC, p. 588.

26 See *In re the Worth Library* [1994] 1 ILRM 161 *per* Keane J, p. 193.

27 *Re Pinion* [1965] Ch 85.

28 See, for example, *National Anti-Vivisection Society* v. *IRC* [1948] AC 31 and *Re Pinion*, op. cit.

29 See Lord Wright in *National Anti-Vivisection Society* v. *Inland Revenue Commissioner*, op. cit., p. 42. In *Re Foveaux* [1895] 2 Ch 501 Chitty J had considered that the abolition of vivisection was charitable because the intention was to benefit the community and it was not for the court to examine whether or not the community would in fact derive any benefit. In coming to the opposite conclusion 50 years later in *National Anti-Vivisection Society* v. *IRC*, the House of Lords repudiated the Chitty J approach stating that the intention of the testator was not determinative of public benefit, this was for the court to decide.

30 *National Anti-Vivisection Society* v. *Inland Revenue Commissioner*, op. cit.

31 *Re Hobourn Aero Components Ltd's Air Raid Distress Fund* [1946] Ch 194.

32 See, for example, *Springhill Housing Action Committee* v. *Commissioner of Valuation* [1983] NI 184.

33 *Gilmour* v. *Coates* [1949] AC 426. Also, see *Trustees of the Congregation of Poor Clares of the Immaculate Conception* v. *The Commissioner of Valuation* [1971] NI 114, p. 169, *per* Lowry L: 'an Order which has no other purpose other than to achieve its own santification by private prayer and contemplation is not an association with charitable objects'.

34 In *Re Wedgewood* [1915] 1 Ch 113 it was held that alleviating the suffering of animals is charitable because of the benefit to the public rather than the animals. See, also, *Re Douglas* (1887) 35 Ch D 472, CA, and *Adamson* v. *Melbourne* [1929] AC 142.

35 *Re Glyn's Will Trusts* (1953), *The Times* 28 March.

36 *Re Grove-Grady* [1929] 1 Ch 557, CA, *per* Lord Hanworth MR.

37 *Thellusson* v. *Woodford* (1799) 4 Ves 227.

38 See, for example, *Re Macduff* [1896] 2 Ch 451, p. 466, *per* Lindley L.J. and *Att-Gen* v. *National Provincial and Union Bank of England* [1924] AC 262, p. 265, *per* Lord Cave LC.

39 *Campbell College* v. *Commissioner of Valuation* [1964] NI 169, HL.

40 *Re Resch's Will Trusts* [1967] 3 All ER 915.

41 See *Income Tax Special Purposes Commissioners* v. *Pemsel*, op. cit., p. 583.

42 Picarda, *Law and Practice Relating to Charities*, p. 621.

43 *Houston* v. *Burns* [1918] AC 337, HL; *Re Jarman's Estate* (1878) 8 Ch D 584; *Re Rilands Estate* [1881] WN 173; *Chichester Diocesan Fund and Board of Finance Inc* v. *Simpson* [1944] AC 341, HL; *A-G for New Zealand* v. *Brown* [1917] AC 393, PC.

44 (1805) 10 Ves 522.

45 Picarda, *Law and Practice Relating to Charities*, p. 221.
46 *James* v. *Allen* (1817) 3 Mer 17; *Re Barnett* (1908) 24 TLR 788; and *Lawrence* v. *Lawrence* (1913) 42 NBR 260.
47 *Re Macduff* [1986] 2 Ch 452; *Re Eades* [1920] 2 Ch 353.
48 *Re Woodgate* (1886) 2 TLR 674.
49 *Re Sidney* (1908) 1 Ch 488.
50 *A-G* v. *National Provincial Bank* [1924] AC 262.
51 *Re Da Costa* [1912] 1 Ch 337; *Vezey* v. *Jamson* (1822) 1 Sim & St 69; *Blair* v. *Duncan* [1902] AC 37; *Houston* v. *Burns* [1918] AC 337; and *Re Davis* [1923] 1 Ch 225.
52 *Kendall* v. *Granger* (1842) 5 Beav 300; *Langham* v. *Peterson* (1903) 87 LT 744.
53 *Re Hewitt* (1883) 53 L.J. Ch 132; *A-G* v. *Whorwood* (1750) 1 Ves Sen 534.
54 *Re Freeman* [1908] 1 Ch 720.
55 *Re Friends Free School* [1909] 2 Ch 675.
56 *Re Best* [1904] 2 Ch 354; *Caldwell* v. *Caldwell* [1921] 91 LJPC 95.
57 Picarda, *Law and Practice Relating to Charities*, p. 621.
58 See *Re Macduff*, op. cit., *per* Stirling J, p. 481 (cited by Picarda, *Law and Practice Relating to Charities*).
59 *Re Eades*, op. cit.
60 *Brewer* v. *McCauley* [1955] 1 DLR 415. Also, *Re Young* (1907) 9 OWR 566 ('needful and worthy institution or institutions, or any needy and worthy individual or individuals'); *Re Street* (1926) 29 OWN 428 ('benevolent institutions'); and *Planta* v. *Greenshields* [1931] 2 DLR 189 ('to aid and help any worthy cause or causes'). *Re Metcalfe* [1947] 1 DLR 567 ('religious, charitable and benevolent purposes').
61 *Re White* [1933] SASR 129 and also *A-G for New South Wales* v. *Adams* (1908) 7 CLR 100; *Re Cole's Estate* (1980) 25 SASR 489.
62 *A.-G. for New Zealand* v. *Brown* [1917] AC 393.
63 See *Re Tetley* [1923] 1 Ch 258, pp. 266–7, as cited in Sheridan, L. A., *Keeton & Sheridan's The Modern Law of Charities* (4th edn), Barry Rose, Chichester. 1992, pp. 4–5.
64 *Re Huyck* (1905) 10 OLR 480.
65 See dicta of Lord Hanworth MR in *Re Watt* [1932] 2 Ch 243, p. 246.
66 See, for example, *Attorney-General* v. *Price* (1907) 24 TLR 763.
67 As in the anti-vivisection cases.

2 Philanthropy and the challenge of social inclusion: the contemporary issues

1 Jenson, J., 'Mapping Social Cohesion: The State of Canadian Research', *Canadian Policy Research Networks*, 1998.
2 Ibid.
3 Beauvais, C. and Jenson, J., 'Social Cohesion: Up-dating the State of the Research', *Canadian Journal of Communication*, 27(2), 2002.
4 See Putnam, R., *Bowling Alone: The Collapse and Revival of American Community*, Simon and Schuster, New York, 2000, p. 19.
5 See Bothwell, J., 'Indicators of a Healthy Civil Society' in Burbridge, J. (edn), *Beyond Prince and Merchant: Citizen Participation and the Rise of Civil Society*, Institute of Cultural Affairs International, Brussels, 1997.
6 See Deakin, N., *In Search of Civil Society*, Palgrave, Hampshire, 2001.
7 See, for example: Cohen, L. and Arato, A., *Civil Society and Political Theory*, MIT Press, Cambridge, 1992; Seligman, A. B., *The Idea of Civil Society*, Princeton University Press, Princeton, N.J., 1992; Putnam, R., 'Bowling Alone: America's Declining Social Capital', *Journal of Democracy*, 6(1), Jan. 1995, pp. 65–78; and Putnam, *Bowling Alone: The Collapse and Revival of American Community*.
8 See *Social Exclusion Unit*, Office of the Deputy Prime Minister, 7th Floor, Eland House, Bressenden Place, London, SW1E 5DU.

9 Burchardt, T., 'The Dynamics of Being Disabled', *Journal of Social Policy*, 29(4), 2000, pp. 645–68.
10 *Vancouver Society of Immigrant and Visible Minority Women* v. *Minister of National Revenue* (1999) 99 DTC 5034, *per* Gonthier J, pp. 5070–1 (see, further, chap. 13).
11 See *The Millennium Development Goals Report 2005*, United Nations, New York, 2005, p. 9.
12 Ibid., p. 20.
13 Ibid., p. 40.
14 Ibid.
15 The Australian Bureau of Statistics (ABS) publication *The Health and Welfare of Australia's Aboriginal and Torres Strait Islander Peoples* (2001) provides the main source of information for this section.
16 Cindy Blackstock, an Aboriginal activist and Executive Director of the First Nations Child and Family Caring Society of Canada wrote in a recent study (*Same Country, Same Lands: 78 Countries Away*) that while Canada as a whole ranks near the top of the UN's Human Development Index, Canada's Aboriginal peoples would rank 78th on the same scale. Much the same could be said of Australia.
17 See, for example, Behrendt, L., *Achieving Social Justice*, The Federation Press, Sydney, 2003.
18 *St John's College, Cambridge* v. *Todington* (1757) 1 Burr 158, *per* Lord Mansfield LC, p. 200.
19 Ibid., pp. 13 and 93. The Bill and Melinda Gates foundation (of which the founding couple are the sole trustees) being a good example. This, the world's biggest and most powerful charity, is free to experiment without being inhibited by accountability for financial loss as it pursues its goal of finding effective vaccines for treating AIDS, malaria and other fatal diseases.
20 See Anheier, H. and Leat, D., *From Charity to Creativity: Philanthropic Foundations in the 21st Century*, Comedia, Stroud, 2002, p. 64.
21 See *Anon*, Duke 133, as cited by Picarda, H., *The Law and Practice Relating to Charities* (3rd edn), Butterworths, London, 1999, p. 306, where a bequest to trustees 'to make seats for poor people to beg in by the highways' was in breach of the law prohibiting begging.
22 See the Foundation Center's *Foundation Yearbook 2004* and further at http://www.effectivephilanthropy.com.
23 See Anheier and Leat, *From Charity to Creativity*, p. 67.
24 See Anheier and Leat, *From Charity to Creativity*, and *Creative Philanthropy: Toward a New Philanthropy for the 21st Century*, 2005.
25 Anheier and Leat, *Creative Philanthropy*, p. 2.
26 Ibid., p. 3.
27 Ibid.
28 Ibid.
29 Ibid.
30 The Pew Charitable Trust, established by family endowments between 1948 and 1979 and based in Philadelphia, states that it serves the public interest by providing information, advancing policy solutions and supporting civic life.
31 Anheier and Leat, *From Charity to Creativity*, p. 153.
32 See Emerson, J. and Twersky, F., *New Social Entrepreneurs: The Success, Challenge and Lessons of Nonprofit Enterprise Creation*, The Roberts Foundations, San Francisco, 1996; Letts, C., Ryan, W. and Grossman, A., 'Virtuous Capital: What Foundations can Learn from Venture Capitalists', *Harvard Business Review*, March/April, 1997, pp. 36–44; Reis, T. and Clohsey, S. J., 'Unleashing New Resources and Entrepreneurship for the Common Good: A Philanthropic Renaissance', in Schluter, A., Then, V. and Walkenhorst, P. (eds), *Foundations in Europe, Society, Management and Law*, Directory of Social Change, London, 2001; Breiteneicher, C. K. and Marble, M. G., 'Strategic Programme Management', in Schluter *et al.*, *Foundations in Europe, Society, Management and Law*.
33 See Reis, T. and Clohsey, S. J., 'Unleashing New Resources and Entrepreneurship for the Common Good', p. 477.

34 See Emerson and Twersky, *New Social Entrepreneurs*; Letts *et al.*, 'Virtuous Capital'.
35 Anheier and Leat, *From Charity to Creativity*, p. 155.
36 Ibid.
37 Ibid.
38 Ibid., p. 10.
39 Ibid., p. 22.
40 Ibid., p. 15.

3 The common law: the emergence of principles, structures and legal functions relating to charities

1 See Seymour, J., '*Parens Patriae* and Wardship Powers: Their Nature and Origins', *Oxford Journal of Legal Studies*, 14(2), 1994, pp. 159–88.
2 As Coke explained:

> The lands were said to come to dead hands . . . for . . . by alienation in mortmaine they lost wholly their escheats and in effect their knights services for the defence of the realme; wards, marriages, reliefes and the like; and therefore was called a dead hand, for that a dead hand yeeldeth no service.

See Coke, C. Litt. 2B; quoted by Delany, V. T. H., *The Law Relating to Charities in Ireland*, Alex Thompson, Dublin, 1962, p. 1.

3 See Clause 43 which provided:

> It shall not be lawful from henceforth to any to give his lands to any religious house and to take the same land again to hold of the same house: nor shall it be lawful to any house of religion to take the lands of any and to have the same of him of whom he received it. If any from henceforth give his lands to any religious house, and thereupon be convict, the gift shall be utterly void, and the land shall accrue to the lord of the fee.

4 See statutes of Henry 111, 1217, of Marlborough 1267; of Edward 1 in 1279 and 1285; of Richard 11 in 1391. Ultimately, the Mortmain Act 1736 was introduced to prohibit devises of land to charity.
5 It was Maitland who first remarked that 'the modern trust developed from the ancient use'.
6 For further information, see Holdsworth, W. S., *History of English Law*, Sweet & Maxwell, London, 1973, vol. 8, pp. 438–9; Also, see Keeton, G. and Sheridan, L. A. 'The Development of the Law of Trusts', in *The Law of Trusts* (12th edn), 1993, pp. 21–35.
7 See, *Attorney General* v. *Wax Chandlers Co.* (1897) LR 6 HL 1, p. 21.
8 Most graphically in the development of trading in 'future options'.
9 *Commissioners for Special Purposes of Income Tax* v. *Pemsel* [1891] AC 531, p. 131.
10 Ibid. ' "Charity" in its legal sense comprises four principal divisions: trusts for . . . etc'.
11 *Oppenheim* v. *Tobacco Securities Trust Co Ltd* [1951] AC 297.
12 See the Companies Act 1862.
13 McGregor-Lowndes, M., 'The Regulation of Charitable Organisations', unpublished PhD thesis, Griffith University, Brisbane, 1994, p. 256.
14 Statute of *Quia Emptores*, 18 Edw. 1 cc. 1–3.
15 '*Cy-près*', a Norman French expression, has generally been interpreted by the courts to mean 'as near as possible'. See Warburton, J., Morris, D. and Riddle, N. F. (eds), *Tudor on Charities* (9th edn), Sweet & Maxwell, London, 2003, p. 444, and *Re Lambeth Charities* (1853) 22 L.J. Ch. 959.
16 *Philpott* v. *St George's Hospital* (1859) 27 Beav 107, p. 111, as cited in Picarda, H., *The Law and Practice Relating to Charities* (3rd edn), Butterworths, London, 1999, p. 302.

17 See Jones, G., *History of the Law of Charity 1532–1827*, Wm. W. Gaunt & Sons, Inc., Holmes Beach, Florida, 1986, p. 10, and also Leonard, E. M., *The Early History of the English Poor Relief*, Cambridge University Press, Cambridge, 1900, p. 9.

18 Statute of Uses 1597, 39 Eliz. 1, c.6.

19 Statute of 43 Eliz. 1 cap. 4. 'The statute was remedial in that it was enacted to cure the widespread misappropriation of funds given to charitable uses and thus to mobilise the resources of private benefaction in the task of national rehabilitation' *per* Brady, J., 'The Law of Charity and Judicial Responsiveness to Changing Need', *Northern Ireland Legal Quarterly*, 27(3), 1976, p. 199. Eventually largely repealed by the Mortmain and Charitable Uses Act 1888.

20 See, for example, *Re Ward* [1941] Ch 308, *per* Mackimmon L.J., p. 310.

21 See, for example, Knight, B., *Voluntary Action*, Home Office, London, 1993.

22 *Royal College of Surgeons of England v. National Provincial Bank Ltd* [1952] AC 631, pp. 650–1.

23 See *Falkland v. Bertie* (1696) 2 Vern 333 *per* Lord Somers LC, p. 342; 23 ER 814, p. 818.

24 See *Re W (a minor) (medical treatment)* [1992] 4 All ER 627, p. 641. Also see *Re X (A Minor) (Wardship: Restriction on Publication)* [1975] 1 All ER 697, 'no limits to that jurisdiction have yet been drawn', *per* Denning L.J., p. 705.

25 *Re X (A Minor)*, op. cit., p. 411.

26 *AG v. Tancred* (1757) Amb 351.

27 *Attorney General v. Skinners Company* (1826) 2 Russ 407.

28 *Moggridge v. Thackwell* (1803) 7 Ves. 36.

29 Ibid., p. 83.

30 *Williams' Trustees v. IRC* [1947] AC 447.

31 *Morice v. The Bishop of Durham* (1804) 9 Ves 405.

32 See also *Kendall v. Grainger* (1842) 5 Beav 302, *per* Lord Langdale MR, and *Dolan v. MacDermott* (1868) LR 3 Ch App 678.

33 *Commissioners for Special Purposes of Income Tax v. Pemsel*, op. cit., p. 583.

34 See the caveat entered by Lord Cave in *AG v. Nat Provincial & Union Bank Ltd.* [1924] AC 262.

35 Ibid., p. 583.

36 *Williams' Trustees v. IRC*, op. cit.

37 See, for example, *Re Hummeltenberg* [1923] 1 Ch 237.

38 See *Note* (1465) YB Pas. 5 Edw. IV, fol. 2, pl. 4.

39 *Gouriet v. Union of Post Office Workers* [1977] 3 All ER 70.

40 *Weir v. Fermanagh County Council* [1913] 1 IR 193.

41 See *Wallis v. Solicitor General for New Zealand* [1903] AC 173, pp. 181–2.

42 In England and Wales the scope of the Attorney General's traditional authority in respect of charities is now largely restricted to cases where criminal prosecutions are being brought on charity related matters and where *cy-près* schemes are being presented before the judiciary. Otherwise the Attorney General has little direct regulatory involvement in the affairs of charities.

43 See *Ludlow Corp. v. Greenhove* (1827) 1 Bli. NS 17, p. 48.

44 See *Attorney General v. Brown* (1818) 1 Swan 265, *per* Lord Eldon, p. 291.

45 See Warburton *et al.*, *Tudor on Charities*, pp. 382–3.

46 More properly described as restitution, or equitable compensation: *Bartlett v. Barclays Bank Trust Co. Ltd.* [1980] Ch 155, *Hubert v. Avens, The Times*, 7 February 2003.

47 *Baldry v. Feintuck* [1972] 1 WLR 552.

48 *Attorney General v. Schonfeld* [1980] 1 WLR 1182.

49 See Gray, B. K., *A History of English Philanthropy: From the Dissolution of the Monasteries to the Taking of the First Census*, Frank Cass & Co. Ltd., London, 1967, p. 38.

50 See Jones, *History of the Law of Charity*, p. 52. Also see Jordan, W. K., *Philanthropy in England 1480–1660: A Study of the Changing Patterns of English Social Aspirations*, George Allen & Unwin Ltd., London, 1958, p. 83.

51 Also known as Gilbert's Act after the Poor Law reformer Sir Thomas Gilbert whose

nine-year campaign to bring such a bill had been repeatedly defeated in the House of Lords.

52 See Owen, D., *English Philanthropy, 1660–1960*, The Belknap Press, Harvard University, Cambridge, Massachusetts, 1964, p. 183.

53 52 Geo. III c. 101.

54 *Re Matter of Bedford Charity* (1819) 2 Swanst. 470; *Attorney-General* v. *Green* (1820) 1 Jac & W 303; *Re Lawford Charity, ex parte Skinner* (1817) 2 Mer 453.

55 By the time this Royal Commission finally completed its mammoth investigation into the abuse of charitable donations it had cost nearly £4 million, produced 40 volumes of reports, scrutinized some 29,000 charities and had recovered at least £13 million in misused or under-utilized assets.

56 The Charity Commissioners constitution, as set out in the First Schedule to the Charities Act 1993, provides for the appointment of a Chief Charity Commissioner and two other Commissioners. The Home Secretary, with Treasury approval, has a discretionary power to appoint a further two Commissioners.

57 Section 1(3) of the Charities Act 1993.

58 See Sir William Grant MR in *Morice* v. *The Bishop of Durham*, op. cit. He then stated that a fixed principle existed in the law of England that purposes deemed to be charitable are those 'which that Statute enumerates' and those 'which by analogies are deemed within its spirit and intendment'. Also see *London University* v. *Yarrow* [1857] 1 De D & J 72, where in reference to the Preamble, Cranworth LC stated that the 'objects there enumerated are not to be taken as the only objects of charity, but are given as instances'.

59 For the constituents of charitable intention see, for example: *In re Lysaght* [1966] Ch 191, pp. 201–3; *In re Woodham's* [1981] 1 WLR 493, p. 500–2; *In re Stewart's Will Trusts* [1983] NI 283, pp. 297–8.

60 See Warburton, J., *et al.* (eds), *Tudor on Charities*, Sweet & Maxwell, London, 1995, p. 9.

61 *Re White* (1893) 2 Ch. 41.

62 Ibid., p. 53.

63 *Mills* v. *Farmer* (1815) 1 Mer. 55.

64 See *Moggridge* v. *Thackwell* (1807) 13 Ves. 416; affirming (1803) 7 Ves. 36, *Re Hill* (1909) 53 SJ 228.

65 *Weir* v. *Crum-Brown* [1908] AC 162.

66 *In re Harwood; Coleman* v. *Innes* [1936] 1 Ch 285.

67 *In re Spence dec'd; Ogden* v. *Shackleton* [1979] Ch 483.

68 See *Attorney General* v. *Pearce* (1740) 2 Atk 87, *per* Lord Hardwicke LC, who declared that it was extensiveness that constitutes a public charity.

69 *Cross* v. *The London Anti-Vivisection Society* [1985] 2 Ch 501, *per* Chitty J, p. 504.

70 *Re Scarisbrick* [1951] Ch 622, pp. 648–9.

71 See, for example, s 1(1) of the Recreational Charities Act 1958: '. . . the principle that a trust or institution to be charitable must be for the public benefit'.

72 *Joseph Rowntree Memorial Housing Association Ltd.* v. *Att-Gen* [1983] Ch 159.

73 *Re Resch's Will Trust, Le Cras* v. *Perpetual Trustee Co Ltd* [1967] 3 All ER 915.

74 *Verge* v. *Somerville* [1924] AC 496, p. 499.

75 See *Re Tree* [1945] 1 Ch 325, 327, *per* Evershed J.

76 See *Verge* v. *Somerville*, op. cit., *per* Lord Wrenbury, p. 499, and *IRC* v. *Baddeley* [1955] AC 572, *per* Lord Simmonds LC, p. 593.

77 See *Trustees of Sir Hj William's Trust* v *IRC* (1944) 27 TC 409, *per* Lawrence L.J., p. 418. Also see *Re Hobourn Aero Components Ltd's Air Raid Distress Fund* [1946] Ch 194 (CA) and *Oppenheim* v. *Tobacco Securities Trust Co. Ltd.*, op. cit., *per* Simons L.J., p. 306.

78 See *Re Drummond* [1914] 2 Ch 91 *per* Eve J, p. 97; *Verge* v. *Somerville*, op. cit., *per* Lord Wrenbury p. 499; *Trustees of Sir Hj William's Trust* v. *IRC*, op. cit., *per* Lawrence L.J., p. 418; *Re Tree*, op. cit., *per* Evershed J, p. 327; *IRC* v. *Baddeley*, op. cit., *per* Lord Simmonds LC, p. 593; and *Davies* v. *Perpetual Trustee Co. Ltd.* [1959] AC 439, *per* Lord Morton, p. 456.

79 See, for example, *Re Tree*, op. cit.
80 See *Re Compton* [1945] Ch. 123 and the 'personal nexus' test.
81 See the 'narrow' and the 'wide' rule in *IRC* v. *Baddeley*, op. cit.
82 See the report of the Goodman Committee, *Charity Law and Voluntary Organisations*, 1976, para. 40.
83 See *IRC* v. *Baddeley*, op. cit., and a class of 'Methodists'.
84 *Springhill Housing Action Committee* v. *Commissioner of Valuation* [1983] NI 184.
85 See *Oppenheim* v. *Tobacco Securities Trust Co. Ltd.*, op. cit., and a maternal relationship.
86 *See Re Tree*, op. cit., and a group of residents.
87 *Re Scarisbrick*, op. cit.
88 See, for example: *A-G* v. *Bucknall* (1741) 2 Atk 328; 26 ER 600; *Issac* v. *Defriez* (1754) Amb 595; and *Brunsden* v. *Woolredge* (1765) Amb 507, 27 ER 327 (Sewell MR).
89 *Issac* v. *Defriez* (1754) Amb. 595.
90 *White* v. *White* (1802) 7 Ves 423, 32 ER 171.
91 *Gillam* v. *Taylor* (1873) LR 16 Eq 581 (Wickens VC).
92 *Spiller* v. *Maude* (1881) 32 Ch.D. 158.
93 *Re Buck* [1896] 2 Ch. 727.
94 *Re Gosling* (1900) 48 WR 300.
95 See *Gibson* v. *South American Stores* (Gath & Chaves) Ltd. [1950] Ch 177; *Re Scarisbrick*, op. cit.; *Dingle* v. *Turner* [1972] AC 601; *Re Cohen* [1973] 1 WLR 415.
96 See, for example, *Vancouver Society of Immigrant and Visible Minority Women* v. *Minister of National Revenue* [1999] SCR 10, *per* Gonthier J.
97 *Trustees of the Londonderry Presbyterian Church House* v. *IRC* [1946] NI 178, p. 183.
98 *AG* v. *Stewart* (1872) LR 14 Eq 17.
99 See *National Anti-Vivisection Society* v. *IRC* [1948] AC 31, *per* Lord Simonds, p. 65.
100 Ibid.
101 See *Trustees of the Londonderry Presbyterian Church House* v. *IRC*, op. cit., p. 183.
102 The effect of the House of Lords ruling in this case was to restrict judicial interpretation of what might constitute a sufficiently 'public' section of the community to satisfy the test.
103 [1895] 2 Ch 501.
104 *National Anti-Vivisection Society* v. *IRC*, op. cit.
105 The leading Irish case in this context is *In re Cranston, Webb* v. *Oldfield* [1898] 1 IR 431.
106 See, for example, *In re the Worth Library* [1994] 1 ILRM 161 where Keane J explained: 'In every case, the intention of the testator is of paramount importance. If he intended to advance a charitable object recognised as such by the law, his gift will be a charitable gift.'
107 See *Oppenheim* v. *Tobacco Securities Trust Co. Ltd.*, op. cit., also *George Drexler Ofrex Foundation Trustees* v. *IRC* [1966] Ch 673; and *IRC* v. *Educational Grants Association Ltd.* [1967] Ch 993.
108 (1976) paras. 38 and 50(b).
109 See Wylie, J. C. W., *Equity and Trusts* (2nd edn), But Butterworths, Dublin, 1998, para. 9.115.
110 *Commissioners of Charitable Donations and Bequests* v. *Sullivan* (1841) 1 Dr & War 501; *Richardson* v. *Murphy* [1903] 1 IR 227.
111 *Re Gavacan* [1913] 1 IR 276.
112 Warburton *et al.*, *Tudor on Charities*, 1995, p. 134.
113 *Knight* v. *Knight* (1840) 3 Beav. 148, p. 172.
114 *Re Koeppler's Will Trusts* [1985] 2 All ER 869.
115 See Warburton, *et al.*, *Tudor on Charities*, p. 163, citing Owen, *English Philanthropy*, p. 71.

4 Alienation, philanthropy and the common law

1 A term that refers to the inherent and essentially feudal duty resting on the King, as

'father of his people', to extend special protection to the interests of the most vulnerable in his kingdom, namely wards, lunatics and charities.

2 *Commissioners for Special Purposes of Income Tax* v. *Pemsel* [1891] AC 531.

3 As explained by the Master of the Rolls Sir William Grant in *Morice* v. *Bishop of Durham* (1804) 32 ER. 656, 9 Ves. J. 399: 'Those purposes are considered charitable which that Statute (the Statute of Charitable Uses 1601) enumerates, or which by analogies are deemed within its spirit and intendment . . .'. See, further, Chap 4.

4 The role of the Charity Commission has led to this becoming an important differentiating theme in the current charity law of England and Wales and other common law jurisdictions such as Australia and Ireland (see, further, Part IV).

5 See, for example, *Vancouver Society of Immigrant and Visible Minority Women* v. *Minister of National Revenue* (1999) 169 DLR (4th) 34, *per* Iacobucci J.

6 Exemplified in the Charity Commission's recent publication CC37, *Charities and Public Service Delivery* (June, 2005), which, in dealing with the fiduciary duties of trustees, warns that government contracts must not be allowed to undermine the independence of trustees.

7 See Radcliffe Commission, *Final Report on the Taxation of Profits and Income* (Cmnd 9474), HMSO, London, 1995, chap. 7. See also *Dingle* v. *Turner* [1972] AC 601 *per* Cross L.J., pp. 624–5.

8 *Commissioners for Special Purposes of Income Tax* v. *Pemsel*, op. cit., p. 572. This approach was endorsed in *McGovern* v. *Attorney General* (1982) 1 Ch. 321, where Slade J commented that 'this relief includes the relief of human suffering and distress' (p. 333).

9 See Charity Commissioners, CC4, *The Public Character of Charities for the Relief of Financial Hardship*, London, 2003.

10 See Hackney, J., 'The Politics of the Chancery', *Current Legal Problems*, 1981, p. 119.

11 *The Abbey Malvern Wells Ltd.* v. *Ministry of Local Government and Planning* [1951] Ch. 728.

12 *Re Resch's Will Trusts* [1969] AC 424.

13 *Re Coulthurst* (1951) Ch. 661.

14 *IRC* v. *Baddeley* [1951] 1 TLR 651, CA, p. 666.

15 Ibid.

16 *In Re Lacy* [1899] 2 Ch 149.

17 *Re de Carteret* [1933] Ch 103.

18 See *Trustees of Mary Clarke* v. *Anderson* [1904] 2 KB 645.

19 *Re Drummond* [1914] 2 Ch. 90.

20 Also, for the purposes of charity, 'poverty' does not include an object to relieve unemployment unless the unemployed person is additionally both poor and in need. See Bright, S., 'Charity and Trusts for the Public Benefit – Time for a Re-Think', *The Conveyancer and Property Lawyer*, vol. 53, 1989, pp. 28–41.

21 *Attorney General* v. *Forde* [1932] N.I. 1, p. 25.

22 *Re Dudgeon* 74 LT (NS) 613.

23 *Re Lucas* (1922) 2 Ch. 52, p. 58.

24 *Re Coulthurst*, op. cit., p. 197, but see p. 000 on gifts for widows.

25 *Russell* v. *Kellett* (1855) 3 Sm & G 264; also see *Jones* v. *Williams* (1767) Amb 651, 27 ER 422.

26 *Attorney-General* v. *Corporation of Exeter* (1827) 2 Russ 45.

27 *AG* v. *Wansay* (1808) 15 Ves 231; *Dawson* v. *Small* (1874) LR 18 Eq 114; *Re Wall* (1889) 42 Ch D 510.

28 *Woodford* v. *Parkhurst* (1639) Duke 70 (378); see also *AG* v. *Price* (1810) 17 Ves 371, 34 ER 143.

29 *Attorney-General* v. *Webster* (1875) LR 20 Eq 483.

30 *Corporation of Reading* v. *Lane* (1601) Duke 81 (361).

31 *Russell* v. *Kellett* (1855) 3 Sm & G 264; see also *Jones* v. *Williams* (1767) Amb 651, 27 ER 422.

32 *Attorney-General* v. *Corporation of Exeter* (1827) 2 Russ 45.

33 *AG* v. *Wansay*, op. cit.; *Dawson* v. *Small* (1874) LR 18 Eq 114; *Re Wall* (1889) 42 Ch D 510.

34 *Re Dudgeon* (1896) 74 LT 613.

35 *Re Coulthurst*, op. cit.

36 *Guinness Trust (London Fund)* v. *West Ham Borough Council* [1959] 1 WLR 233.

37 *A-G* v. *Painter-Stainers' Co* (1788) 2 Cox Eq Cas 51.

38 Note that in *Re Courtauld-Thomson Trusts* (1954) *The Times*, 18 December, the gift of Dorneywood estate for use 'as an official residence for the Prime Minister or a Minister of the Crown nominated by him' was almost certainly wrongly held to be charitable. As explained with admirable brevity in *Keeton & Sheridan*: 'There is no public benefit in free housing for well-to-do-people or for one minister rather than another' Sheridan, L.A., *Keeton & Sheridan's The Modern Law of Charities* (4th edn), Barry Rose, Chichester, 1992, p. 188.

39 *A-G for Northern Ireland* v. *Ford* [1932] NI 1.

40 *Re Lewis* [1953] Ch 115.

41 See, for example, *Attorney-General* v. *Matthews* where a gift 'to the poor generally' was held to be valid.

42 See, for example, *Dingle* v. *Turner* [1972] AC 601.

43 Charitable intent being itself exposed to an objective test; see, for example *Re Pinion* [1965] Ch 85, where such an intent did not prevent the court from objectively viewing the gift as non-charitable.

44 See, for example, *Re Owens* [1929] 37 OWN 97 and 'very poor people'.

45 See, for example, *Gibson* v. *South American Stores (Gath and Chaves) Ltd.* [1950] Ch 177, CA, where the form of words 'necessitous and deserving' was interpreted as disclosing the donor's primary objective to confer a benefit upon persons in a 'necessitous' state.

46 See, Picarda, H., *The Law and Practice Relating to Charities* (3rd edn), Butterworths, London, 1999, p. 36.

47 *Re Cohen* (1919) 36 TLR 16.

48 *Perpetual Trustee Co Ltd* v. *John Fairfax & Sons Pty Ltd* (1959) 76 WN NSW 226.

49 See *Incorporated Council for Law Reporting for England and Wales* v. *Attorney General* [1972] 1 Ch 73, p. 102.

50 *Re Ward* [1941] Ch 308.

51 *Whicker* v. *Hume* (1858) 7 HLC 124.

52 *Royal Choral Society* v. *IRC* [1943] 2 ALL ER 101.

53 *Incorporated Society* v. *Richards* (1841) 4 Ir Eq R 177.

54 *R* v. *Newman* (1684) 1 Lev 284.

55 See *A-G* v. *Flood* (1816) Hayes and Jo App xxi, p. xxxviii.

56 *Smith* v. *Kerr* [1902] 1 Ch 774, CA.

57 *Royal College of Surgeons of England* v. *National Provincial Bank, Ltd.* [1952] AC 631.

58 *Re Mellody* [1918] 1 Ch 228.

59 *Yates* v. *University College London* (1873) 8 Ch App 454; (1875) LR 7 HL 438; *Re British School of Egyptian Archaeology* [1954] 1 WLR 546.

60 *Re Berridge* (1890) 63 LT 470, CA; *Re Corbett* (1921) 17 Tas. LR 139.

61 *Reagan* (1957) 8 DLR (2d) 541.

62 *A-G* v. *Sepney* (1804) 10 Ves 22.

63 *Corrymeela Community* v. *Commissioner of Valuation* VR/1/1967.

64 *Lylehill Young Farmers Club* v. *Commissioner of Valuation* VR/7/1981; *Trustees of the Agricultural Research Institute* v. *Commissioner of Valuation* VR/81+82/1967.

65 *Institution of Civil Engineers* v. *IRC* [1932] 1 KB 149; *Re Lambert* [1967] SASR 19.

66 *Re Koettgen's Will Trusts* [1954] Ch 252.

67 *Re Elmore* [1968] VR 390.

68 *Re Hamilton-Grey* (1938) 38 SRNSW.

69 *Royal Choral Society* v. *Inland Revenue Commissioners* (1943) 2 All ER 101, p. 104.

70 *Re Cranstoun* (1932) 1 Ch. 537.

71 *Re Holburne* (1885) 53 LT 212, and see *Re Town and Country Planning Act 1947, Crystal*

Palace Trustees v. *Minister of Town and Country Planning* [1951] Ch 132; and *Abbott* v. *Fraser* (1874) LR 6 PC 96.

72 *Re Spence* (1938) Ch. 96.

73 *Re Hamilton-Grey* (1938) 38 SR (NSW) 262; and *Re Hopkins' Will Trusts* [1965] Ch 669.

74 *Royal Choral Society* v. *Inland Revenue Commissioners* (1943) 2 All ER 101.

75 *IRC* v. *Glasgow Musical Festival Association* [1926] SC 920; *Shillington* v. *Portadown Urban Council* [1911] 1 IR 247.

76 *Re Levien* [1955] 3 All ER 35.

77 *Re Delius, Emmanuel* v. *Rosen* [1957] Ch 299.

78 *Re Shakespeare Memorial Trust, Earl Lytton* v. *A-G* [1923] 2 Ch 398, *Associated Artists* v. *Inland Revenue Commissioners* (1956) 1 WLR 752.

79 *Keren Kayemeth Le Jisroel* v. *Inland Revenue Commissioners* (1931) 48 TLR 459, p. 477. But also see *Thornton* v. *Howe* (1862), 54 ER, 1042, 31 Beav 14 where, in a doubtful ruling, the court held that a trust for the printing, publishing and propagation of the sacred writings of the late Joanna Southcote (who claimed to have been made pregnant by the Holy Ghost and was to give birth to the second Messiah) was a valid charitable trust for a religious purpose.

80 *Re South Place Ethical Society, Barralet* v. *Attorney General* [1980] 1 WLR 1565; (1980) 124 SJ 774; [1980] 3 All ER 918.

81 *Re South Place Ethical Society, Barralet* v. *Attorney General* (1980) 3 All ER 918, p. 924.

82 *Application for Registration as a Charity by the Church of Scientology (England and Wales)*, Charity Commissioners Decision, 17 November 1999, p. 24.

83 *Fellowship of Humanity* v. *County of Almeda* 153 Cal. App. 2d673 (1957), formally rejected in the *Church of Scientology* Case, op. cit.

84 See the ruling of the House of Lords in *Farley* v. *Westminster Bank* (1939) AC 430, where a trust for 'parish work' was denied charitable status because the form of words was too all–encompassing.

85 *Morice* v. *Bishop of Durham* (1805) 9 Ves 399.

86 *Re Foster* [1939] 1 Ch 22.

87 *Thornton* v. *Howe* (1862), 31 Beav 14.

88 See *Re Lysaght, Hill* v. *Royal College of Surgeons of England* [1966] Ch 191, [1965] 2 All ER 888, which concerned a trust to establish a medical scholarship unavailable to both Roman Catholics and Jews.

89 Ibid, at p. 20.

90 *Application for Registration as a Charity by the Church of Scientology (England and Wales)*, p. 24.

91 *Church of the New Faith* v. *Commissioner for Pay Roll Tax* (1983) 49 ALR 65.

92 *R* v. *Registrar General ex parte Segerdal* (1970) 2 QB 697.

93 *Funnell* v. *Stewart* (1996) 1 WLR 288.

94 See, for example, *Vancouver Regional FreeNet Association* v. *Minister of National Revenue* [1996] 137 DLR (4th) 206, where the court held that the provision of a free publicly accessible Internet service to a particular community was a charitable purpose.

95 See, for example, *Re Lucas* (1922) 2 Ch 52, where the court was of the view that a gift to old people of a parish would fail unless the court implied poverty into the gift.

96 *Baddeley* v. *IRC* [1955] AC 572, 585.

97 *Re Hadji Daeing Tahira binte Daeing edelleh's Estate* (1947) 14 MLJ 62, p. 63 (Singapore CA).

98 *Re Sanders' Will Trusts* [1954] Ch 265.

99 *Re Niyazi's Will Trusts* [1978] 1 WLR 910.

100 *Joseph Rowntree Memorial Trust Housing Association Ltd.* v. *Attorney General* [1983] Ch 159, 171 (see also, *Re Dunlop* [1984] NI 408).

101 *Re Scarisbrick* (1951) Ch. 622, p. 639.

102 See *National Anti-Vivisection Society* v. *IRC* [1948] AC 31, 65, *per* Lord Simonds; and also *McGovern* v. *A-G* [1982] Ch 321, *per* Slade J.

103 This is a strict legal requirement for charitable status. See, for example, dicta of Russell L.J. in *Re Grove-Grady* [1929] 1 Ch 557.

104 *Re Compton* [1945] Ch 123.
105 *In re Gulbenkian's Settlements* [1970] AC 508.
106 *Re Compton*, op. cit., Ch 123, p. 131.
107 *Spencer* v. *All Souls College* (1762) Wilm 163; and *Attorney General* v. *Sidney Sussex College* (1869) LR 4 Ch App 722.
108 *Re Koettgen's Will Trusts* [1954] Ch 252.
109 *Re Shaw* [1957] 1 WLR 729, p. 737.
110 See *Incorporated Council for Law Reporting for England and Wales* v. *Attorney General* [1972] 1 Ch 73, *per* Buckley L.J., who expressed the view of the court that education must 'extend to the improvement of a useful branch of human knowledge and its public dissemination' (p. 102).
111 See *The Abbey, Malvern Wells Ltd* v. *Ministry of Local Government and Planning* [1951] Ch 728, where it was said that 'it is well established that education need not be provided free of charge in order to be charitable'.
112 See *Attorney-General* v. *Lord Lonsdale* (1827) 1 Sim 105.
113 See *Re Mariette* [1915] 2 Ch 284; and *Re Geere's Will Trusts (No. 2)* [1954] CLY 388.
114 See *Brunyate* (1945) 61 LQR 268, p. 273.
115 See *Re Pinion* [1965] Ch 85; and *Sutherland's Trustees* v. *Verschoyle* 1968 SLT 43.
116 See *Commissioner of Valuation* v. *Trustees, Newry Christian Brothers* [1971] NI 114.
117 *Trustees of the Congregation of Poor Clares* v. *Commissioner of Valuation* [1971] NI 174.
118 *Gilmour* v. *Coats* [1949] A.C. 426. But also see *Decisions of the Charity Commissioners*, vol. 3, HMSO, London, January 1995, pp. 11–17, which records that the Charity Commissioners did register an enclosed community of Anglican nuns, the Society of the Precious Blood, following amendments to the community's constitution.
119 See Martin, J., *Hanbury & Martin, Modern Equity* (14th edn), 1993, p. 420.
120 See Lord Simonds in *Williams* v. *IRC* [1947] AC 447 and *IRC* v. *Baddeley* [1955] AC 572, p. 615; and Lord Somervell in *IRC* v. *Baddeley*, op. cit., p. 592 (although note the quite different conclusion reached by Lord Reid in *Baddeley*, pp. 612–13).
121 *Oppenheim* v. *Tobacco Securities Trust Co. Ltd.* [1951] AC 297.
122 Ibid.
123 *IRC* v. *Baddeley* [1955] AC 572, p. 590.
124 See *Re Dunlop*, op. cit., *per* Carswell J, p. 426.
125 Following the decision in *I.R.C.* v. *Baddeley* [1955] AC 572.
126 See *Re Nottage* [1985] 2 Ch 649, where a gift to encourage 'mere sport and recreation' was denied charitable status.
127 *Clancy* v. *Commissioner of Valuation* [1911] 2 IR 173.
128 *Commissioner of Valuation* v. *Lurgan Borough Council* [1968] NI 104.
129 *Shillington* v. *Portadown UDC* [1911] IR 247, pp. 156–7.
130 See *Armstrong* v. *Reeves* (1890) 25 LR Ir 325; *Swifte* v. *Colam* (1909) unreported, *per* Meredith MR; and *Swifte* v. *The Attorney-General* [1912] 1 IR 133, *per* Barton J.
131 See the issues raised by the law's recognition of charities for animal welfare (e.g. *University of London* v. *Yarrow* (1857) 1 De G & J 72; *Re Douglas* (1887) 35 Ch D 472; *Re Cranston* [1898] 1 IR 431; *Re Wedgwood* [1915] 1 Ch 113 (CA); *Re Grove-Grady* [1929] 1 Ch 557 (CA); *Re Moss* [1949] 1 All ER 495).
132 *Re Grove-Grady*, op. cit., Ch 557, p. 582.
133 See, for example, *Trustees of the Londonderry Presbyterian Church House* v. *IRC* [1946] NI 178, p. 183.
134 *In re the Worth Library* [1995] 2 IR 301; [1994] ILRM 161.
135 *Re Vancouver Regional FreeNet Association* v. *Minister of National Revenue* (1996) 137 DLR (4th) 206.
136 See RR1a, *Recognising New Charitable Purposes*, 2001, para 2.3.
137 See *Society of Immigrant & Visible Minority Women* v. *Minister of National Revenue*, op. cit.
138 See Brady, J., 'The Law of Charity and Judicial Responsiveness to Changing Need', *Northern Ireland Legal Quarterly*, 27(3), 1976, p. 201.

139 See Knight, B., *Voluntary Action: Report for the Home Office* (1993), p. 301.
140 *McGovern* v. *Attorney-General* [1981] 3 All ER 493.
141 Ibid. Also see, *N.D.G. Neighbourhood Association* v. *Revenue Canada* 88 DTC 6279 which concerned a neighbourhood association the activities of which involved campaigning on such issues as government cutbacks, transportation changes, conversion of areas into condominiums and improving roads (see, further, Chap. 13).
142 *McGovern* v. *Attorney General*, op. cit., p. 354.
143 *In re Income Tax Acts (No 1)* [1930] VLR 211.
144 See *Inland Revenue Commissioners* v. *Baddeley* [1955] 1 All ER 525, where a gift of land to trustees for the moral, social and physical well-being of a community was found to be too vague to qualify as a charitable gift.
145 See, for example, *Attorney-General (NSW)* v. *Cahill* [1969] 1 NSWR 85.
146 *Inland Revenue Commissioners* v. *Oldham Training and Enterprise Council* (1996) STC 1218.

5 The 'public benefit' test and social inclusion: the roles of government and charity in a common law context

1 See Preamble to the Charitable Uses Act 1601 (also referred to as 'the Statute of Elizabeth 1') 43 Eliz. 1. c.4.
2 *Income Tax Special Purposes Commissioners* v. *Pemsel* [1891] AC 531.
3 The rule is to the effect that to be charitable a purpose must either be specifically stated in the Preamble to the Charitable Uses Act 1601 or be capable of being construed as coming within its spirit and intendment.
4 See McIntosh, M., 'Poverty, Charity and Coercion', *Journal of Interdisciplinary History*, 35(3), 2005, pp. 457–79.
5 See the *Oxford English Dictionary* where 'impotent' is defined as 'physically weak; without bodily strength; unable to use one's limbs; helpless, decrepit'.
6 See, for example, the 'homes of rest' cases (e.g. *Re Estlin* (1903) 72 L.J. Ch. 667; *Re James* [1932] 2 Ch. 25; *Re Chaplin* [1933] Ch 115; and *Re Dean's Will Trusts* [1950] 1 All ER 882) which suggest that residential establishments used for convalescence or for the convenience of those visiting hospitalized relatives would fit within the 'impotent' category.
7 *Re Glyn* (1950) 66 TLR 510.
8 *Re Robinson* (1951) Ch. 198.
9 Ibid., p. 200.
10 *Re Lewis* [1955] Ch 104.
11 *Joseph Rowntree Memorial Trust Housing Assoc. Ltd.* v. *A-G* [1983] Ch 159.
12 Ibid., p. 171.
13 Statute of Pious Uses 1634, 10 Car. 1 Sess. 3 cap. 1.
14 See, *Joseph Rowntree Memorial Trust Housing Assoc. Ltd.* v. *A-G*, op. cit., at 174C–D, *per* Gibson J, p. 79. In Australia, see *Downing* v. *Commissioner of Taxation* (1971) 125 CLR 185, where Walsh J observed that 'the object of the amelioration clause is to benefit persons whose lot needs improvement' (p. 194).
15 *Verge* v. *Somerville* [1924] AC 496.
16 *A-G* v. *Duke of Northumberland* (1877) 7 Ch D 745.
17 England and Wales: *Wright* v. *Hobert* (1723) 9 Mod. 64; *R* v. *Special Commissioners of Income Tax, ex parte University College of North Wales* (1909) 78 LJKB 576. Ireland: *Barrington's Hospital* v. *Commissioner of Valuation* [1957] IR 299; *Campbell College, Belfast (Governors)* v. *Commissioner of Valuation for Northern Ireland* [1964] 1 WLR 912. Australia: *Verge* v. *Somerville*, op. cit.; *Re Resch's Will Trusts* [1969] 1 AC 514.
18 *Morice* v. *Bishop of Durham* (1805) 9 Ves. 399; 10 Ves. 522; 32 ER 947.
19 *Incorporated Council for Law Reporting for England and Wales* v. *Attorney General* (1971) 3 All ER 1029, p. 1036.
20 In Australia, see *Re Tasmanian Electronic Commerce Centre Pty Ltd and Federal Commissioner of*

Taxation [2004] AATA 521 and *Re The Triton Foundation and Federal Commissioner of Taxation* [2003] AATA 408.

21 *Commissioners of Inland Revenue* v. *Yorkshire Agricultural Society* (1928) KB 611.
22 *Crystal Palace* v. *Minister of Town Planning* (1951) Ch. 132.
23 See Lansley, J., 'Changing Concepts of Charity 1700–1900', paper presented to NCVO conference, Birmingham, September 2000; as cited by Deakin, N., *In Search of Civil Society*, Palgrave, London, 2001, p. 28.
24 See, for example, *Re Good* (1905) 2 Ch. 60 and *Re Gray* (1925) Ch. 362.
25 *Inland Revenue Commissioners* v. *City of Glasgow Police Athletic Association* (1953) AC 380.
26 Ibid., p. 391.
27 *Re Corbyn* (1941) Ch. 400.
28 *Inland Revenue Commissioners* v. *City of Glasgow Police Athletic Association*, op. cit.
29 Ibid., p. 391.
30 *Mahony* v. *Duggan* (1883) 11 LR Ir. 26.
31 Ibid., p. 264.
32 *Re Cohen* (1919) 36 TLR 16.
33 Ibid., p. 17.
34 See Duke, G., *Law of Charitable Uses* (1676) 109; edn Bridgman, R. W. (1805) 136; as cited by Picarda, H., *The Law and Practice Relating to Charities* (3rd edn), Butterworths, London, 1999, p. 141.
35 *Incorporated Council of Law Reporting for England and Wales* v. *A-G* [1972] Ch. 73.
36 See [1983] Charity Commission Reports, paras 28–34, as cited by Picarda, *Law and Practice Relating to Charities*, p. 141.
37 In Northern Ireland, gifts to promote peace and reconciliation have consistently been refused charitable status.
38 *Camille and Henry Dreyfus Foundation Ltd.* v. *IRC* [1954] Ch 672.
39 *Re Hood* [1931] 1 Ch 240 CA.
40 *Clancy* v. *Valuation Commissioners* [1911] 2 IR 173.
41 See, respectively, *Buell* v. *Gardner* 83 Misc 513 (1914) and *Farewell* v. *Farewell* (1892) 22 OR 573.
42 *Re Hillier*, [1944] 1 All ER 528.
43 *Re Chaplin* [1933] Ch 115.
44 See, for example, Bean, P. and Melville, J., *Lost Children of the Empire*, Unwin Hyman, London, 1989, and Platt, A., *The Child Savers*, University of Chicago Press, Chicago, 1969.
45 Dr Barnardo established his first home for orphans and abandoned children in Stepney in 1870. By his death in 1905 there were nearly 8,000 children in 96 residential homes.
46 The National Society for the Prevention of Cruelty to Children was founded in 1884 as an extension of its members' original concern for the prevention of cruelty to animals.
47 *Jackson* v. *Attorney General* (1917) 1 IR 332.
48 *Re Sahal's Will Trusts* (1958) 1 WLR 1243.
49 See Deakin, *In Search of Civil Society*.
50 Unlike mutual benefit associations that were established for member benefit: see, for example, *Nuffield (Lord)* v. *Inland Revenue Commissioners* (1946) 175 LT 465.
51 See, for example, *Re Clergy Society* (1856) 2 K & J 615, which concerned the Society for Promoting Christian Knowledge and the Church Missionary Society.
52 See, for example, Gordon, L., *Mary Wollstonecraft: A New Genus*, Little Brown, London, 2004.
53 See Carpenter, M., *Reformatory Schools for the Perishing and Dangerous Classes and for the Prevention of Juvenile Delinquency*, 1851.
54 Organizations set up for the mutual benefit of members have, of course, consistently been refused charitable status: see, for example, *Nuffield (Lord)* v. *Inland Revenue Commissioners*, op. cit.
55 See Spencer, H., *Man versus the State*, D. Appleton, New York, 1896.

56 See Gray, K., *Philanthropy and the State*, 1908.

57 See Webb, S. and Webb, B., *The Prevention of Destitution*, Longmans, London 1911.

58 See, for example, observations made by G. B. Shaw (1850–1956) in *The Intelligent Woman's Guide to Socialism, Capitalism, Sovietism, and Fascism*.

59 *IRC* v. *Baddeley* [1955] AC 572.

60 As stated in the memorandum accompanying the draft Bill.

61 See Warburton, J., Morris, D. and Riddle, N. F. (eds), *Tudor on Charities* (9th edn), Sweet & Maxwell, London, 2003, p. 122, citing RR4 *The Recreational Charities Act 1958*, 2000, para. A8.

62 *Springhill Housing Action Committee* v. *Commissioner of Valuation* [1983] NI 184.

63 See Bromley, B. and Bromley, K. 'The Historical Origins of the Definition of Religion in Charity Law', paper presented to ISTR conference, Dublin, July 2000; cited by Deakin, *In Search of Civil Society*, p. 26.

64 See Beveridge, W. H., *Voluntary Action: A Report on Methods of Social Advance*, Allen and Unwin, London, 1948. See also Wolfenden, J., *The Future of Voluntary Organisations*, Croom Helm, London, 1978, and the Home Office, *The Government and the Voluntary Sector*, HMSO, London, 1978.

65 See *Report of the Committee on the Law and Practice Relating to Charitable Trusts* (Cmd. 8710), HMSO, London, 1952, p. 8, as cited in Sheridan, L. A., *Keaton & Sheridan's The Modern Law of Charities* (4th edn), Barry Rose, Chichester, 1992, p. 2.

66 See Home Office, *Efficiency Scrutiny of Government Funding of the Voluntary Sector, Profiting from Partnership*, HMSO, London, 1990.

67 Charity Commission 6, *Charities for The Relief of Sickness* (1996).

68 *Re Resch's Will Trusts*, op. cit.

69 Ibid., p. 540–1.

70 *Re Roadley* [1930] 1 Ch 524.

71 *A-G* v. *Belgrave Hospital* [1910] 1 Ch 73.

72 *Re Adams* [1968] Ch 80.

73 See, for example, *Re Frere* [1951] Ch 27 and *Re Perreyman* [1953] 1 All ER 223. Also, see *Re Hart, Whitman* v. *Eastern Trust Co* [1951] 2 DLR 30 and *Kytherian Association of Queensland* v. *Sklavos* [1959] ALR 5.

74 *Re Resch's Will Trusts*, op. cit.

75 *Re Dunlop* [1984] NI 408. See, also, Dawson, N., *'Old Presbyterian Persons' – A Sufficient Section of the Public?* [1987] Conv. 114.

76 *Re Dunlop*, op. cit., p. 414.

77 See, for example, Salaman, L. and Anheier, H., *Defining the Nonprofit Sector: A Cross-National Analysis*, Johns Hopkins Nonprofit Sector Series 4, Manchester University Press, Manchester, 1997.

78 See *Report of the Committee on the Law and Practice Relating to Charitable Trusts* (Cmnd. 8710). This report acknowledged in the introduction its debt to Beveridge and the concern that 'financial difficulties have led to a widely-felt need to obtain the greatest advantage from the funds available and to adjust and develop the relationship between voluntary action and the government and public authorities' (p. 1).

79 In Scotland the Charities Act 1960, in the Republic of Ireland the Charities Act 1961 and in Northern Ireland the Charities Act 1964.

80 The Rowntree Charitable Trust, in keeping with other organizations, has had to hive off its non-charitable activities (in this case, research undertaken for the purpose of challenging government policy) to a quite separately established organization set up for that purpose, in order to protect the charitable status of the initial trust.

81 See, for example, Foster, C. and Plowden, J., *The State Under Stress*, Open University Press, Buckingham, 1996, for an assessment of the strategic significance of government policy at this time.

82 See the Commission on the Future of the Voluntary Sector in England, *Meeting the Challenge of Change: Voluntary Action into the 21st Century*, NCVO Publications, London,

1996 (also referred to as the Deakin report), and Kendall, J. and Knapp, M., *The Voluntary Sector in the UK*, Manchester University Press, Manchester, 1996.

83 See, for example, Pattie, C., Seyd, P. and Whiteley, P., *Citizenship in Britain*, Cambridge University Press, 2004, which draws attention to the Millennium Fund and the Russell Commission on volunteering as examples of government initiatives to promote the participation of volunteers in community projects.

84 See, for example, the Labour Party Review of the Voluntary Sector, *Building the Future Together: Labour's Policies for Partnership between Government and the Voluntary Sector*, 1997, and the Deakin and Kemp reports, each of which endorsed the contribution made by voluntary organizations to the democratic process.

85 In Northern Ireland, such involvement led to many housing estates being controlled by paramilitary factions.

86 In 1997, there were 187,000 charities registered with the Charity Commission and perhaps a further 200,000 organizations, groups, etc., that were not.

87 See the Deakin report, op. cit., and the Commission on the Future of the Voluntary Sector in Scotland, *Head and Heart*, SCVO, Edinburgh, 1997 (also referred to as the Kemp report), p. 47, para. 6.5.5.

88 See Charity Commission 37 and *Charities and Contracts* (CC 37), September 2003.

89 See the Deakin report, op. cit.

90 See, Knight, B., *Voluntary Action: Report for the Home Office*, HMSO, London, 1993, pp. 297–8.

91 See the Deakin report, op. cit., pp. 13–14.

92 See *Report of the Committee on the Law and Practice Relating to Charitable Trusts* (Cmnd. 8710), 1952 (the Nathan report), p. 12, para. 53.

93 See the Deakin report, op. cit., p. 50, para. 2.2.21.

94 The *Scottish Compact* was published in October 1998, the English Compact *Getting it Right Together* and the *Compact for Wales* were both published in November 1998. In Northern Ireland, *Building Real Partnership – Compact between Government and the Voluntary and Community Sector in Northern Ireland*, was laid before Parliament in December 1998.

95 *Building Real Partnership*, where the view is expressed that 'short-term contracts may threaten independence and the ability to speak out or campaign'.

96 See Perri 6 and Randon, A., *Liberty, Charity and Politics: Non-Profit Law and Freedom of Speech*, Dartmouth, Aldershot, 1995, pp. 5–6. Also note the observation made in the New Zealand case of *Re Collier* [1998] 1 NZLR 81, regarding the non-charitable status of trusts for the benefit of political parties, that this 'appears to be the agreed position throughout the common law world', *per* Hamond J, p. 90.

97 See the Nathan report, op. cit., p. 12, para. 53.

98 Note that charities may campaign against certain laws provided their goal is to educate the public to do voluntarily that which they may otherwise be statutorily required to do. For example, the purpose in *Jackson* v. *Phillips* (1867) 96 Mass. (14 Allen) 539 was to end slavery, not by changing the law, but by changing public sentiment through education.

99 See *Baldry* v. *Feinbuck* [1972] 1 WLR 552; (1971) 115 SJ 965; [1972] 2 All ER 81, and *Webb* v. *O'Doherty and Others* (1991) 3 Admin. LR 731, *The Times*, 11 February 1991, respectively.

100 See, further, Perri and Randon, *Liberty, Charity and Politics*.

101 See *National Anti-Vivisection Society* v. *IRC* [1948] AC 31, as applied in *Re Jenkin's Will Trusts* [1966] Ch. 249.

102 *National Anti-Vivisection Society* v. *IRC*, op. cit., p. 62.

103 *McGovern* v. *Attorney General* [1982] 1 Ch 321.

104 *Re Koeppler's Will Trusts* (1984) Ch. 243.

105 *Molloy* v. *Commissioner of Inland Revenue* [1981] 1 NZLR 688.

106 See Dal Pont, G., *Charity Law in Australia and New Zealand*, Oxford University Press, Melbourne, 2000, p. 205.

107 See Hackney, J. 'The Politics of Chancery', in *Current Legal Problems*, Stevens & Sons, University College, London, vol. 1 (1948), v. 49, pt 1, 1981, pp. 113–131.

108 See [1989] Charity Commission Report para. 31.

109 Ibid., para. 32.

110 *Joseph Rowntree Memorial Trust Housing Assoc. Ltd.* v. *A-G*, op. cit.

111 *Anglo-Swedish Society* v. *IRC* (1931) 16 TC 34, *Re Strakosch* [1949] Ch. 529 and *Buxton* v. *Public Trustee* (1962) 41 TC 235.

112 See Warburton *et al.*, *Tudor on Charities*, p. 61, citing [1983] Charity Commission Report, para. 15 ff.

113 See for example [1988] Charity Commission Report, para. 24.

114 *Att-Gen* v. *Ross* [1986] 1 WLR 252.

115 See RR1, *The Review of the Register of Charities*, 2001, pt 2.

116 See RR8, *The Public Character of Charities*, 2001.

117 See RR3, *Charities for the Relief of Unemployment*, 1999. Following *IRC* v. *Oldham Training and Enterprise Council* [1996] STC 1218, the relief of unemployment became charitable under the fourth *Pemsel* head whereas previously it was confined to the first, which required the unemployed to also be poor.

118 See RR1, *The Promotion of Urban and Rural Regeneration*, 1999.

119 Ibid.

120 Warburton *et al.*, *Tudor on Charities*, pp. 102–3.

121 See RR5, *The Promotion of Community Capacity Building*, 2000.

122 See 4 Charity Commission, Dec. 1995, pp. 1–7.

123 See 3 Charity Commission, Dec. 1995, pp. 7–10

124 See CC9a, *Political Activities and Campaigning by Local Community Charities*, 1997, and CC9, *Political Activities and Campaigning by Charities*, 1999.

125 See Charity Commission Discussion Paper, *The Promotion of the Voluntary Sector for the Benefit of the Public*, 2001.

126 See Charity Commission Discussion Paper, *Promoting the Efficiency and Effectiveness of Charities and the Effective Use of Charitable Resources*, 2001.

127 See Charity Commission Guidance, *Charities and Social Investment*, 2002.

128 See Charity Commission, *The Promotion of Human Rights*, 2002.

6 Legal functions relating to social inclusion in a modern regulatory environment for charities

1 *Income Tax Special Purposes Commissioners* v. *Pemsel* [1891] AC 531.

2 See Mitchell, C. and Moody, S., (eds), *Foundations of Charity*, Hart Publishing, Oxford, 2000.

3 See, for example, Leiter, J., *Structural Isomorphism in Australian Non-Profit Organizations*, Working Paper No. CPNS 28, Centre of Philanthropy and Nonprofit Studies, QUT, Brisbane, Australia, 2005.

4 See Ontario Law Reform Commission, *Report on the Law of Charities*, Ontario, 1996, and further at chap. 12.

5 See the Charity Law Reform Committee report *Inquiry into the Definition of Charities and Related Organisations*, Canberra, June 2001, and further at chap. 9.

6 See the Working Party on Charities and Sporting Bodies, *Report on the Accountability of Charities & Sporting Bodies*, 1997, and further at chap. 10.

7 See the Department of Equality and Law Reform *Report of the Advisory Group on Charities/Fundraising Legislation*, November 1996, and further at chap. 8.

8 See Panel on the Nonprofit Sector, *Strengthening Transparency, Governance, Accountability of Charitable Organisations*, final report to Congress and the Nonprofit Sector, Washington, 2005.

9 See, for England and Wales: the National Council for Voluntary Organizations, *For the Public Benefit? A Consultation Document on Charity Law Reform*, London, 2001, and

Private Action, Public Benefit, a Review of Charities and the Wider Not-For-Profit Sector, London, September 2002. See, for Scotland: the Scottish Charity Law Review Commission report, *Charity Scotland*, Edinburgh, 2001. See, for Northern Ireland: the Charities Branch, Voluntary & Community Unit, Department for Social Development, *Consultation on the Review of Charities Administration and Legislation in Northern Ireland*, Belfast, 2005.

10 See *The Laws of Barbados*, vol. VIII, title XVIII, chap. 243: 'Charities'.

11 See Sir William Grant MR in *Morice* v. *The Bishop of Durham* (1804) 9 Ves 405. He then stated that a fixed principle existed in the law of England that purposes deemed to be charitable are those 'which that Statute enumerates' and those 'which by analogies are deemed within its spirit and intendment'. Although the 1601 Act, and therefore also its Preamble, did not necessarily have any direct application to other common law nations, the principles and case law did extend to shape the development of their charity law (see Picarda, H., *The Law and Practice Relating to Charities* (3rd edn), Butterworths, London, 1999, pp. 14–19).

12 See, for example, *Vancouver Regional Free Net Association and Minister of National Revenue* (1996) 137 DLR (4th) 206.

13 In Ireland the test is subjective: see, for example, *In re the Worth Library* [1994] 1 ILRM 161 and further at chap. 9.

14 See *Attorney General* v. *Pearce* (1740) 2 Atk 87, *per* Lord Hardwicke LC, who declared that it was extensiveness that constitutes a public charity.

15 See, UN, foreword to *The Millennium Development Goals Report*, 2005, where the Secretary General explains:

> The eight Millennium Development Goals range from halving extreme poverty to halting the spread of HIV/AIDS and providing universal primary education – all by the target date of 2015. They form a blueprint agreed by all the world's countries and all the world's leading development institutions. . . .

16 *National Anti-Vivisection Society* v. *IRC* [1948] AC 31.

17 See Warburton, J., Morris, D. and Riddle, N. F. (eds), *Tudor on Charities*, (9th edn), Sweet & Maxwell, London, 2003, pp. 6–7.

7 International benchmarks for charity law as it relates to social inclusion

1 In the eighteenth century, Captain Cook considered he was entitled to take possession of the continent and all its creatures and resources in the name of the British Crown. The full ownership of the continent remained vested in Great Britain until transferred to the government of Australia when the latter acquired Dominion status.

2 See Article 11 as reinforced by the Preamble to the Treaty of Waitangi 1840.

3 See, for example, the UN Declaration of Indigenous Peoples 1993.

4 See, for example, the United Nations Convention on the Rights of the Child 1989.

5 See, also, The Hague Convention on Protection of Children and Co-operation in Respect of Intercountry Adoption 1993 and the United Nations Declaration on Social and Legal Principles relating to the Protection and Welfare of Children with Special Reference to Foster Placement and Adoption Nationally and Internationally 1986.

6 See *Gaudiya Mission* v. *Brahmachary* [1997] 4 All ER 957, p. 963.

7 The Human Rights Act 1998, incorporating the Convention, came into force in the UK on 2 October 2000 (see, further, chap. 8).

8 For a fuller discussion, see Warburton, J. and Cartwright, A., 'Human Rights, Public Authorities and Charities', *The Charity Law Practice Review*, 6(3), 2000.

9 *Foster* v. *British Gas* [1990] 3 All ER 897.

10 See Warburton, J., Morris, D. and Riddle, N. F. (eds), *Tudor on Charities* (9th edn), Sweet & Maxwell, London, 2003, p. 393.

11 See *National Union of Teachers* v. *Governing Body of St Mary's Church of England (Aided) Junior School* [1997] 3 CMLR 630, and also see *R* v. *Panel on Take-overs and Mergers, ex p Datafin plc* [1987] 1 QB 815.

12 *Olson* v. *Sweden (No 1)* (1988) 11 EHRR 299.

13 *R* v. *Registrar General Ex p. Segerdal* [1970] 2 QB 697.

14 See, for example, *Steel and Morris* v. *the United Kingdom* (application no. 68416/01) (2005).

15 See, for example: Canada and the Canadian Charter of Rights and Freedoms, where the freedom of association has become an entrenched right (see, further, chapter 13); the USA and the First Amendment to the US Constitution which reads:

> Congress shall make no law respecting an establishment of religion, or prohibiting the free exercise thereof; or abridging the freedom of speech, or of the press; or the right of the people peaceably to assemble, and to petition the government for a redress of grievances.

(See, further, chap. 12).

16 As does the Helsinki Accords of the Organization (former Conference) on Security and Cooperation in Europe (OSCE). Also, see the Freedom of Association and Protection of the Right to Organize Convention, 1948 (No. 87) and the Right to Organize and Collective Bargaining Convention, 1949 (No. 98).

17 *Sidiropoulos and Others* v. *Greece* (26695/95) 27 EHRR (1998).

18 Ibid., para. 40.

19 See, for example, *Young, James and Webster* v. *the United Kingdom* (1982) 4 EHRR 38, where the court stressed the importance of ensuring 'the fair and proper treatment of minorities' and held that the 'closed shop' was a violation of Article 11.

20 *The Socialist Party of Turkey and Others* v. *Turkey* (1998) 27 EHRR 51.

21 See, also, *Refah Partisi (Welfare Party) and Others* v. *Turkey* (2002) 35 E.H.R.R. 3, pp. 77–8.

22 *Partidul Communistilor (Nepeceristi) and Ungureanu* v. *Romania* (application no. 46626/99), (2005).

23 *Wilson and Palmer* v. *United Kingdom* (2002) 35 EHRR 20.

24 See *National Union of Belgian Police* v. *Belgium* (1975) 1 EHRR 578, para. 39.

25 *Refah Partisi* v. *Turkey*, App. Nos 41340/98 and 41342/98, 13 February 2003.

26 See, also, *Ezelin* v. *France*, 26 Apr. 1996 (No. 202), 14 E.H.R.R. 362, para. 62.

27 *RSPCA* v. *Attorney General and Others* [2002] 1 WLR 448.

28 The debate as to whether *McGovern* v. *Att-Gen* [1982] Ch 321 would now be decided differently, in the light of the Human Rights Act 1998, continues.

29 *Bowman* v. *United Kingdom* (1998) 26 EHRR 1.

30 *Open Door and Dublin Well Woman* v. *Ireland* (1992) 15 EHRR 244.

31 *Steel and Morris* v. *The United Kingdom*, op. cit.

32 *Southwark LBC* v. *St Brice* [2002] EWCA Civ 1138, [2002] 1 WLR 1537.

33 Citing *Kjeldsen, Busk Madsen and Pedersen* v. *Denmark* (1976) 1 EHRR 711, para. 56.

34 As expressed by the ECHR in *National Union of Belgian Police* v. *Belgium*, op. cit.

35 *Dudgeon* v. *United Kingdom* (1981) 4 EHRR 149.

36 See, for example, *Tsirlis and Kouloumpas* v. *Greece* (1997) 25 EHRR 198. Also, see the *Belgian Linguistic Case* (1968) (No 2) 1 EHRR 252, where the ECHR held that there must be an objective and reasonable justification for differential treatment and this will only exist where there is a 'legitimate aim' for the action and where the action taken is 'proportionate' to that aim.

37 For a fuller discussion, see Quint, F. and Spring, T., 'Religion, Charity Law and Human Rights', *The Charity Law & Practice Review*, 5(3), 1999, pp. 153–86.

38 *Lithgow* v. *United Kingdom* (1986) 8 EHRR 329.

39 *Fredin* v. *Sweden* (1991) 13 EHRR 784.

40 *Abdulaziz, Cabales and Balkandali* v. *United Kingdom* (1985) 7 EHRR 471.

41 See *Van Raalte* v. *Netherlands* (1997) 24 EHRR 503, where again the ECHR ruled that a

difference in treatment based on gender was not justified under the Convention and that the State had breached the applicant's Article 14 rights taken in conjunction with Article 1 of the First Protocol.

42 Quint and Spring, 'Religion, Charity Law and Human Rights', p. 169.
43 *Thlimmenos* v. *Greece* (2000) 31 EHRR 4121, para. 44.
44 Ibid.
45 *Moreira de Azevedo* v. *Portugal* (19990) 13 EHRR 721.
46 *Airey* v. *Ireland* (1979) Series A No 32, 2 EHRR 305.
47 See *Dombo Beheer BV* v. *Netherlands* (1993) 18 EHRR 213, para. 33.
48 *Steel and Morris* v. *The United Kingdom*, op. cit.
49 See *Kroon* v. *Netherlands* (1994) 19 EHRR 263.
50 See *Airey* v. *Ireland*, op. cit.
51 See *Re W and B; Re W (Care Plan)* [2001] EWCA Civ 757, as reported in 31 Family Law 581.
52 See *Olson* v. *Sweden (No 1)*, op. cit., where it is explained that to be justifiable such interference must be 'relevant and sufficient; it must meet a pressing social need; and it must be proportionate to the need'.
53 See, for example, *Buchberger* v. *Austria*, Application No. 32899/96, 20 December 2001.
54 See, for example, *TP and KM* v. *United Kingdom* [2001] 2 FLR 549. Also, see *Re M (Care: challenging decision by local authority)* [2002] FLR 1300.
55 *Smith and Grady* v. *United Kingdom* (2000) 29 EHRR 548.
56 *Goodwin* v. *United Kingdom* (2002) 35 EHRR 447.
57 *Malone* v. *United Kingdom* (1984) 7 EHRR 14.
58 *Halford* v. *United Kingdom* (1997) 24 EHRR 523. Also, see, *Niemietz* v. *Germany* (1992) 16 EHRR 97.
59 See *Malone* v. *United Kingdom*, op. cit., para. 79; as cited in Wadham, J., Mountfield, H. and Edmundson, A., *Blackstone's Guide to The Human Rights Act 1998* (3rd edn), Oxford, Oxford University Press, 2003, p. 163.
60 See Gunn, T. J., 'Adjudicating Rights of Conscience Under the European Convention on Human Rights' in Van der Vyver, J.D. and Witte, J.D. (eds), *Religious Human Rights in Global Perspective: Legal Perspectives*, Martinus Nijhoff, The Hague, 1996.
61 Ibid., p. 311.
62 *Kokkinakis* v. *Greece* (A/260-A) (1994) 17 EHRR 397.
63 *Manoussakis* v. *Greece* (18748/91) (1996) 21 EHRR CD3.
64 Ibid., para. 48.

8 Charity law and social inclusion in England and Wales

1 Established in 1997 as part of the Cabinet Office, the Unit moved to the Office of the Deputy Prime Minister in May 2002. Its brief is described as 'working to create prosperous, inclusive and sustainable communities for the 21st century'. See, further, at http://www.socialexclusionunit.gov.uk.
2 See Charity Commission, *Annual Report*, 2005.
3 See Wright, K., 'Generosity vs. Altruism: Philanthropy and Charity in the United States and United Kingdom', *Voluntas: International Journal of Voluntary and Nonprofit Organizations*, 12(4), 2002, p. 401.
4 The Joseph Rowntree Charitable Foundation is a social policy research and development charity that funds research projects designed to increase understanding of the causes of social difficulties in the UK.
5 See the Centre for Analysis of Social Exclusion, London School of Economics, *Policies towards Poverty, Inequality and Exclusion since 1997*, 2005. Report findings are published in Hills, J. and Stewart, K. (eds), *A More Equal Society? New Labour, Poverty, Inequality and Exclusion*, The Policy Press, Bristol, 2005.
6 Barnardo's, established in 1866, is the UK's largest children's charity.

7   See Barnardo's, *Then and Now*, 2005. Note, also, the End Child Poverty Now coalition of charities claim that 3.6 million children are still living in poverty and that infant mortality rates are 70 per cent higher in low-income areas than in more affluent areas.

8   Poverty is interpreted for charity law purposes in a flexible manner – see Charity Commission booklet CC4.

9   See Barnardo's, *Then and Now*, p. 9; citing Department for Work and Pensions, 2002.

10 See The Home Office, *After Stephen Lawrence*, HMSO, 1999. This report presented the findings of an inquiry led by Sir William Macpherson into the murder of Stephen Lawrence in 1993. Among the principal findings was the extent of 'institutional racism' in the Metropolitan Police service.

11 See Ms Fiona Mactaggart on introducing the Charities Bill in May 2005.

12 Statute of Charitable User 1601, 43 Eliz. 1, c.4.

13 Kelley, T., 'Rediscovering Vulgar Charity – A Historical Analysis of America's Tangled Nonprofit Law', *Fordham Law Review*, 73(6) May 2005, pp. 2437–99.

14 The author is grateful to Paul Bater for his observations on this matter.

15 See *Income Tax Special Commissioners v. Pemsel* [1891] AC 531.

16 This rule provides that even though a purpose cannot be defined as coming under one of the established heads of charity, it will nonetheless be construed as charitable if it can be interpreted as falling within the 'spirit or intendment' of the Preamble to the 1601 Act.

17 See *Inland Revenue Commissioners v. Baddeley* [1955] AC 572.

18 See *Report of the Committee on the Law and Practice Relating to Charitable Trusts* (Cmnd. 8710), 1952 (the Nathan report).

19 See *Government Policy on Charitable Trusts in England and Wales* (Cmnd. 9538), 1955.

20 See the Charities Act (NI) 1964.

21 See the Charities Act 1961.

22 See Ford, P., 'Public Benefit Versus Charity: A Scottish Perspective', in Mitchell, C. and Moody, S. (eds), *Foundations of Charity*, Hart Publishing, Oxford, 2005, pp. 205–48.

23 Despite recommendations made in the Nathan report, op. cit., that the time had come to introduce a statutory definition of 'charity', albeit along the lines of the *Pemsel* classification.

24 See *Efficiency Scrutiny of the Supervision of Charities* 1987 (the Woodfield report).

25 See *Charities: A Framework for the Future* (Cmnd. 694), 1989, paras 2.07–2.17. Thereby ignoring the recommendation made by the National Council of Social Services (later the NCVO) in the report of the Goodman Committee, *Charity Law and Voluntary Organisations*, 1976, (the Goodman report) that it was time for a statutory restatement of charitable purposes.

26 *Charities: A Framework for the Future*, para. 2.11.

27 See *For the Public Benefit? A Consultation Document on Charity Law Reform*, NCVO Charity Law Reform Advisory Group, London, January 2001. In Scotland the law is now to be found in the Charities and Trustee Investment (Scotland) Act 2005 as a result of *Charity Scotland*, the report of the Scottish Charity Law Review Commission, 2001. In Northern Ireland the law remains largely framed by the Charities Act (NI) 1964, which was closely modelled on the Charities Act 1960, as supplemented by the Charities (NI) Order 1987; though new legislation is imminent and consultation on establishing a Charity Commission is underway.

28 *Re King* [1923] 1 Ch. 243.

29 See, for example, *Anglo-Swedish Society v. Commissioners of Inland Revenue* (1931) 16 TC 34.

30 See, for example, s. 1(1) of the Recreational Charities Act 1958: 'the principle that a trust or institution to be charitable must be for the public benefit'.

31 *The Report of the Commission on the Future of the Voluntary Sector*, NCVO, 1996 (the Deakin report).

32 *Att.-Gen. of the Cayman Islands v. Wahr-Hansen* [2000] 3 All ER 642

33 Charity Commission RR7, *The Independence of Charities from the State*, London, 2001.

34 See Charity Commission CC37, *Charities and Contracts*, London, September 2003.
35 See Charity Commission, *Policy Statement on Charities and Public Service Delivery* (June 2005), p. 2. Also, see Charity Commission RR7, op. cit., in which, however, there is a notable lack of cited case law. The case of *Construction Industry Training Board* v. *A-G* [1973] Ch 173 suggests that ministerial control is not incompatible with charity status (the author is grateful to Paul Bater for drawing this to his attention).
36 See, Charity Commission and Applications for Registration of (i) Trafford Community Leisure Trust and (ii) Wigan Leisure and Culture Trust (21 April 2004).
37 The author is grateful to Paul Bater for drawing this to his attention.
38 See Charity Commissioners, RR8, *The Public Character of Charity*, London, 2001, p. 2.
39 Charity Commissioners, RR1a, *Recognising New Charitable Purposes*, London, 2001.
40 Charity Commissioners, RR2, *Promotion of Urban and Rural Regeneration*, London, 1999.
41 Charity Commissioners, RR3, *Charities for the Relief of Unemployment*, London, 1999.
42 Charity Commissioners, RR5, *The Promotion of Community Capacity Building*, London, 2000.
43 See Warburton, J., Morris, D. and Riddle, N. F., Thomson (eds), *Tudor on Charities* (9th edn), Sweet & Maxwell, London, 2003, p. 103.
44 The author is grateful to Gareth Morgan for the information illustrating the wide use of alternative legal structures.
45 The Charity Commission liaises with the Inland Revenue at the pre-registration stage in difficult cases and, since the latter must accept the Commission's registration as conclusive of charitable status for tax purposes, if it disagrees with the decision to register it has to challenge that decision at this stage.
46 The Charities Act 1993, s. 16.
47 Ibid., s. 32.
48 See, for example, *Re Hummeltenberg* [1923] 1 Ch 237.
49 See, for example, *Gaudiya Mission* v. *Brahmachary* [1997] 4 ALL ER 957.
50 See *Re Le Cren Clarke* [1996] 1 All ER 715.
51 See (1993) 1 Ch. Com. Dec., paras 4 *et. seq.*
52 Continued under the Charities Act 1993, s. 3(1).
53 Committee of Public Accounts, *Charity Commission: Regulation and Support of Charities*, 28th Report, HC Session 1997–8, The Stationery Office, London, 1998, p. 10: a position that has at times left it open to the challenge that it does not give sufficient attention to its statutory regulatory duties: see, for example, Wilkinson, H. W., 'The Charity Commission: Regulation and Support of Charities', 148 NLJ 752, 1998.
54 See *A Generous Society*, the Home Office, 2005.
55 *Varsani* v. *Jesani* [1999] Ch 219.
56 Gareth Morgan has helpfully explained 'commercial participator' to the author as follows: where a business participates in a form of cause-related marketing, whereby it promises a contribution to charity for each item sold, the business is a commercial participator for the purposes of Part II of Charities Act 1992.
57 The distinction between professional fundraisers and commercial participation, as defined in the 1992 Act, is that the main business of the former is fundraising whereas the business of the latter is not fundraising but making a promised contribution to charity out of the proceeds of business.
58 See Charity Commissioners, CC20, *Charities and Fund-Raising*, London, 2002.
59 See Charity Commissioners, CC35, *Charities and Trading*, London, 2001.
60 See the Goodman report, op. cit.
61 See the Commission on the Future of the Voluntary Sector in England, *Meeting the Challenge of Change: Voluntary Action into the 21st Century*, NCVO Publications, London, 1996, p. 50, para. 2.2.21.
62 The *Scottish Compact* was published in October 1998, the English Compact *Getting it Right Together* and the *Compact for Wales* were both published in November 1998. In Northern Ireland, *Building Real Partnership – Compact between Government and the Voluntary*

and Community Sector in Northern Ireland was laid before Parliament in December 1998. Subsequently local compacts have been agreed and a new Compact Plus introduced (2005). See, further, at http://www.compact.org.uk.

63 See, for example, the Deakin report, op. cit.

64 Charity Commission, *Policy Statement on Charities and Public Service Delivery* (June 2005), p. 2. Also, see, Charity Commission RR7, *The Independence of Charities from the State*, London, 2001, and *Charities and Contracts* (CC37).

65 The author is grateful to Paul Bater for drawing this to his attention.

66 See, for example, *The Gdansk Hospice Fund* [1990] Charity Commission Report 7, para. 32. See, further, Picarda, H., 'Charity overseas and the public benefit' in *The Law and Practice Relating to Charities*' (3rd edn) Butterworths, London, 1999, pp. 27–9.

67 *Camille & Henry Dreyfus Foundation Inc.* v. *Inland Revenue Commissioners* [1954] Ch. 672.

68 See, Charity Commission, *Report*, 1963, para. 72.

69 *McGovern* v. *A-G* [1982] Ch. 321: the court's ruling – that it has no means of determining whether the outcome of policy change would be beneficial or otherwise – being equally applicable to the position of such an aid-giving charity.

70 See, further, the EU consultation in July 2005 on draft recommendations to member states on a code of conduct for nonprofit organizations.

71 See Charity Commissioners, CC60, *The Hallmarks of a Well-Run Charity*, London, 1999.

72 See, Warburton *et al.*, *Tudor on Charities*, p. 173.

73 See, for example, *National Anti-Vivisection Society* v. *IRC* [1948] AC 31 and *McGovern* v. *A-G*, op. cit., *per* Slade J, pp. 336–7.

74 See Charity Commissioners, CC9, *Political Activities and Campaigning by Charities*, London, 1997. Also, see comments by the Commission released in 2004 during the Charities Bill discussions (at http://www.charity commission.gov.uk).

75 *Commissioners for Special Purposes of Income Tax* v. *Pemsel* [1891] AC 531.

76 The Human Rights Act 1998, s. 1(1), makes it unlawful for any public authority to act in a manner that breaches a Convention right or freedom as defined in Articles 2–12 of the Convention, Articles 1–3 of the First Protocol and Articles 1 and 2 of the Sixth Protocol as read with Articles 16–18 of the Convention.

77 See *A and others* v. *Secretary of State for the Home Department, X and another* v. *Secretary of State for the Home Department* [2004] UKHL 56.

78 See NCVO, *For the public benefit? A consultation document on charity law reform.*

79 See Cabinet Office Strategy Unit, *Private Action, Public Benefit: A Review of Charities and the Wider Not-For-Profit Sector*, London, 2002.

80 See Home Office, *Charities and Not-for-Profits: A Modern Legal Framework*, London, 2003.

81 See Home Office, *Charities Bill*, London, 2004, and revised Bill introduced in House of Lords, 18 May 2005.

82 See *The Report of the Commission on the Future of the Voluntary Sector*, National Council for Voluntary Organizations, London, 1996.

83 Contrary to the position taken in the previous government White Paper, *Charities: A Framework for the Future* (Cmnd 694), 1989.

84 The provision of recreational facilities in the interests of social welfare will continue to be recognized as charitable under the Recreational Charities Act 1958.

85 See Charity Commissioners, RR8, *The Public Character of Charity*, London, 2001, as revised in *Public Benefit – The Legal Principles*, 2005.

86 According to the Regulatory Impact Assessment published at the same time as the draft bill, charities will not have to pay to use the tribunal although they will have to pay any legal fees unless awarded costs in the absence of the suitor's fund proposed to but rejected by the government.

87 See *Public Collections for Charitable, Philanthropic and Benevolent Purposes*, Home Office, London, 2003.

88 The sector, led by the Institute of Fundraising, established the Buse Commission in 2003, under the chairmanship of Rodney Buse, to review the scope for the charity

sector to establish a self-regulatory framework for charity fundraising. It released its initial report in January 2004.

89 See Barnardo's, *Then and Now*.

90 See, also, Charity Commissioners, RR1a, *Recognising New Charitable Purposes*, London, 2001.

9 Charity law and social inclusion in Ireland

1 Statute of Pious Uses 1634 (10 Car. 1, Sess. 3, c. 1).

2 Statute of Charitable Uses 1601 (43 Eliz. 1, c. 4).

3 The population of the State increased by over 290,000 persons between 1996 and 2002 to reach its highest level since 1871, according to *Census 2002 – Preliminary Report*. The number of immigrants now exceeds the number of emigrants by a considerable margin. Ireland is thus, for the first time in its recent history, becoming a country of immigration.

4 Under the Belfast (Good Friday) Agreement 1998.

5 See, further, O'Halloran, K., *Charity Law*, Round Hall Sweet & Maxwell, Dublin, 2000; O'Halloran, K. and Fitzgerald, E., 'Country Report for Ireland: NGO Laws and Regulations', for the *International Reporter of Not-for-Profit Law*, ICNL, Washington, D.C., 2002, vol. 1, pp. 1–33.

6 See, for example, the National Anti-Poverty Strategy 1997.

7 As expressed by an Taoiseach:

> Voluntary activity forms the very core of all vibrant and inclusive societies . . . Particularly in a time of great change in our country, we must work hard to protect and enhance the spirit of voluntary participation and we must see this as a key social goal.

See Dept of Social Welfare, *Supporting Voluntary Activity: A White Paper on a Framework for Supporting Voluntary Activity and for Developing the Relationship between the State and the Community and Voluntary Sector*, Stationery Office, Dublin, 2000, Foreword.

8 See Donoghue, F., Anheier, H. and Salamon, L., *Uncovering the Nonprofit Sector in Ireland*, Johns Hopkins University/National College of Ireland, 1999.

9 Revenue Commissioners, 2000.

10 Irish Charities Tax Reform Group, 2000.

11 The Department of Finance indicated that unemployment had reached 3.9 per cent in March 2001.

12 See, for example, two studies carried out by the independent Economic and Social Research Institute for the Department of Social Welfare and the Combat Poverty Agency, *Poverty in the 1990s – Evidence from the Living in Ireland Survey* and *A Review of the Commission on Social Welfare's Minimum Adequate Income*, both published in December 1996. These studies provide a wide variety of very useful information on poverty levels in Ireland.

13 See Piaras Mac Éinrí, *Immigration into Ireland: Trends, Policy Responses, Outlook*, ICMS, 2001, where it is noted that in the period 1995–2000, approximately a quarter of a million persons (constituting a 7 per cent increase in the population) migrated to Ireland, of whom about half were returning Irish.

14 Since 1995, asylum seekers have probably constituted no more than 10 per cent of all foreign immigrants to Ireland but have presented a considerable challenge to Irish social inclusion policies.

15 See *National Action Plan Against Poverty and Social Exclusion*, Office for Social Inclusion, First Annual Report, Implementation of Plan 2003–4.

16 See *Report of the Committee on Fundraising Activities for Charitable and Other Purposes*, Stationery Office, Dublin, 1990, (also known as the Costello report) and *Report of the Advisory*

Group on Charities/Fundraising Legislation, Department of Equality and Law Reform, Dublin, 1996. Also, see Department of Social Welfare, *Supporting Voluntary Activity: A Green Paper on the Community Voluntary Sector and its Relationship with the State*, Stationery Office, Dublin, 1997 (the 'Green Paper') and *Supporting Voluntary Activity: A White Paper for Supporting Voluntary Activity and for Developing the Relationship between the State and the Community and Voluntary Sector*, 2001 (the 'White Paper'). Also, a report from the Law Society (2002), as well as the Arthur Cox-led Review (2002).

17 *Agreed Programme of Government*, Dublin, June 2002.

18 See Ahern D., Minister for Social, Community and Family Affairs, in Dept of Social Welfare, *Supporting Voluntary Activity: A White Paper on a Framework for Supporting Voluntary Activity and for Developing the Relationship between the State and the Community and Voluntary Sector*, Stationery Office, Dublin, 2000, foreword.

19 Statute of Charitable Uses 1601, op. cit.

20 Statute of Pious Uses 1634, op. cit.

21 *Incorporated Society v. Richards*, 3 Ir. Eq. Rep. 177.

22 *Income Tax Special Commissioners v. Pemsel* [1891] AC 531.

23 For example, whereas a properly constituted registered charity from outside the jurisdiction may fundraise in Ireland it will not qualify for charitable exemption from Irish taxes because the Revenue Commission will not recognize as charitable an organization that is not 'established' in Ireland.

24 See the Valuation (Ireland) Acts 1852 and 1854. Note, however, that the Poor Relief (Ireland) Act 1838 has now been repealed and replaced by the Valuation Act 2001.

25 The leading Irish case in this context is *In re Cranston, Webb v. Oldfield* [1898] 1 IR 431.

26 *In re the Worth Library* [1994] 1 ILRM 161.

27 See, for example, s. 1(1) of the Recreational Charities Act 1958: 'the principle that a trust or institution to be charitable must be for the public benefit'.

28 See *Jackson v. Attorney General* (1917) 1 IR 332 and *Moore v. The Pope* (1919) 1 IR 316.

29 Delany, H., *Equity and the Law of Trusts in Ireland*, Round Hall Sweet & Maxwell, Dublin, 1996, p. 252.

30 *In re the Worth Library*, op. cit.

31 Specifically overruling, by a majority of three to two, the decision in *Inland Revenue Commissioners v. Broadway Cottages Trust* [1955] Ch 20.

32 See *Inland Revenue Commissioners v. Broadway Cottages Trust*, op. cit.; also see *In re Gulbenkian's Settlements* [1970] AC 508.

33 See *Kilroy v. Parker* [1966] IR 309.

34 See *In the matter of Davoren dec'd; O'Byrne v. Davoren and Coughlan*, unreported, High Court, Budd J., 13 May 1994.

35 *Re Koettgen's Will Trusts* [1954] Ch 252.

36 See Keane J in *Re Worth Library*, op. cit., reference made to: *In re Shaw, Public Trustee v. Day* [1957] 1 WLR 729, 737, dicta of Harman J doubted; *Re Hopkins' Will Trusts, Naish v. Francis Bacon Society Inc* [1965] Ch 669, 680, dicta of Wilberforce J approved.

37 *Re Worth Library*, op. cit.

38 Citing as his authority *Re Scowcroft, Ormrod v. Wilkinson* [1898] 2 Ch 638, 642.

39 See *Attorney General v. Marchant* (1866) LR 3 Eq 424.

40 This was acknowledged by O'Higgins CJ in *Norris v. A-G* [1984] IR 36.

41 *O'Hanlon v. Logue* [1906] IR 247. See also: *Arnott v. Arnott (No 2)* [1906] 1 IR 127; and *Rickerby v. Nicholson* [1912] 1 IR 343, p. 347, where Ross J declared that 'according to our law a bequest for a religious purpose is *prima facie* charitable'.

42 The Statute of Chantries 1547 led to gifts for the saying of masses being deemed illegal in England and Wales but it never applied to Ireland where the validity of such gifts was recognized (See *Commissioners of Charitable Donations and Bequests v. Walsh* (1828) 7 Ir Eq R 34n and *Read v. Hodgins* (1844) 7 Ir Eq R 17).

43 In *Gilmour v. Coats* [1949] AC 426 the House of Lords took the view that the subjective approach had no relevance to trusts for religious purposes.

44 See *Re Hetherington* [1989] 2 All ER 129, where it was finally confirmed that such gifts are *prima facie* charitable.
45 See, for example, *Cocks* v. *Manners* (1871) LR 12 Eq 574, p. 585, where the view of the English courts towards a gift for a closed Dominican convent was expressed by Sir John Wickens V-C as follows:

> A voluntary association of women for the purpose of working out their own salvation by religious exercises and self-denial seems to me to have none of the requisites of a charitable institution, whether the word 'charitable' is used in its popular sense or in its legal sense.

46 *Re Howley* [1940] IR 109.
47 *Gilmour* v. *Coats*, Op. cit.
48 *Re Cranston* [1898] 1 IR 431, pp. 446–7.
49 *Attorney-General* v. *Becher* [1910] 2 IR 251.
50 *Stillington* v. *Portadown UDC* [1911] 1 IR 247. See, also, *Re Ni Brudair*, High Court 1976 No 93 Sp (Gannon J) 5 Feb 1979.
51 *Re Worth Library*, Op. cit.
52 He referred to *Carne* v. *Long* (1860) 2 De GF & J 75 and also to *Re Prevost* [1930] 2 Ch 383.
53 See *Barrington's Hospital* v. *Commissioner of Valuation* [1957] IR 299; *Re McCarthy* [1958] IR 311; *Gleeson* v. *Attorney General*, High Court 1972, No 2664 SP (Kenny J) 6 April 1973.
54 See the Trustee Act 1893 and the Charity Act 1961.
55 See the Companies Acts 1963 and 1990.
56 *Regulating Better*, Government White Paper, 2004.
57 http://www.revenue.ie.
58 See *Re Denley's Trust Deed* [1969] 1 Ch 373. Also, see, Byrne R., and McCutcheon J. P., *The Irish Legal System* (3rd edn), Butterworths, Dublin, 1996, paras 3.54–3.60.
59 See the Costello report, op. cit.
60 See *Report of the Advisory Group on Charities/Fundraising Legislation*, Department of Equality and Law Reform, November 1996.
61 See ss. 11 and 12 of the Companies (Amendment) Act 1982 as amended by s. 245 of the 1990 Act.
62 See *Revenue Commissioners* v. *Sisters of Charity of the Incarnate Word* [1998] 2 IR 553, where Geoghegan J agreed with the Revenue Commissioners that the exemptions in ss. 333 and 334 Income Tax Act 1967 (now consolidated as ss. 207 and 208 TCA 1997) only applied to charities which were established in Ireland.
63 The VAT laws and the discretionary powers of the Revenue Commissioners are constrained by the parameters of the European Union's Sixth Council Directive on VAT (77/388/EEC (as amended)) which sets out the structure for a common system of VAT throughout the EU.
64 In *Valuation Tribunal decision, Rehab Lotteries Ltd* v. *Commissioner of Valuation* (Appeal No. VA89/229, 1991), it was contended that organizing and running lotteries on behalf of charities, to facilitate their fundraising, was not in itself a charitable purpose. The Tribunal refuted this argument and held that third parties who facilitate fundraising on behalf of charities are viewed as doing so as agents of those charities, are thereby fully complicit in the charitable purposes of those charities and therefore entitled to charitable exemption from rates.
65 Ss. 63 and 64 of the Poor Relief (Ireland) Act 1838 having been repealed by the 2001 Act.
66 See *Representative Church Body* v. *Attorney-General* [1988] IR 19.
67 See *In re Prescott* [1990] 2 IR 342.
68 Under s. 52 of the Courts and Court Officers Act 1995, resulting in a virtual doubling of the number of schemes framed by the Board.

69 See, for example, the 'White Paper', op. cit. Also, see, the 'Green Paper', op. cit. Note that 'partnership' is used in Ireland in different senses in relation to the social economy; see, for example, the principles set out in chapter II of *Partnership 2000* and in *A Framework for Partnership – Enriching Strategic Consensus through Participation* (NESF 1997).
70 See, for example, the Deakin report, op. cit.
71 *Colgan* v. *Independent Radio and Television Commission, Ireland and the Attorney General* [1999] 1 ILRM 22.
72 Ibid., pp. 24–5.
73 See *Re Royal Kilmainham Hospital* [1966] IR 451 and *Re The Worth Library* [1995] 2 IR 301.
74 See *In re the Worth Library* [1995] 2 IR 301.
75 See *Swifte* v. *Att-Gen for Ireland (No. 2)* [1912] 1 IR 133.
76 For example, Article 40.6 declares the right of citizens to express freely their convictions and opinions.
77 It has promoted a number of specific campaigns, mainly in the area of raising public awareness, such as the 1998 *A Part of Ireland Now* campaign on refugees and immigrants in Ireland.
78 See *Establishing a Modern Framework for Charities*, Dublin, 2003.
79 Ibid., p. 15.

10 Charity law and social inclusion in Australia

1 In 'real' terms (i.e. after adjustment for changes in prices), equivalized disposable household income for all people, on average, increased by 12 per cent between 1994–5 and 2000–1 while the real mean income of low-income people increased by 8 per cent, the increase spread reasonably evenly over the period. The real mean income of middle-income and high-income people increased by 12 per cent and 14 per cent respectively.
2 Saunders, P., *The Meaning and Measurement of Poverty: Towards an Agenda for Action*, Submission to the Senate Community Affairs References Committee Inquiry into Poverty and Financial Hardship, Social Policy Research Centre, University of New South Wales, 2003.
3 Dickey, B., *No Charity There: A Short History of Social Welfare in Australia* (2nd edn), Allen and Unwin, Sydney, 1987.
4 Lyons, M., *Third Sector. The Contribution of Nonprofit and Cooperative Enterprises in Australia*, Allen and Unwin, Crows Nest, 2001.
5 CPNS, *Current Issues Information Sheet* 2005/2, ATO Data: *Deductible Gift Recipients*, available at http://www.bus.qut.edu.au/research/cpns/howwecanhelp/documents/DGR11-QCFPhilProj.pdf.
6 Australian Bureau of Statistics, *Non-Profit Institutions Satellite Account*, Cat No. 526.0, Canberra, 2002.
7 Salamon, L.M., Sokolowski, S.W. and List, R., *Global Civil Society: An Overview*, The Johns Hopkins Comparative Nonprofit Sector Research Project, Baltimore, 2003.
8 Australian Government, *Giving Australia: Research of Philanthropy in Australia, Summary of Findings*, Canberra, October 2005.
9 Australian Bureau of Statistics, *Non-Profit Institutions Satellite Account*.
10 Australian Bureau of Statistics, *Measures of Australia's Social Progress, Multiple Disadvantage*, 21 April 2004, updated 18 March 2005, available at http://www.abs.gov.au.
11 Arthuson, K., 'Editorial Special Issue on Social Inclusion', *Australian Journal of Social Issues*, 39(1), p. 4, February 2004.
12 Reference Group on Welfare Reform, *Participation Support for a More Equitable Society. Full Report*, Department of Family and Community Services, Canberra, 2000.
13 Ibid., p. 3.

14 Commonwealth of Australia, *Building a Simpler System to Help Jobless Families and Individuals*, Canberra, 2002, pp. 5 and 7.
15 Saunders, P., *Can Social Exclusion Provide a New Framework for Measuring Poverty?*, SPRC Discussion Paper No. 127, October 2003, p. 5.
16 The Australian Bureau of Statistics (ABS) publication *The Health and Welfare of Australia's Aboriginal and Torres Strait Islander Peoples* (2001) provides the main source of information for this section. Also, see Australian Bureau of Statistics, *Measures of Australia's Social Progress, Multiple Disadvantage*.
17 Evidence given during *Trustees of the Indigenous Barristers' Trust: The Mum Shirl Fund v. FC of T* (2002) ATC 5055 by the Director of the Centre of Aboriginal Economic Policy Research at the Australian National University. The Centre is a multi-disciplinary Social Sciences Research Centre at the ANU that focuses on Indigenous Australian economic policy and economic development issues, including social justice and the socio-economic status of Indigenous Australians. Also, see Hunter, B., *Indigenous Self-Employment: Miracle Cure or Risky Business?*, CAEPR Discussion Paper 176 (1999), CAEPR, ANU, Canberra.
18 See *Trustees of the Indigenous Barristers' Trust: The Mum Shirl Fund v. FC of T*, op. cit.
19 See ATO, *Non-Profit News Service*, No. 0031.
20 See the Hon. John Howard MP, Prime Minister, 'Inquiry into Charitable and Related Organisations', press release, 18 September 2000, at http://www.pm.gov.au.
21 Sheppard, I., Fitzgerald, R. and Gonski, D., *Inquiry into the Definition of Charities and Related Organisations*, 2001, at http://www.cdi.gov.au.
22 *Chesterman v. Federal Commissioner of Taxation* [1925] 37 CLR 317.
23 *The Perpetual Trustee Co. Ltd. v. Federal Commissioner of Taxation* [1931] 45 CLR 224 *per* Starke J, p. 232.
24 Chesterman, M., 'Foundations of Charity Law in the New Welfare State', *The Modern Law Review*, 62(3), 1999.
25 See, for example, the Trusts Act 1973 (Qld.), the Charities Act 1978 (Vic.) and the Charitable Trusts Act 1962 (WA).
26 43 Eliz. 1, c.4.; this act is a modification of a prior Statute of Uses in 1597, 39 Eliz. I, c.6. The Statute of Charitable Uses 1601 has been repealed with reservations that it will not affect the general law of charity in the Australian Capital Territory: Imperial Acts Application Act 1986 (ACT) s. 4(5), New South Wales: Imperial Acts Application Act 1969 (NSW) s. 8 and Queensland: Trusts Act 1973 s. 103(1). It is not in force in Victoria, but remains in force in the other jurisdictions.
27 Adopted in Queensland, South Australia, Tasmania and Western Australia.
28 *Income Tax Special Purposes Commissioners v. Pemsel* [1891] All ER Rep 28. For application of *Pemsel* to estate duty see *Chesterman v. Federal Commissioner of Taxation* [1926] AC 128; to rates see *Salvation Army (Victoria) Property Trust v. Fern Tree Gully Corp.* (1952) 85 CLR 159; *Ashfield Corp. v. Joyce* [1978] AC 122.
29 Australian Taxation Office, *Income Tax and Fringe Benefits Tax: Charities*, TR 2005/21 & 22, dated 21 December 2005.
30 Queensland, South Australia, Tasmania and Western Australia follow the pattern of the Recreational Charities Act 1958 (UK).
31 Associations Incorporation Act 1984 (NSW); Associations Incorporation Act 1981 (Vic); Associations Incorporation Act 1981 (Qld); Associations Incorporation Act 1985 (SA); Associations Incorporation Act 1987 (WA); Associations Incorporation Act 1964 (Tas); Associations Incorporation Act 1991 (ACT); Associations Act 2003 (NT).
32 Fundraising Appeals Act 1998 (Vic); Charitable Fundraising Act 1991 (NSW); Collections for Charitable Purposes Act 1939 (SA); Collections for Charities Act 2001 (Tas); Collections Act 1966 (Qld); Charitable Collections Act 1940 (WA); Collections Act 1959 (ACT).
33 *Bathurst City Council v. PWC Properties* (1998) 195 CLR 566 concerned a church carpark and the previous case was *Commissioner of Land Tax (NSW) v. Joyce* (1974) 132 CLR 22.

34 See, ATO, *Draft Taxation Ruling* TR 1999/D21, para. 8.

35 *Bathurst City Council* v. *PWC Properties*, op. cit.

36 *Re Compton* [1945] 1 Ch 123 and *Oppenheim* v. *Tobacco Securities Trust Co Ltd* [1951] AC 297.

37 *Congregational Union of New South Wales* v. *Thistlethwayte* (1952) 87 CLR 375.

38 ATO, *Income Tax and Fringe Benefits Tax: Charities*, TR 1999/D21.

39 ATO, *Income Tax and Fringe Benefits Tax: Charities*, TR 2003/5.

40 ATO, *Income Tax and Fringe Benefits Tax: Charities*, TR 2005/21.

41 *Metropolitan Fire Brigade Board* v. *The Commissioner of Taxation* (1990) 27 FCR 279; *Mines Rescue Board* (NSW) v. *The Commissioner of Taxation* (2000) 101 FCR 91; *Ambulance Service of New South Wales* v. *The Deputy Commissioner of Taxation* (2003) 130 FCR 477.

42 *Central Bayside Division of General Practice Ltd* v. *Commissioner of State Revenue* [2005] VSCA 168.

43 Ibid., para. 21.

44 *Attorney General (NSW)* v. *Satwell* [1978] 2 NSWLR 200.

45 *Southwood* v. *AG* [1998] 40 LS Gaz R 37.

46 *The Church of the New Faith* v. *The Commissioner of Pay-Roll Tax (Victoria)* (1983) 154 CLR 120.

47 *Tasmanian Electronic Commerce Centre Pty Ltd* v. *FC of T* (2005) 142 FCR 371; 2005 ATC 4219; (2005) 59 ATR 10.

48 *FC of T* v. *The Triton Foundation* 2005 ATC 4891; (2005) 60 ATR 451.

49 *Aboriginal Hostels Ltd* v. *Darwin City Council* (1985) 75 FLR 197; *Flynn and others* v. *Mamarika and others* (1996) 130 FLR 218.

50 *Toomelah Co-operative Limited* v. *Moree Plains Shire Council* [1996], unreported Land and Environment Court of New South Wales, Stein J.

51 *Public Trustee* v. *Attorney-General of New South Wales* (1997) 42 NSWLR 600.

52 S. 103 of the *Trusts Act 1973* (Qld); s. 69C of the *Trustee Act 1936* (SA); s. 5 of the *Charitable Trusts Act 1962* (WA) and s. 4 of the *Variation of Trusts Act '1994* (Tas).

53 *Re Inman* [1965] V.R. 258; *Sir Moses Montefiore Jewish Home* v. *Howell and Co, (No.7) Pty Ltd* [1984] 2 N.S.W.L.R. 406 and Victoria, 'Report on Charitable Trusts', Chief Justice's Law Reform Committee, Melbourne, 1965, p. 26; Ford, H. A. J., 'Dispositions for Purposes', in Finn, P. (edn), *Essays in Equity*, Law Book Company Limited, Sydney, 1985, p. 168.

54 Associations Incorporation Act 1984 (NSW); Associations Incorporation Act 1981 (Vic); Associations Incorporation Act 1981 (Qld); Associations Incorporation Act 1985 (SA); Associations Incorporation Act 1987 (WA); Associations Incorporation Act 1964 (Tas); Associations Incorporation Act 1991 (ACT); Associations Act 2003 (NT).

55 Refer correspondence with Fair Trading Offices at http://www.bus.qut.edu.au/research/cpns/whatweresearch/usefullinks.jsp#stats.

56 Lyons, *Third Sector*.

57 The public register is available at http://www.business.gov.au.

58 Industry Commission, Charitable Organizations in Australia, Report No. 45, 16 June 1995, Australian Government Publishing Service, Melbourne, pp. 306–9.

59 Ibid., p. 307.

60 Ibid., p. 309.

61 Costello, P. *Tax Reform – Not a New Tax – A New Tax System*, August 1988, Treasury, Canberra, pp. 114–15.

62 Ibid., pp. 280 and 286.

63 Ibid., pp. 288–9.

64 Letter contained in ATO submission to the Inquiry available at http://www.cdi.gov.au/html/public_submissions.htm.

65 Ibid., p. 293.

66 Refer to their website (http://www.ato.gov.au) for publications such as *CharityPack* and other fact sheets and comprehensive taxation rulings on the matters such as TR2005/21 and 22.

67 See Victorian Legal and Constitutional Committee, 'A Report to Parliament on the Law Relating to Charitable Trusts', Victorian Government Printer, Melbourne, 1989, p. 77.

68 Fundraising Appeals Act 1998 (Vic); Charitable Fundraising Act 1991 (NSW); Collections for Charitable Purposes Act 1939 (SA); Collections for Charities Act 2001 (Tas); Collections Act 1966 (Qld); Charitable Collections Act 1940 (WA); Collections Act 1959 (ACT).

69 Industry Commission, *Charitable Organisations in Australia*, Report No 45, AGPS, Canberra, 1995, p. 210; Sheppard *et al.*, *Inquiry into the Definition of Charities and Related Organisations*.

70 The first Act to impose a tax on income (dividends) was Tasmania's Real and Personal Estate Duty Act 1880. However, South Australia was the first state with the Taxation Act 1884 and the Commonwealth's income tax provisions closely followed the state's exemption provision in s. 23 of Income Tax Assessment Act 1936 (Cth).

71 Howard, J., 'Community-Business Partnership Develops New Initiatives to Promote Philanthropy', press release, 30 March 2001, available at http://www.pm.gov.au.

72 S43 85ATC 343 and Commissioner of Taxation, *Taxation Determination* 93/185.

73 For example the Charitable Funds Act 1990 (Qld.), s. 6.

74 Trusts Act 1973 (Qld.), s. 105; Charities Act 1978 (Vic.), ss. 2 and 3; Charitable Trusts Act 1962 (WA), s. 7.

75 *Attorney General* v. *Sherborne Grammar School* (1854) 18 Beav 256.

76 Charitable Trusts Act 1993 (NSW), s. 9(1).

77 Trusts Act 1973 (Qld), s. 105; Trustee Act 1936 (SA), s. 69B(1); Variation of Trusts Act 1994 (Tas), s. 5(3); Charities Act 1978 (Vic), s. (2)(1).

78 In other recent cases similar tardiness is apparent: *Re Anzac Cottages Trust* [2000] QSC 175; *Roman Catholic Trusts Corp. for Diocese of Melbourne* v. *Att. Gen.* (Vic) [2000] VSC 360.

79 Williams J., *Re Application by Perpetual Trustees Queensland Ltd*, No. 4239 of 1999, para. 15.

80 *Re Inman*, op. cit.; *Sir Moses Montefiore Jewish Home* v. *Howell and Co, (No.7) Pty Ltd*, op. cit., and Victoria, 'Report on Charitable Trusts', 1965, p. 26; Ford, 'Dispositions for Purposes', p. 168.

81 Dal Pont, G., *Charity Law in Australia and New Zealand*, Oxford University Press, Melbourne, 2000, p. 388.

82 Industry Commission, *Charitable Organisations in Australia*, Report No 45, AGPS, Canberra, 1995, pp. 221–30.

83 McGregor-Lowndes, M. and Turnour, M., 'Recent Developments in Government Community Service Relations: Are You Really My Partner?' *The Journal of Contemporary Issues in Business and Government*, 9(1), 2003, pp. 31–42.

84 *Central Bayside Division of General Practice Ltd* v. *Commissioner of State Revenue*, op. cit.

85 See ATO, *Draft Taxation Ruling* TR 1999/D21, para. 43.

86 See *Aboriginal Hostels Ltd.* v. *Darwin City Council*, op. cit., and also *Flynn* v. *Mamarika* (1996) 130 FLR 218.

87 *Northern Land Council* v. *The Commissioner of Taxes* [2002] NCTA 11; *Alice Springs Town Council* v. *Mpweteyerre Aboriginal Corporation* (1997) 139 FLR 236; *Dareton Local Aboriginal Land Council* v. *Wentworth Council* 9 (1995) 89 LGERA 120.

88 *Toomelah Co-operative Limited* v. *Moree Plains Shire Council*, op. cit.

89 Australia, 'Report on the Problems and Needs of Aboriginals on the New South Wales Queensland Border', Human Rights Commission, June 1988.

90 See ATO, *Draft Taxation Ruling*, TR 1999/D21, p. 7.

91 See *Re Vancouver Regional FreeNet Association* v. *Minister of National Revenue* (1996) 137 DLR (4th) 206.

92 Johns, G. and Roskam, J., *The Protocol: Managing Relations with NGOs*, IPA, Melbourne, April 2004.

93 See *Trustees of the Indigenous Barrister's Trust: The Mum Shirl Fund* v. *FC of T*, op. cit.

94 Ibid.

95 See, for example, *Attorney-General (NSW)* v. *Cahill* [1969] 1 NSWR 85.
96 See *Latvian Co-operative Society* v. *Commissioner of Land Taxes (Vic)* (1989) 20 ATR 3641.
97 See *Trustees of the Indigenous Barrister's Trust: The Mum Shirl Fund* v. *FC of T*, op. cit. Citing in support: *Re Mathew* [1951] VLR 226, p. 232; *Re Bryning* [1976] VR 100, pp. 101–2; *Aboriginal Hostels Ltd* v. *Darwin City Council*, op. cit., pp. 211–12; *Tangentyere Council Inc* v. *Commissioner of Taxes (NT)* (1990) 99 FLR 363, pp. 369–71 (although cf. *Commissioner of Taxes (NT)* v. *Tangentyere Council Inc* (1992) 102 FLR 470); and *Alice Springs Town Council* v. *Mpweteyerre Aboriginal Corporation*, op. cit., pp. 252–4.
98 For a summary of the provisions refer to Australian Parliamentary Library, Terrorism Law Brief at http://www.aph.gov.au/library/intguide/LAW/TerrorismLaws.htm.
99 For example: the Age Discrimination Act 2004 (Cth), Racial Hatred Act 1995 (Cth), Disability Discrimination Act 1992 (Cth), and the Sex Discrimination Act 1984 (Cth).
100 For example, the Anti-Discrimination Act 1977 (NSW).
101 Income Tax Assessment Act 1997, s. 50–50 ITAA 97.
102 Ibid., s. 30–15 ITAA 97 – ancillary funds are excluded, but they can only disburse grants to other DGRs.
103 Commissioner of Taxation, *Taxation Ruling* 2355.
104 Sheppard *et al.*, *Inquiry into the Definition of Charities and Related Organisations*.
105 Board of Taxation, *Consultation on the Definition of a Charity*, 2003.
106 Costello, P., 'Final Response to the Charities Definition Inquiry', press release, no. 31, 11 May 2004.

11 Charity law and social inclusion in New Zealand

1 See Tennant, M., *Paupers and Providers: Charitable Aid in New Zealand*, Allen & Unwin, Wellington, 1989, cited in Dal Pont, G., *Charity Law in Australia and New Zealand*, Oxford University Press, 2000, p. 78 ff. Also, see Thompson, D., *A World without Welfare: New Zealand's Colonial Experiment*, Auckland University Press, Auckland, 1998.
2 The 2001 census reveals a population consisting of: European, 70 per cent; Maori, 8 per cent; Asian, 5.7 per cent, Pacific Islander 4.4 per cent, other 0.5 per cent and mixed 7.8 per cent; of whom 80 per cent are resident in towns.
3 See the 1991 Budget document *Welfare that Works* and Shipley, H. J., *Social Assistance: Welfare that Works*, Government Printer, Wellington, 1991.
4 See, for example, St John, S., *Redesigning the Welfare State in New Zealand*, conference paper presented at School of Social Work and Social Policy, University of Queensland, Brisbane, 4–5 October 2001.
5 See, for example: Dalziel, P., 'New Zealand's Economic Reform Programme was a Failure', unpublished manuscript, Christchurch, 1999; Easton, B., *The Commercialisation of New Zealand*, Auckland University Press, Auckland, 1997, and *In Stormy Seas: The Post-War New Zealand Economy*, University of Otago Press, Dunedin, 1997; Jesson, B., *Only Their Purpose is Mad*, The Dunmore Press, Wellington, 1999; and Kelsey, J., *Rolling Back the State*, Bridget Williams Books, Wellington, 1993, and *The New Zealand Experiment* (2nd edn), Auckland University Press/Bridget Williams Books, Auckland, 1997.
6 See Human Rights Commission, *Human Rights In New Zealand Today / Ngā Tika Tangata O Te Motu* (the Status report), 2004.
7 See, for example, Commissioner for Equal Employment Opportunity, *Framework for the Future: Equal Employment Opportunities in New Zealand*, Christchurch, 2004.
8 See Hawke, G. and Robinson, D., (eds.) *Performance Without Profit: The Voluntary Sector in New Zealand*, Institute of Policy Studies, Wellington, 1993.
9 See Working Party on Charities and Sporting Bodies, *Report to the Minister of Finance and the Minister of Social Welfare*, 1989, p. 88; as cited in Dal Pont, *Charity Law in Australia and New Zealand*, p. 4.
10 See, ZeroWaste, a New Zealand Trust, at http://www.zerowaste.co.nz.
11 The Treasury, 2001, p. 62.

12 See Statistics of New Zealand, *Census of Population and Dwellings*, Wellington, 1996.
13 See the Policy Advice Division of the Inland Revenue Department, *Taxation of Maori Organisations Discussion Document*, 2001.
14 See the Status report, op. cit.
15 From media statement made by the Hon. Judith Tizard, Associate Minister of Commerce, announcing the new legislation on 14 April 2005.
16 See Thompson, *A World Without Welfare*.
17 Statute of Charitable Uses, 43 Eliz. 1 cap. 4.
18 This rule provides that even though a purpose cannot be defined as coming under one of the established heads of charity, it will nonetheless be construed as charitable if it can be interpreted as falling within the 'spirit or intendment' of the Preamble to the 1601 Act.
19 See *Income Tax Special Commissioners* v. *Pemsel* [1891] AC 531.
20 For further information on the legislative history see Dal Pont, *Charity Law in Australia and New Zealand*, p. 78 ff.
21 See Dal Pont, *Charity Law in Australia and New Zealand*, p. 81.
22 See Rickett, C., 'A Statutory Charitable Trust', *New Zealand Law Journal*, March 2000, pp. 59–61, which examines the statutory transformation of the New Zealand Railways Staff Welfare Society into the New Zealand Railways Staff Welfare Charitable Trust, notwithstanding its member-benefit purpose.
23 The Income Tax Act 2004, the Tax Administration Act 1994 and the Estate and Gift Duties Act 1968 are technically amended by the 2005 Act to refer as appropriate to 'registered charities' and to the 'Charity Commission' and appropriate amendments are made to the Incorporated Societies Act 1908.
24 The report of the Working Party on Charities and Sporting Bodies, 1989, concluded that changing the definition of a charity was not the way to determine eligibility for preferential taxation treatment and that the current common law definition of charity and charitable purposes should apply in the meantime.
25 See *Oppenheim* v. *Tobacco Securities Trust Co Ltd* [1951] AC 297.
26 See, for example, *New Zealand Society of Accountants* v. *Commissioner of Inland Revenue* [1986] 1 NZLR 147.
27 Policy Advice Division of the Inland Revenue Department, *Taxation of Maori Organisations*.
28 *Commissioner of Inland Revenue* v. *Medical Council of New Zealand* [1997] 2 NZLR 297 (CA).
29 See Rickett, 'A Statutory Charitable Trust', p. 60.
30 See, for example, *Molloy* v. *Commissioner of Inland Revenue* [1981] 1 NZLR 688.
31 See the Treasury, *Guidelines for Contracting with Non-Government Organisations for Services Sought by the Crown*, 2001.
32 See *Centrepoint Community Growth Trust* v. *Commissioner of Inland Revenue* [1985] 1 NZLR 673.
33 See, for example, *New Zealand Society of Accountants* v. *Commissioner of Inland Revenue* [1986] 1 NZLR 147, p. 157, *per* Somers J.
34 Companies Reregistration Act, 1994, s. 3.
35 Section 89 of the Tax Administration Act 1994.
36 Sections 32, 58 and 89 of the Tax Administration Act 1994.
37 See Property Law and Equity Reform Committee, *Report on the Charitable Trusts Act 1957*, Department of Justice, Wellington, 1979, p. 2.
38 Section 23 of the Incorporated Societies Act 1908.
39 The Accountability of Charities and Sporting Bodies Working Party (established in 1995 under the auspices of Philanthropy New Zealand) prepared a *Report on the Accountability of Charities and Sporting Bodies* in April 1997, which advocated a self-regulatory approach based on a code of practice for voluntary organizations. The code was to address governance, programmes for standards of service, organizational integrity, management practices and human resources, accountability for funds (including fundraising and financial accounting) and communication of information to the public.

40 See the Institute of Chartered Accountants of New Zealand, *Financial Reporting by Voluntary Sector Entities* (R-120) 1999. The purpose of this bulletin was to provide 'guidance on the application of generally accepted accounting practice and recommendations as to good external reporting practice by not for profit and voluntary sector entities'. It does not have the authority of a financial reporting standard but would be guidance to members of the Institute preparing or auditing accounts for charities.

41 The Report of the Committee of Experts on Tax Compliance, 1998, recommended that the law and practice relating to the income tax exemption for amateur sports bodies should be reviewed.

42 See, for example, *Re Goldwater (deceased)* (1967) NZLR 754.

43 *Auckland Medical Aid Trust* v. *Commissioner of Inland Revenue* [1979] 1 NZLR 382; as cited in Sheridan, L. A., *Keeton & Sheridan's The Modern Law of Charities* (4th edn), Barry Rose, Chichester, 1992, p. 170. But also see *Molloy* v. *Commissioner of Inland Revenue* op. cit.

44 The report by the Committee of Experts on Tax Compliance, 1998, proposed that income from continuous and regular commercial activities of a charity that are unrelated to the charitable purpose for which they have been given a tax exemption should be taxed on the net income derived from those activities.

45 *Re Tennant* [1996] 2 NZLR 633.

46 *Commissioner of Inland Revenue* v. *Medical Council of New Zealand*, op. cit., p. 314.

47 *Molloy* v. *Commissioner of Inland Revenue*, op. cit.

48 However, under section 38 of the Charitable Trusts Act 1957 the term 'charitable purpose' means a number of purposes '*whether or not* they are beneficial to the community or to a section of the community' [emphasis added]. Given that the Charities Commission will require charitable entities to demonstrate 'public benefit' (Charities Act 2005 s. 5 (2)(a) the purpose of a trust, society or institution is a charitable purpose under this Act '*if the purpose would satisfy the public benefit requirement* apart from the fact that the beneficiaries of the trust, or the members of the society or institution, are related by blood;' [emphasis added] this may conflict with section 38 of the Charitable Trusts Act 1957 and therefore constitute a constraint on social inclusion for any minority group that is not a significant part of the community. The author is grateful to Michael Gousmett for this observation.

49 See *Educational Fees Protection Society Inc.* v. *Commissioner of Inland Revenue* [1992] 2 NZLR 115.

50 See Inland Revenue Department, Policy Advice Division, *Tax and Charities*, Wellington, 2001.

51 The Working Party issued its first report on 28 February 2002 and its second on 31 May 2002.

52 See the *Report to the Minister of Finance and the Minister of Social Welfare* (the 'Russell report') which recommended the following functions for a Charities Commission: registration, monitoring, advice and support to the sector, assistance to charitable organizations in being accountable to the public, co-ordination of information within the sector and providing advice to government regarding the charitable sector.

53 See Dal Pont, G., 'The Charities Bill', *The New Zealand Law Journal*, March 2005, p. 55.

54 The document also considered the merits of establishing a Charities Commission.

55 See Dal Pont, 'The Charities Bill', p. 57.

56 The *marae* is the sacred open meeting area that is associated with a traditional meeting house. It is the customary focal point for meetings, discussions, funerals and for welcoming visitors to the area.

57 See the Status report, op. cit.

12 Charity law and social inclusion in the United States

1 The Model Nonprofit Corporation Act was passed in 1964, and versions of it are

currently in effect in Alabama, the District of Columbia, New Jersey, North Dakota, Texas, Virginia and Wisconsin. The Revised Model Nonprofit Corporation Act 1987, based loosely on California law, has been passed with varying amounts of modification in Alaska, Arizona, Colorado, Georgia, Hawaii, Idaho, Indiana, Maine, Minnesota, Mississippi, Missouri, Montana, Nebraska, North Carolina, Oregon, South Carolina, Tennessee, Utah, Vermont, Washington, West Virginia and Wyoming. See Fremont-Smith, M., *Governing Nonprofit Organisations: Federal and State Law and Regulation*, Cambridge, Mass., Belknap Press, Harvard University Press, 2004, app. tbl. 3, pp. 514–17.

2 Panel on the Nonprofit Sector, *Strengthening Transparency Governance Accountability of Charitable Organizations: A Final Report to Congress and the Nonprofit Sector*, June 2005.
3 Ibid., p. 22.
4 Amerindian and Alaska natives (1 per cent).
5 Native Hawaiian and other Pacific Islander (0.2 per cent).
6 Protestant 52 per cent, Roman Catholic 24 per cent, Mormon 2 per cent, Jewish 1 per cent, Muslim 1 per cent, other 10 per cent, none 10 per cent (2002 estimates).
7 English 82.1 per cent, Spanish 10.7 per cent, other Indo-European 3.8 per cent, Asian and Pacific Island 2.7 per cent, other 0.7 per cent (2000 census).
8 5.1 per cent (2005, estimate).
9 3.2 per cent (2005, estimate).
10 See the National Centre for Charitable Statistics, a programme of the Centre of Nonprofits and Philanthropy at the Urban Institute, at http://nccsdataweb.urban.org/PubApps/profile1.php?state=US.
11 Staff of Joint Commission On Taxation, 18th Cong., *Description of Present Law Relating to Charitable and Other Exempt Organisations and Statistical Information Regarding Growth and Oversight of the Tax-Exempt Sector*, 2004, available at http://www.house.gov/jct/x–44–04.pdf.
12 American Association of Fund-Raising Counsel [AAFRC], 2000, as cited by Wright, K., in 'Generosity vs. Altruism: Philanthropy and Charity in the United States and United Kingdom', *Voluntas: International Journal of Voluntary and Nonprofit Organisations*, 12(4), 2002, p. 401. It is claimed that in recent years the level of charitable contribution has increased yet further: reaching $260 billion or 2.5 per cent of GDP in 2005 (see Cornwell, R., 'This Golden Age of Philanthropy', *The Independent*, 27 June 2006, p. 27).
13 Independent Sector, *The New Nonprofit Almanac and Desk Reference*, 2002.
14 See Brody, E., 'Charities in Tax Reform: Threats to Subsidies Overt and Covert', *Tennessee Law Review*, 66, 1999, pp. 687–763. As cited in Reich, B., 'A Failure of Philanthropy: American Charity Shortchanges the Poor, and Public Policy is Partly to Blame', *Stanford Social Innovation Review*, Winter 2005.
15 See Salamon, L. M. and Geller, S. L., *Nonprofit Governance and Accountability*, The Johns Hopkins Nonprofit Listening Post Project Communiqué No. 4, 2005, p. 13.
16 See US Census Bureau, 'Poverty in the United States', 2005.
17 See Berry, J., 'A Needless Silence: American Nonprofits and the Right to Lobby', Berry, J., and Arons, D. F., *A Voice for Nonprofits*, Brookings Institution, Tufts University, 2005. Also, see Council on Foundations at http://www.cof.org.
18 See the United States Census Bureau, 2003. The largest tribes are the Cherokee, Navajo, Choctaw, Sioux, Chippewa, Apache, Blackfeet, Iroquois and Pueblo: eight out of ten are of mixed blood and by 2100 that figure will rise to nine of ten.
19 On 31 January 1876, the United States government ordered all Native Americans into reservations.
20 As recently as the 1970s, the Bureau of Indian Affairs was still actively pursuing a policy of 'assimilation', the goal of which was to eliminate the reservations and steer Indians into mainstream US culture.
21 (1938) 304 US 144.
22 Ibid., p. 152.
23 See Revenue Ruling 68–70, 1968–1 C.B. 248, online: Taxlinks at http://www.taxlinks.com/rulings/1968/revrul68–70.htm: 'This organisation's activities are

designed to eliminate prejudice and discrimination in the community by various means. Its lectures and forums are intended to educate potential employers in the advantages of hiring qualified workers without regard to race or creed.' They also arranged interviews with potential employers for qualified workers.

24 See Revenue Ruling 68–655, 1968–1 C.B. 248, online: Taxlinks at http://www.taxlinks.com/rulings/1968/revrul68–655.htm:

> By education [*sic*] the public about integrated housing and conducting intensive neighborhood educational programs to prevent panic selling because of the introduction of a non-white resident into a formerly all-white neighborhood, the organisation is striving to eliminate prejudice and discrimination and to lessen neighborhood tensions. By making mortgage loans to families that cannot obtain such loans commercially but that otherwise are considered desirable residents, the organisation is trying to break down the barriers of prejudice and gain acceptance of integrated housing within the community. It accomplishes this same objective by purchasing homes and reselling or leasing them on an open occupancy basis to families that will be compatible to a neighborhood and demonstrate the feasibility of integrated communities. By stabilizing the neighborhood, the organisation is combatting potential community deterioration.

25 See Revenue Ruling 68–15, 1968–1 C.B. 244, online: Taxlinks at http://www.taxlinks.com/rulings/1968/revrul68–15.htm:

> The work of the organisation's committees is charitable since it is designed to contribute directly to lessening neighborhood tensions, eliminating prejudice and discrimination, and combatting community deterioration and juvenile delinquency. The dissemination of information to residents of the community and other interested people of the city at large is educational because the material instructs the public on subjects useful to the individual and beneficial to the community.

The Ruling also established that the group did not engage in propaganda, attempt to influence legislation, or intervene in political campaigns.

26 See Revenue Ruling 68–438, 1968–2 C.B. 209, online: Taxlinks at http://www.taxlinks.com/rulings/1968/revrul68–438.htm:

> The organisation's activities of investigating the existence of discrimination and seeking compliance with applicable laws directly contribute to the elimination of prejudice and discrimination, the defense of human and civil rights secured by law, and the lessening of neighborhood tensions. The information that is disseminated to individuals and groups within the community through the organisation's publication program and speakers' bureau instructs the public on subjects useful to the individual and beneficial to the community.

It was also noted that the group did not 'engage in economic boycotts, reprisals, or picketing', nor did it attempt to influence legislation or disseminate propaganda.

27 See *Democracy in America* (1835), trans. G. Lawrence, HarperCollins New York,: 'In every case, at the head of a great new undertaking, where in France you would find the government or in England some territorial magnate, in the US you are sure to find an association', 1988 (p. 513).

28 An approach continued by President George Bush in his 'thousand points of light' policy and currently by his son in his 'faith based initiative'.

29 See, generally, Minnow, M., 'Public and Private Partnerships: Accounting for the New Religion', 116 Harv. L. R. 1229 (2003).

30 See Lipman, H., 'Health-Conversion Funds Hold $16 Billion in Assets', *Chronicle of*

Philanthropy, 4 May 2000, p. 12, and Grantmakers in Health, *A Profile of New Health Foundations*, Washington, D.C., 2003.

31 See Corbet, C., 'Stewardship of Public Assets Under Nonprofit Conversion Models: New York's Empire Blue Cross Blue Shield Case Study', *Nonprofit Management & Leadership*, 16(2), 2005, p. 153.

32 As envisioned by the National Association of Attorneys General and described in its 'Model Legislation on Conversion of Nonprofit Health Care Entities to For-Profit Status' (1998).

33 The Independent Sector is a nonprofit, nonpartisan coalition of approximately 500 national public charities, foundations, and corporate philanthropy programmes, collectively representing tens of thousands of charitable groups in every state across the nation.

34 Consisting of 24 members who are distinguished leaders from public charities and private foundations from around the country.

35 See, for example, Trattner, W. I., *From Poor Laws to Welfare State: A History of Social Welfare in America* (6th edn), free Press, 1998.

36 See Kelley, T., 'Rediscovering Vulgar Charity: An Historical Analysis of America's Tangled Nonprofit Law', *Fordham Law Review*, 73(6), pp. 3437–99.

37 The Constitution was drawn up on 17 September 1787 and took effect on 4 March 1789.

38 See *Roberts* v. *United States Jaycees*, 1984.

39 *NAACP* v. *Alabama ex rel. Patterson*, 357 U.S. 449 (1958).

40 See *Boy Scouts of America* v. *Dale*, 530 U.S. 640 (2000), holding that the Boy Scouts had a constitutional right to exclude a homosexual member because of their disagreement with his way of life. Both the majority and the dissent recognized that the relevant standard was whether the Boy Scouts had an expressive agenda that would be compromised by allowing homosexual men to participate in the organization.

41 See Fisch, E. L., 'The *Cy-près* Doctrine and Changing Philosophies', *Michigan Law Review*, 51, 1953, pp. 377–83.

42 *Jackson* v. *Phillips*, 96 Mass. 539, 556 (1867), quoted in Fremont-Smith, *Governing Nonprofit Organisations*, p. 119.

43 See Hopkins, *The Law of Tax Exempt Orgs* (6th edn) as cited by Kelley, 'Rediscovering Vulgar Charity'.

44 See, Scrivener, G., '100 Years of Tax Policy Changes Affecting Charitable Organisations', in Gies, D., *et al.* (eds), *The Nonprofit Organisation, Essential Readings*, 46, 1990; as cited by Kelley, 'Rediscovering Vulgar Charity'.

45 See *Scripture Press Foundation* v. *US* 285 F.2d 800 (Ct. Cl. 1961); *American Ins. For Economic Research* v. *United States*, 302 F.2d. 934 (Ct. Cl. 1962); *Elisian Guild, Inc.* v. *United States*, 292 F. Supp. 219 (D. Mass. 1968); and *Living Faith, Inc.* v. *Comm'r*, 60 TCM 710 (1990).

46 Fremont-Smith, *Governing Nonprofit Organisations*.

47 IRC, s. 170 (c)(2).

48 *Bob Jones University* v. *United States*, 461 US 574 (1983).

49 *Fire Insurance Patrol* v. *Boyd*, 120 Pa. 624, 643 (1888). Other cases where charitable status was similarly upheld, as cited by Kelley, 'Rediscovering Vulgar Charity': *Patterson Rescue Mission* v. *High*, 64 NJL 116, 118–119, 44 A. 974, 975, 1899 (home for aged and disabled men which paid for its running costs by requiring residents to manufacture and sell firewood); *House of Refuge* v. *Smith*, 140 Pa. 387, 1891 (juvenile correction home where employed residents contributed to running costs); *Trustees of Academy of Protestant Episcopal Church* v. *Taylor*, 150 Pa. 565, 1892 (school, open to the public, charging students to cover running costs); *Contributors to Pennsylvania Hospital* v. *Delaware County*, 169 Pa. 305, 1895 (profit from sale of convalescent farm produce used to maintain hospital); and *Trustees of Kentucky Female Orphan School* v. *City of Louisville*, 36 SW 921 (Ky. Ct. of App.), 1896 (revenue from service users paid for upkeep of school).

50 As a result, 48 states have passed laws adopting the distinction between private foundations and public charities and prohibiting private foundations from being controlled by
substantial donors, holding certain investments, dealing with insiders, etc.

51 Rev. Rul. 72–369, 1972–2 C.B. 245.

52 Treas. Reg. § 1.501 (c)(3)–1 (c)(1).

53 (7th Cir., Feb. 10, 1999). The Seventh Circuit then held that the Internal Revenue
Service had improperly revoked an organization's charitable tax exemption on the
grounds that the organization's net earnings had inured to the benefit of a professional
fundraising company it hired despite the fact that only $2.3 million from a total of
$28.8 million raised by the company ever reached the organization.

54 See Kelley, 'Rediscovering Vulgar Charity'.

55 See Treasury Reg. s. 1.50 (c) (3)–1 (d)(2).

56 See *Vidal* v. *Girard's Executor* 43 US (2 How.) 127 (1844), where it was found that the
English Chancellor was able to exercise the enforcement of charitable trusts independently of the Statute of Uses 1601, and so the power existed in American law.

57 See Fishman, J. J., 'The Development of Nonprofit Corporation Law and an Agenda
for Reform', *Emory Law Journal*, 34, 1985, pp. 619–83, esp. p. 631.

58 See *Stegemeier* v. *Magness*, 728 A.2d 557 (Del. 1999) for a judicial ruling describing the
difference between trust and corporate standards.

59 Two states (South Carolina and West Virginia) had adopted charity commissions similar to the Charity Commission of England and Wales, but they later repealed the
authority setting up the commissions, in part because they were too cumbersome and
expensive.

60 See I.R.S., *Search for Charities, Online Version of Publication 78*, at http://www.irs.gov/char-
ities/page/0,id=15053,00.html. It might be added that an organization is perfectly
free to set itself up as a charity and undertake charitable activities and need never be
known to the IRS unless it also chooses to seek tax-exemption status and/or becomes
incorporated.

61 There have been proposals to tighten the definition of public charity, or simply to force
all public benefit organizations to abide by the same strict self-dealing rules that currently apply only to private foundations (see *Charity Oversight and Reform: Keeping Bad
Things from Happening to Good Charities Before the Senate Comm. On Finance*, 108th Cong.
(2004), available at http://finance.senate.gov/sitepages/hearing062204.html.

62 IRC, s. 509 (a)(2).

63 IRC s. 509 defines private foundation. There are also 'private operating foundations'
that actually spend all the income on their endowment each year on charitable activities; but the principal distinction in the Code is between the public charities and the
private foundations.

64 IRC s. 4940(d),(e).

65 There are over 50,000 foundations in the US with $448 billion in assets in 1999
(somewhat less now). When the federal government launched its War on Poverty
foundations' assets were then valued at less than $30 billion. The Bill and Melinda
Gates Foundation started in 1999 with $21 billion is now the biggest US foundation.
John Walters, publisher of *Philanthropy*, estimates that foundation assets alone may
easily grow to between $4 trillion and $5.9 trillion by 2035 ('Come the Revolution',
Philanthropy, July–Aug 1999, pp. 25–6).

66 See Fremont-Smith, *Governing Nonprofit Organisations*, p. 267; cited in Panel on the
Nonprofit Sector, p. 26.

67 Organizations other than private foundations with annual gross receipts of $25,000 or
less, houses of worship and specific related institutions, specified governmental instru-
mentalities, and other organizations relieved of this requirement by authority of the
IRS are excluded from this requirement.

68 Form 990, 990-EZ, or 990-PF.

69 See, for example, the recent IRS settlement reached with the former trustees of

Hawaii's wealthiest charity, commonly known as the Bishop Estate, following the effective intervention of the Attorney General of Hawaii to halt the widespread abuse by the trustees of the charity's assets worth between $6 billion and $10 billion.

70 Scandals involving organizations such as the United Way, New Era Fund and NAACP have led to much concern about the ability of underfunded and understaffed state Attorney General offices to oversee charities.

71 See Fishman, 'The Development of Nonprofit Corporation Law', pp. 617–39.

72 Panel on the Nonprofit Sector, op. cit., p. 26.

73 It is anticipated that the IRS will soon make public the results of its first three market segment studies, conducted in 2002. Between 100 and 150 501(c)(6) trade associations, 501(c)(5) labour unions and 501(c)(7) social clubs were randomly chosen by the IRS to provide detailed information about their compliance and their use of IRS resources.

74 See, Howard, C., *The Hidden Welfare State: Tax Expenditures and Social Policy in the United States*, Princeton University Press, Princeton, 1997. As cited by Wright, 'Generosity vs. Altruism', p. 410.

75 Ibid.

76 See Clotfelter, C., 'Tax-Induced Distortions in the Voluntary Sector', *Case Western Law Review*, 39 (1988/1989), pp. 663–94.

77 See Weisbrod, B., 'The Pitfalls of Profits', *Stanford Social Innovation Review* (Winter 2004).

78 I.R.C. s. 170 (2000). The exception is organizations that test for public safety.

79 See I.R.C. s. 2055(d) (2000).

80 See, Fremont-Smith, *Governing Nonprofit Organisations*, pp. 174–86. She explains that:

> [the] doctrine is now generally accepted as part of the common or statutory law of all of the states except Alaska, and North Dakota, although in Hawaii and Nevada it has been recognised only in dictum, while South Carolina uses the doctrine of 'deviation' in its stead.

81 See the *Matter of Multiple Sclerosis Service Organisation of New York, Inc.*, 68 NY 2d 32 (1986).

82 See, further, at http://www.raffa.com/Interior/s_frame.htm.

83 *Village of Schaumberg* v. *Citizens for a Better Environment*, 444 U.S. 620 (1980).

84 Treas. Reg. s. 1.501(c)(3)–1(d)(e)(1).

85 *B.S.W. Group Inc.* v. *Commissioner* 70 TC 352, 356–7 (1978).

86 See, Grønbjerg, K. A. and Rathgeb Smith, S., 'Nonprofit Organisations and Public Policies in the Delivery of Human Services', *Philanthropy and the Nonprofit Sector in a Changing America*, 139 (1999), 149–50.

87 Salamon and Geller, *Nonprofit Governance and Accountability*, pp. 152–3.

88 See the National Association of Attorneys General, 'State Regulation of Charitable Trusts and Solicitations', Committee on the Office of Attorney General, Washington, 1977. Also see Fishman, 'The Development of Nonprofit Corporation Law', p. 699.

89 See *Jackson* v. *Phillips* 96 Mass 539 (1867), where the court upheld as charitable a gift to be used to 'create a public sentiment that will put an end to negro slavery in this country'. Gray J found the purpose to be within the spirit and intendment of the Preamble being analogous to the relief or redemption of prisoners or captives.

90 The leading case on this matter is the 1966 IRS ruling in relation to the lobbying activities of the Sierra Club.

91 Nonprofits that cannot offer a tax deduction to their contributors – such as labour unions and trade associations – regulated under ss. 501(c)(5) and 501(c)(6), are free to engage in unlimited lobbying.

92 See Reich, 'A Failure of Philanthropy', p. 9.

93 Ibid.

94 See, for example, *Walz* v. *Tax Commission of the City of New York*, 397 US 664 (1970).

95 See Brown, *Giving USA 2005*, the Annual Report on Philanthropy for the Year 2004, cited by Reich, 'A Failure of Philanthropy', p. 8.

96 See Simon, K. and Irish, L., *A Public Benefit Commission for the United States?* A discussion document for the Senate Finance Committee, Roundtable Discussion, 22 July 2004.
97 See US Department of the Treasury Antiterrorist Financing Guidelines: *Voluntary Best Practices for U.S.-Based Charities*, available at http://www.treas.gov/press/releases/docs/tocc.pdf.
98 See Silk, T., 'Corporate Philanthropy and Law in the United States: A Practical Guide to Tax Choices and an Introduction to Compliance with Anti-Terrorism Laws', *International Journal of Not-for-Profit Law*, 6, available at http://www.icnl.org/JOURNAL/vol6iss3/ar_silk.htm; Council on Foundations, Comments on US Department of the Treasury Antiterrorist Financing Guidelines: *Voluntary Best Practices for U.S.-Based Charities*, available at http://www.cof.org/files/Documents/Legal/Treasury_Comments_06.03.pdf.
99 Also, see The Financial Action Task Force on Money Laundering, *Combating the Abuse of Nonprofit Organizations: International Best Practices*, October 2002.
100 Senate Finance Committee staff discussion draft, 108th Cong., *Tax-Exempt Governance Proposals* 7 (2004).
101 Mark W. Everson, Commissioner of Internal Revenue, testimony before the US Senate Finance Committee, 22 June 2004 and 5 April 2005.

13 Charity law and social inclusion in Canada

1 See The Joint Regulatory Table, *Strengthening Canada's Charitable Sector: Regulatory Reform*, 2003.
2 See Hall, M., Barr, C., Easwaramoorthy, M., Wojciech Sokolowski, S. and Salamon L., *The Canadian Nonprofit and Voluntary Sector in Comparative Perspective* (the Johns Hopkins report), the Johns Hopkins Comparative Nonprofit Sector Project, Johns Hopkins University, 2005, executive summary, p. 6.
3 Mainly comprising the Indian, Métis and Inuit communities.
4 Ethnic groups are as follows: British Isles origin 28 per cent; French origin 23 per cent; other European 15 per cent; American Indian 2 per cent; other, mostly Asian, African, Arab 6 per cent; and of mixed background 26 per cent (2001 census).
5 Religious backgrounds are as follows: Roman Catholic 42.6 per cent, Protestant 23.3 per cent (including United Church 9.5 per cent, Anglican 6.8 per cent, Baptist 2.4 per cent, Lutheran 2 per cent), other Christian 4.4 per cent, Muslim 1.9 per cent, other and unspecified 11.8 per cent, none 16 per cent (2001 census).
6 See Ontario Law Reform Commission, *Report on the Law of Charities*, Toronto, 1997.
7 The Johns Hopkins report, op. cit., at executive summary, p. 6.
8 See, for example, Sharpe, D., *A Portrait of Canada's Charities: The Size, Scope and Financing of Registered Charities*, Canadian Centre for Philanthropy, Toronto, 1994, and Day, K. M. and Devlin, R. A., *The Canadian Nonprofit Sector*, Canadian Policy Research Network and Kahanoff Foundation, Ottawa, 1996. More recently, see the National Survey of Non-Profit Voluntary Organisations at http://www.nonprofitscan.ca/Files/nsnvo/nsnvo_report_english.pdf.
9 See Canadian Centre for Philanthropy, Non-Profit Sector Research Initiative, Volunteer Canada, Canadian Heritage, Health Canada, Human Resources Development Canada, and Statistics Canada, *Caring Canadians, Involved Canadians: Highlights from the 1997 National Survey of Giving, Volunteering and Participating*, Ministry of Industry, Ottawa, 1998.
10 Ibid., p. 13.
11 In 1867, the confederation process initiated under the British North American Act made 'Indians and Lands reserved for Indians' a federal responsibility within the new Dominion of Canada. This process included treaties with indigenous people and led to the Indian Act 1876, under which all indigenous people were made wards of the federal government.

12 Nunavut came into being on 1 April 1999, through the division of the Northwest Territories, as a result of two agreements: the Nunavut Political Accord, and the Nunavut Land Claims Agreement.

13 See Census statistics for 2001: the population of Nunavut has increased by 8.1 per cent since the last census in 1996, a growth rate which is twice the national average.

14 See, for example, the *Royal Commission on Aboriginal Peoples: Looking Forward, Looking Back*, Ottawa, 1996.

15 *Native Communications Society of BC* v. *Minister of National Revenue* [1986] 3 F.C. 471, p. 483.

16 See, for example, Zweibel, E., 'A Truly Canadian Definition of Charity and a Lesson in Drafting Charitable Purposes: A Comment in *Native Communications Society of B.C. v. M.N.R.*' (1987), 26 *Estates and Trusts Reports* 41.

17 See, for example, the National Council of Welfare, *The 2003 Report Card on Child Poverty in Canada, Urban Poverty in Canada: A Statistical Profile* (17 April 2000) and Canadian Policy Research Networks, *Does a Rising Tide Lift All Boats?*, 2002.

18 See *Child Poverty Profile 1998*, a special report in the National Council of Welfare's annual series *Poverty Profile*, which uses Statistics Canada's *Survey of Consumer Finances and Survey of Labour and Income Dynamics* to track the changes in poverty rates in Canada. New data was released on 24 November 2005. The one in six number remains accurate. See http://www.campaign2000.ca/rc/index.html.

19 See *Urban Poverty in Canada: A Statistical Profile* (17 April 2000).

20 See National Council of Welfare, *Poverty Profile 2001*, Autumn 2004.

21 See, for example, Omidvar, R. and Richmond, T., *Immigrant Settlement and Social Inclusion in Canada*, The Laidlaw Foundation, Toronto, 2003.

22 See *Canada Trust Co.* v. *Ontario Human Rights Commission* (1990) 69 DLR (4th) 321.

23 See the Canada Customs and Revenue Agency, CPS – 021, *Registering Charities that Promote Racial Equality*, 2003.

24 See Hay, D., *A New Social Architecture for Canada's 21st Century*, 2004. Also, see Richmond, T., *Social Inclusion as Policy: Challenges and Opportunities*, Laidlaw Foundation, Dec 2004, vol 7, no 2.

25 The Prime Minister, on introducing the document entitled *An Accord Between the Government of Canada and the Voluntary Sector*, released in December 2001.

26 See the Johns Hopkins report, op. cit., chap. 1, p 8.

27 See *Income Tax Special Commissioners* v. *Pemsel* [1891] AC 531.

28 See *Vancouver Society of Immigrant and Visible Minority Women* v. *Minister of National Revenue* (1999) 169 DLR (4th) 34, SC.

29 The author is grateful to Blake Bromley for bringing this point to his attention.

30 See rulings in cases such as *Native Communications Society of British Columbia* v. *M.N.R.*, op. cit., and *Vancouver Society of Immigrant and Visible Minority Women v. M.N.R.*, op. cit.

31 Act to Amend the Income Tax, SC 1950, c.40.

32 See *Report of the Royal Commission on Taxation*, Ottawa, 1966.

33 Income Tax Act Reforms 1972, SC 1970–71–72, c 63.

34 See the Department of Finance, *Charities and the Canadian Tax Treatment of Charities: A Discussion Paper*, Ottawa, 1975.

35 SC 1976–77, c. 4.

36 c. 45.

37 See the Department of Finance, *Charities and the Canadian Tax System: A Discussion Paper*, Ottawa, 1983.

38 See Revenue Canada, *A Better Tax Administration in Support of Charities 1990: A Discussion Paper*, Ottawa, 1990.

39 The Voluntary Sector Roundtable, established in 1995 and consisting of 12 national umbrella organizations, commissioned an independent panel of inquiry to consider how best to promote accountability and governance in the voluntary sector. This Panel (known as the Broadbent Panel) issued its report in 1999, recommending a move towards the English model 'the model we have proposed bears a resemblance to the

Charity Commission of England and Wales' (p. 56) and is available at http://www-
.web.net/vsr-trsb.

40 Following the release of the Broadbent Panel report, voluntary sector members and
federal officials met in three groups, called 'Joint Tables', to make recommendations on
sector/government relationships, to strengthen the voluntary sector's capacity, and to
improve regulations and legislation. The Joint Tables issued their combined report in
August 1999.

41 The Joint Accord Table developed two Codes of Good Practice: the *Code of Good
Practice on Policy Dialogue*, intended to encourage voluntary sector participation in the
public policy process; and the *Code of Good Practice on Funding*, intended to guide the
funding aspect of the relationship between the voluntary sector and the Government
of Canada and reinforce reciprocal accountability.

42 S.C. 2001, c. 4, brought into effect on 1 June 2001.

43 R.S.C. 1985, c. I–21

44 The author is grateful to Blake Bromley for bringing this to his attention.

45 See Revenue Canada, Information Circular CPS – 022 – *Political Activities*, 2003,
para. 4.

46 *Canada Trust Co.* v. *Ontario Human Rights Commission* (1990) 69 DLR (4th) 321.

47 See Ontario Law Reform Commission, *Report on the Law of Charities*, Toronto, 1997.

48 Income Tax Act, s. 149.1(1). See, also, s. 501(c)(3) of the Internal Revenue Code, 26
USC, which requires an organization to be 'explicitly organised for exclusively
charitable purposes'.

49 *Vancouver Society of Immigrant and Visible Minority Women* v. *M.N.R.* [1999] 1 S.C.R. 10,
para. 194.

50 Ibid., p. 33.

51 See the Johns Hopkins report, op. cit., p. 22.

52 *Tawich Development Corporation* v. *Deputy Minister of Revenue of Quebec*, 2001 D.T.C. 5144.

53 *Alberta Institute of Mental Retardation* v. *The Queen* [1987] 2 C.T.C. 70, 87 D.T.C. 5306
(F.C.A.).

54 See s. 501(c)(3) of the Internal Revenue Code (see p. 000).

55 See the Federal Court of Appeal decision in *Earth Fund* v. *Canada (Minister of National
Revenue)* (2002), [2003] 2 C.T.C. 10; (2002), 57 D.T.C. 5016, para. 30 ff., available at
http://www.canlii.org/ca/cas/fca/2002/2002fca498.html.

56 Note that s. 501(c)(3) of the Internal Revenue Code also specifies certain purposes as
having tax-exempt status.

57 *Everywoman's Health Centre Society* v. *Canada* [1991] 2 C.T.C. 320, 92 D.T.C. 6001
(F.C.A.).

58 See the Johns Hopkins report, op. cit, p. 36.

59 Blake Bromley, note to author, 22 January 2006.

60 See Wayne, S., Canadian Council for International Co-operation, *A Profile of Planned
Giving and Endowments within the Canadian International NGO Community*, 1999, at http://
www.ccic.ca/e/docs/002_od_profile_of_planned_giving_and_endowments.pdf.

61 As stated, tax exemption applies to all not-for-profit organizations, not just charities.
There are a large number of organizations (some 90,000 according to the NSNVO)
that do fundraising of some sort but are not registered charities. Some government-
operated foundations (e.g., Trillium Foundation in Ontario and Wild Rose Foundation
in Alberta) make grants to not-for-profit organizations whether or not they are
registered charities.

62 Para. 149.1(1)(e) of the Act. Note: the disbursement quota provisions related to
charities changed in July 2005 through a provision that was tacked onto the bill implementing the Joint Regulatory Table provisions. The 80 per cent rule that applied to
charitable organizations (as opposed to foundations) has now been supplemented by
complex provisions.

63 According to the Joint Round Table report, an average of five or ten are deregistered

for cause. More than 90 per cent are deregistered for failure to file the annual report, with the remainder being voluntary deregistrations or annulments.

64 The July 2005 amendments expanded the information that is available, so that the Charities Directorate will now release reasons for its registration decisions, positive and negative.

65 See subsections 149.1(2), (3) and (4) of the Income Tax Act 1985. Note: intermediate sanctions were introduced in 2005 as a result of the recommendations of the Joint Regulatory Table.

66 Joint Regulatory Table, *Strengthening Canada's Charitable Sector*, chap. 5, p. 3.

67 See the Income Tax Act, 1985, s. 91(3).

68 For a discussion of the provincial role in regulating charities, see Ontario Law Reform Commission, *Report on the Law of Charities*, OLRC, Toronto, 1996, pp. 385–92.

69 See *Vancouver Society of Immigrant and Visible Minority Women* v. *Minister of National Revenue, op. cit, per* Iacobucci, J at p 95.

70 A tax credit is a deduction from tax otherwise payable, while a tax deduction reduces income upon which tax is levied. The credit is therefore of identical value to all taxpayers making annual gifts of the same value.

71 16 per cent is the lowest federal tax rate in Canada, while 29 per cent is the highest. Each province also imposes taxes, using a system which is essentially a mirror of the federal system, but with lower rates.

72 *Alberta Institute of Mental Retardation* v. *The Queen*, op. cit. Also, see *Gull Bay Development Corp.* v. *The Queen* [1984] Ex. C.R. 159, 62 DTC 1099, where the income from a logging company was directed towards the economic and social welfare of residents in the Gull Bay Indian Reserve; held charitable.

73 See Quebec Law Reform Commission, op. cit., chap. 11, p. 7.

74 *Earth Fund* v. *Canada (Minister of National Revenue)*, op. cit. Note, also, that post the Voluntary Sector Initiative a 5 per cent tax was imposed on unrelated business rising to 100 per cent if there is repeated business (see s. 188.1).

75 Note: the rules related to umbrella organizations changed in autumn 2005. See Customs and Revenue Agency's website (http://www.cra-arc.gc.ca) for a new policy which extends recognition to umbrella organisations that represent other charities.

76 See, for example, the Canada Customs and Revenue Agency, CPS – 012, *Benefits to Aboriginal Peoples of Canada*, 1997.

77 *Lewis* v. *Doerle* (1898), 25 OAR 206 (CA).

78 See *Re Oldfield Estate (No. 2)* [1949] 2 DLR 175 (Manitoba).

79 See *Camille & Henry Dreyfus Foundation Inc.* v. *Inland Revenue Commissioners* [1954] Ch. 672, which suggests it is necessary for an international aid charity to also generate benefit within the UK jurisdiction (see, further, chapter 8).

80 See *McGovern* v. *Attorney-General* [1982] Ch. 321 [1981] 3 All ER 493.

81 *Re Laidlaw Foundation* (1985) 13 DLR (4th) 491 (Ont. HCJ).

82 *Re Vancouver Regional Free Net Association and Minister of National Revenue* (1996) 137 DLR (4th) 206 Federal Court of Appeal. Also, see *Everywoman's Health Centre Society* v. *Canada*, op. cit.

83 See Income Tax Act s. 149.1(6.2).

84 Revenue Canada has revised, somewhat, its rules relating to the 10 per cent threshold. See Revenue Canada, Information Circular CPS – 022 – *Political Activities*, 2003, para. 8.

85 *Re Co-operative College of Canada and Saskatchewan Human Rights Commission* (1975) 64 DLR (3rd) 531 (Saskatchewan CA). See, also, Revenue Canada, Information Circular 87–1 *Registered Charities – Ancillary and Incidental Political Activities*, 1987; RC4107 – *Registered Charities: Education, Advocacy and Political Activities*, 2000; and CPS – 022 – *Political Activities*, 2003 (replacing 87–1).

86 However, see also *Scarborough Community Legal Services* v. *The Queen*, [1985] 1 C.T.C. 98, 85 D.T.C. 5102 (F.C.A.), where it was found that political activities in the form of

participation in rallies and work to change municipal by-laws would not invalidate charitable purposes because they were non-essential and incidental to other charitable activities.

87 *NDG Neighbourhood Association* v. *Minister of National Revenue* (1988) 30 ETR 99.
88 Ibid.
89 *Alliance for Life* v. *M.N.R.* [1999] CarswellNat 625 (F.C.A.). See, also, *Alliance for Life* v. *M.N.R.* [1999] 3 F.C.R.
90 See Bridge, R., *The Law of Advocacy for Charitable Organisations: The Case for Change*, Institute for Media, Policy and Civil Society, Vancouver, 2000. For an example of critical judicial comment on this field see the decision of Strayer J. A. of the Federal Court of Appeal in *Human Life International in Canada Inc.* v. *The Minister of National Revenue*, (1998) F.C. 202 (C.A.). Also, see Drache, A., *Canadian Taxation of Charities and Donations*, where he states that 'the problem of charities and political activity [which includes advocacy] has been a serious one for at least ten years'. Carswell, Toronto, 1999, pp. 1–15.
91 It should be noted, however, that Revenue Canada has relaxed its rules relating to public awareness campaigns. See CPS – 022, op. cit., para. 7.
92 Ibid., p. 19.
93 See Boyle, F., *Charitable Activity Under the Canadian Income Tax Act: Definition, Process and Problems*, a background paper for the Voluntary Sector Roundtable, 1997, p. 28.
94 The Broadbent report, op. cit.
95 An argument not accepted by the Federal Court of Appeal in *Alliance for Life* (1999). Bob Wyatt, in correspondence with the author, adds:

> Note that there is a dispute in Canada as to whether the activities of charities in terms of advocacy are, in fact, constrained by the legislation and interpretations or by the widespread lack of understanding by charities of what they can and cannot do. The commentary cited predates the change in the political-activity policy – a byproduct of the Voluntary Sector Initiative process. While there are still limitations, it is questionable whether charities are, in fact, badly hampered in what they can do, so long as they can demonstrate that the political activity is related to the charitable objects and remains incidental and ancillary.

96 For suggested intermediate sanctions, see the Joint Regulatory Table, *Strengthening Canada's Charitable Sector*, executive summary, p. 3.
97 *Tawich Development Corporation* v. *Deputy Minister of Revenue of Quebec*, op. cit.
98 Revenue Canada will regard the requirement as satisfied where a band demonstrates that it performs functions and provides services in a manner generally exhibited by a government. Examples of such activities would be if the band has been involved in negotiating land treaties (or has negotiated a settlement agreement with Canada) or if the band provides community, health, safety and education services to its members. See, also, Revenue Canada, Information Circular CPS-023, *Applicants Assisting Ethnocultural Communities*, 2005.
99 *Native Communications Society of B.C.* v. *Minister of National Revenue* [1980] 2 CTC 170 [1986] 3 FC 471 (Fed. CA).
100 *Vancouver Society of Immigrant and Visible Minority Women* v. *M.N.R.* [1999] 1 S.C.R. 10, 2 C.T.C. 85 (F.C.A.); a decision upheld by the Supreme Court of Canada in 1999.
101 See Revenue Canada, Policy Statement CPS – 012, *Benefits to Aboriginal Peoples of Canada*, 1997.
102 See Joint Regulatory Table, *Strengthening Canada's Charitable Sector*, chap. 3, p. 25.
103 Bromley, B., 'Voluntary Sector Initiative Methodology', conference paper, Ottawa, 5–6 December 2005, p. 7.
104 As Blake Bromley has pointed out:

Post the Voluntary Sector Initiative there is now an internal review process prior to going to court. However, registration denials still go to the Federal Court of Appeal. If a charity is assessed an interim sanction such as the tax on unrelated business, this can now be appealed to the Tax Court rather than having no appeal other than to the Federal Court of Appeal.

(Note to author, 22 January 2006.)

105 *Re Strakosch* [1949] 1 Ch. 529 (C.A.).
106 See the Canada Customs and Revenue Agency, CPS – 021, *Registering Charities that Promote Racial Equality*, 2003. Note that in 1983 the Charity Commission in England and Wales reconsidered the *Re Strakosch* decision in light of social and legislative change, and determined that it should no longer be followed.
107 See *Slaight Communications Inc.* v. *Davidson* (1989) 59 DLR (4th) 416 (SCC).
108 *Wren* [1945] OR 778, [1945] 4 DLR 674 (HCJ).
109 *Canada Trust Co.* v. *Ontario Human Rights Commission*, op. cit.
110 See *Report on the Law of Charities*, Ontario Law Reform Commission, 1996, chap. 8, p. 21.
111 The Canadian Multiculturalism Act 1985 and the Canadian Race Relations Foundation Act 1991 have also set benchmarks for legislation at provincial and territorial level.
112 *Toronto Volgograd Committee* v. *M.N.R.* [1988] 1 C.T.C. 365, 88 D.T.C. 6192 (F.C.A.).
113 See, Bromley, B., *Reflections on Charities and the Anti-Terrorism Act*, statement to Special Committee on the Anti-Terrorism Act, 20 June 2005.
114 See *Report on the Law of Charities*, Ontario Law Reform Commission, 1996.
115 *Vancouver Society of Immigrant and Visible Minority Women* v. *M.N.R.*, 1 S.C.R. 10 (1999).
116 See, for example, Drache, A., *Broadening the Definition of Charity*, at http://www.queensu.ca/sps/courses/mpa880/broadening_the_definition_of_c.php.
117 See Broadbent Commission report, *Building on Strength: Improving Governance and Accountability on Canada's Voluntary Sector*, at http://www.pagvs.com.
118 See Joint Regulatory Table, *Strengthening Canada's Charitable Sector*, recommendation 13.
119 See *Report on the Law of Charities*, p. 152.
120 See Joint Regulatory Table, *Strengthening Canada's Charitable Sector*, recommendation 21.
121 Ibid., recommendation 28.
122 An alternative view has been expressed to the author by Bob Wyatt:

The recent changes in policy relating to ethnocultural organisations, along with the 2000 policy on community economic development could, if adopted by the sector and funders, go quite a way to achieve this. In other words, I think an argument could be made that the framework is already there and it's the sector's fault that we're not acting on it.

123 See the Johns Hopkins report, op. cit., p. 33.

Conclusion

1 See Charity Commission and Applications for Registration of (i) Trafford Community Leisure Trust and (ii) Wigan Leisure and Culture Trust (21 April 2004).
2 See the decision of the Supreme Court of the state of New York (20 June 2005) in the Empire Blue Cross Blue Shield case and the ensuing related initiative by the New York state legislature.
3 See Grant Makers in Health, *A Profile of New Health Foundations*, Washington, D.C., 2003, which reports on 165 such conversions with assets of over $16.4 billion.
4 See Anheier, H. and Leat, D., *From Charity to Creativity: Philanthropic Foundations in the 21st Century*, Comedia, Stroud, 2002.
5 See, further, at http://www.communityfoundations.org.uk/.

6 Anheier and Leat, *From Charity to Creativity*, p. 149.

7 See *Vancouver Society of Immigrant and Visible Minority Women* v. *Minister of National Revenue* (1999) 169 D.I.R. (4th) 34, SC, where a minority group established to provide mutual support for immigrant women failed to gain charitable status because their purposes could be construed as permitting political rather than exclusively educational activities.

8 *McGovern* v. *A-G.* [1982] Ch. 321, where the court ruled that it had no means of determining whether the outcome of policy change would be beneficial or otherwise.

9 A 'self-serving' requirement not unlike that which guides the public benefit test in relation to animals, i.e. it is not enough that the animal benefits; as far as charity law is concerned that is simply the means for achieving a benefit (opportunity to practise compassion) for mankind.

10 *McGovern* v. *A-G.* [1982] Ch. 321. The court's ruling – that it has no means of determining whether the outcome of policy change would be beneficial or otherwise – being equally applicable to the position of such an aid-giving charity.

11 Variously attributed to inbreeding, intergenerational abuse of alcohol, inherent genetic weakness or other such essentially eugenic attitudes. In fact a combined American-Australian Research team from Monash University, the Menzies School of Health Research in the Northern Territory and the University of Mississippi has done extensive autopsies on the kidneys of whites, Afro-Americans, Native Americans and Indigenous Australians. They discovered a common link among many people with fatal kidney and heart disease that crosses over race, has nothing to do with weak genes but is certainly associated with poverty. The common link is being born a low birthweight baby, which results in kidneys having a much reduced capacity to process sugar leaving the adult prone to diabetes, heart disease and other illnesses.

12 See Harvard University's Indian Economic Development Project, led by Professor Stephen Cornell.

13 See, for example, *Re Royal Kilmainham Hospital* [1966] IR 451, which concerned a hospital established in Dublin by Charles II in 1684 for the support and maintenance of old soldiers of 'our army in Ireland' (see, further, chap. 9).

14 *Vancouver Regional Free Net Association* v. *Minister of National Revenue* [1996] 137 DLR (4th) 206.

Index